Infectious Disease
Emergencies

T0177901

Infectious Disease Emergencies

Edited by

Arjun S. Chanmugam, MD, MBA

Professor of Emergency Medicine
Johns Hopkins University School of Medicine
Baltimore, Maryland

Andrew H. Bissonette, MD

Fellow, Emergency Medicine and Internal Medicine
Henry Ford Hospital
Detroit, Michigan

Sanjay V. Desai, MD

Associate Professor of Medicine
Johns Hopkins University School of Medicine
Baltimore, Maryland

Shannon B. Putman, MD

Assistant Professor of Emergency Medicine
Johns Hopkins University School of Medicine
Baltimore, Maryland

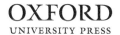

OXFORD
UNIVERSITY PRESS

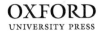

Oxford University Press is a department of the University of Oxford. It furthers
the University's objective of excellence in research, scholarship, and education
by publishing worldwide. Oxford is a registered trade mark of Oxford University
Press in the UK and certain other countries.

Published in the United States of America by Oxford University Press
198 Madison Avenue, New York, NY 10016, United States of America.

Library of Congress Cataloging-in-Publication Data
Names: Chanmugam, Arjun S., editor. | Rothman, Richard, MD, editor. | Desai, Sanjay V., editor. |
Putman, Shannon B., editor.
Title: Infectious disease emergencies / edited by Arjun S. Chanmugam, Richard Rothman,
Sanjay V. Desai, Shannon B. Putman.
Other titles: Infectious disease emergencies (Chanmugam)
Description: Oxford ; New York : Oxford University Press, [2016] |
Includes bibliographical references and index.
Identifiers: LCCN 2016002340 | ISBN 9780199976805 (alk. paper) | ISBN 9780199976829 (e-ISBN)
Subjects: | MESH: Communicable Diseases | Emergencies
Classification: LCC RC112 | NLM WC 100 | DDC 616.9/0425—dc23
LC record available at http://lccn.loc.gov/2016002340

9 8 7 6 5 4 3 2 1
Printed by Webcom Inc., Canada

Contents

Section VIII Gastrointestinal Infections

Section IX Genitourinary Infections

Section X Skin and Soft Tissue Infections

Section XI Bone and Joint Infections

Section XV Antibiotic Resistance

Series Preface

Emergency physicians care for patients with any condition that may be encountered in an emergency department. This requires that they know about a vast number of emergencies, some common and many rare. Physicians who have trained in any of the subspecialties—cardiology, neurology, obstetrics and gynecology, and many others—have narrowed their fields of study, allowing their patients to benefit accordingly. The Oxford University Press *Emergencies* series has combined the very best of these two knowledge bases, and the result is the unique product you are now holding. Each handbook is authored by an emergency physician and a subspecialist, allowing the reader instant access to years of expertise in a rapid access, patient-centered format. Together with evidence-based recommendations, you will have access to their tricks of the trade as well as the combined expertise and approaches of a subspecialist and an emergency physician.

Patients in the emergency department often have quite different needs and require different testing from those with a similar emergency who are in-patients. These stem from different priorities; in the emergency department, the focus is on quickly diagnosing an undifferentiated condition. An emergency occurring to an in-patient may also need to be newly diagnosed, but usually the information available is more complete and the emphasis can be on a more focused and in-depth evaluation. The authors of each Handbook have produced a guide for you wherever the patient is encountered, whether in an out-patient clinic, urgent care, emergency department, or on the wards.

A special thanks should be extended to Andrea Knobloch, Senior Editor for Medicine at Oxford University Press, for her vision in bringing this series to press. Andrea is aware of how new electronic media have impacted the learning process for physician-assistants, medical students, residents, and fellows, yet, at the same time, she is a firm believer in the value of the printed word. This series contains the proof that such a combination is still possible in the rapidly changing world of information technology.

Over the last 20 years, the Oxford Handbooks have become an indispensable tool for those in all stages of training throughout the world. This new series will, I am sure, quickly grow to become the standard reference for those who need to help their patients when faced with an emergency.

Jeremy Brown, MD
Series Editor
Associate Professor of Emergency Medicine
The George Washington University Medical Center

Preface

The history of medicine can be linked to the battle against infectious disease. A striking historical example is found within the Edwin Smith papyrus, which describes the management of 48 medical cases dating to about 1600 BCE. Impressively, this ancient document may date back much further, as the writings are often attributed to Imhotep, the great architect and chief physician from the Old Kingdom, 3000–2500 BCE. Within the papyrus are instructions on a number of medical and surgical interventions, but the inclusion of treating and preventing infection figures prominently. The struggle against infection is indeed almost as old as the history of human kind.

The challenges of preventing, diagnosing, and treating infection continue to be a significant part of medical practice today. In the acute care setting, especially emergency departments, urgent care centers, and hospitals, diagnosing and treating infectious diseases is a prime concern. Providing the correct antibiotic or medical intervention after recognizing that an infection is present can be a complicated and often time-consuming process. One of the key steps to correctly managing an infection is to have an understanding of the causes, the associated recommended therapies, and the typical disease course. This can be even more challenging in the acute setting where time limitations and comorbidities complicate matters.

Although there are a number of excellent references available to medical practitioners, a concise text that rapidly summarizes the key points of various infectious diseases, especially as it relates to acute care management, is still in demand. The battle against infectious disease will likely be ongoing, as new antibiotics and chemotherapeutics are introduced, as organisms develop resistance, and other defense mechanisms evolve along with new microbial threats. A succinct reference that provides a rapid understanding of the basic interventions and basic process to manage infections can only help to formulate appropriate initial strategies. In the emergency department, in urgent care centers, in hospitals, and in clinicians' offices, having such a reference could make a difference in making the correct diagnosis and starting the proper treatment in a timely fashion.

The practice of medicine will likely always include a need to consider infectious processes as they contribute to the morbidity and mortality of our patients. To that end, we designed this reference to be used by clinicians everywhere and to be one more effective reference tool in the battle against infectious disease.

Acknowledgments

With thanks to Dr. Richard Rothman for his guidance and contributions to this book.

Contributors

Kevin Alexander, MD
Fellow, Cardiovascular Diseases
Brigham and Women's Hospital
Boston, Massachusetts

Trisha Anest, MD, MPH
Emergency Physician
Baltimore, Maryland

Annie Antar, MD, PhD
Clinical Fellow, Division of Infectious Diseases
Johns Hopkins University School of Medicine
Baltimore, Maryland

Michael Arce
Department of Emergency Medicine
UMass Memorial Medical Center
Worcester, Massachusetts

Kamna Balhara, MD
Assistant Professor of Emergency Medicine
UT Health Science Center
San Antonio, Texas

Hasan E. Baydoun
Department of Orthopaedics
Massachusetts General Hospital
Boston, Massachusetts

Jamil D. Bayram
Associate Professor of Emergency Medicine
The Johns Hopkins University School of Medicine
Baltimore, Maryland

Alexander Billioux
Department of Medicine
Johns Hopkins University
Baltimore, Maryland

Andrew H. Bissonette, MD
Fellow, Emergency Medicine and Internal Medicine
Henry Ford Hospital
Detroit, Michigan

Sarah Carle, MD
Emergency Physician
Baltimore, Maryland

Mary P. Chang, MD, MPH
Assistant Professor of Emergency Medicine
University of Texas Southwestern Medical
Center
Dallas, Texas

Arjun S. Chanmugam, MD, MBA
Professor of Emergency Medicine
Johns Hopkins University, School of Medicine
Baltimore, Maryland

Sneha A. Chinai, MD, FACEP
Assistant Professor of Emergency Medicine
Associate Director, Emergency Medicine
   Residency Program
Department of Emergency Medicine
University of Massachusetts Medical School
Worcester, Massachusetts

Ryan Circh, MD
Emergency Physician University of Maryland
   Baltimore Washington Medical Center
Baltimore, Maryland

Lisa Cuttle, MD
Emergency Physician
Knoxville, Tennessee

M. DeAugustinas, MD
Emergency Physician
California

Sanjay V. Desai, MD
Associate Professor of Medicine
Johns Hopkins University, School of Medicine
Baltimore, Maryland

Andrea Dugas, MD, PhD
Assistant Professor of Emergency Medicine
Johns Hopkins University, School of Maryland
Baltimore, Maryland

Michael Ehmann, MD, MPH, MS
Instructor
Department of Emergency Medicine
The Johns Hopkins University
   School of Medicine
Baltimore, Maryland

Swathi Eluri
Fellow, Gastroenterology
University of North Carolina
Chapel Hill, North Carolina

Caren Euster, MD
Assistant Professor of Emergency Medicine
The Johns Hopkins University
   School of Medicine
Baltimore, Maryland

Matthew Finn
Fellow, Cardiovascular Diseases
Columbia University
New York, New York

Alida Gertz, MD, MPH
The Everett Clinic
Seattle, Washington

Kevin Gibbs, MD
Assistant Professor of Pulmonary, Critical Care,
    Allergy, and Immunologic Medicine
Wake Forest University
Winston-Salem, North Carolina

Bachar Hamade, MD, MSc
Chief Resident, Department of Emergency Medicine
Johns Hopkins University, School of Medicine
Baltimore, Maryland

Bhakti Hansoti, MBChB, MPH
Assistant Professor of Emergency Medicine
Johns Hopkins University, School of Medicine
Baltimore, Maryland

Michelle Henggeller, MD
Department of Emergency Medicine
The Johns Hopkins Howard County General
    Hospital
Columbia, Maryland

John Holst, DO, RDMS, RDCS
Emergency Medicine Ultrasound Director
Essentia Health Systems, St. Mary's Hospital
Duluth, Minnesota

Gabrielle Jacquet, MD, MPH, FACP
Assistant Professor,
Boston University School of Medicine
Director, Global Health, Dept. of Emergency
    Medicine
Assistant Director, Global Health, Boston
    University School of Medicine
Affiliate Faculty, Boston University Center for
    Global Health and Development
Boston, Massachusetts

Clare Kelleher
Department of Medicine
University of North Carolina
Chapel Hill, North Carolina

Basem F. Khishfe, MD
Department of Emergency Medicine
Cook County Stroger Hospital
Chicago, Ilinois

Amanda Elizabeth Kiely, M.D.
Assistant Professor
Department of Ophthalmology
The Johns Hopkins University School of Medicine
Baltimore, Maryland

Eili Y. Klein, PhD
Associate Professor
Department of Emergency Medicine
The Johns Hopkins University School of Medicine
Baltimore, Maryland

Ajar Kocher
Fellow, Cardiovascular Diseases
Duke University
Durham, North Carolina

Bharati Kocher, MD
Fellow, Gastroenterology
University of North Carolina at Chapel Hill
Chapel Hill, North Carolina

Joshua Lupton, MD
Resident
Department of Emergency Medicine
The Johns Hopkins University School of Medicine
Baltimore, Maryland

David Mabey, MD
Department of Emergency Medicine
Ultrasound Education Intermountain Medical
    Center
Murray, Utah

Tyler Martinez, DO
Emergency Physician
Phoenix, Arizona

Monica Mix
Johns Hopkins University
Baltimore, Maryland

Dana Mueller
Mary's Center
Washington D.C.

Timothy Niessen, MD, MPH
Assistant Professor of Medicine
Johns Hopkins University
Baltimore, Maryland

Lawrence Page, DDS, PhD
Periodontist
Ellicott City, Maryland

Susan Peterson, MD
Assistant Professor of Emergency Medicine
Johns Hopkins University School of Medicine
Baltimore, Maryland

Shannon B. Putman, MD
Assistant Professor of Emergency Medicine
Johns Hopkins University, School of Medicine
Baltimore, Maryland

Sri Raghavan, MD, PhD
Clinical Fellow, Hematology/Oncology
Dana-Farber Cancer Institute
Boston, Massachusetts

Rod Rahimi, MD, PhD
Fellow, Division of Pulmonary and Critical Care
    Medicine
Massachusetts General Hospital
Harvard Medical School
Boston, Massachusetts

Staci Reintjes, DO
Emergency Physician
Saint Luke's Health Care System in
    Kansas City, Missouri

Elizabeth Rosenblatt, MD
Fellow, Gastroenterology
University of Washington
Seattle, Washington

Richard Rothman, MD, PhD
Professor of Emergency Medicine
The Johns Hopkins University School of Medicine
Baltimore, Maryland

Sudip Saha, MD
Cardiology Fellow
Beth Israel Deaconess Medical Center
Boston, Massachusetts

Sarina Sahetya, MD
Postdoctoral Fellow
Pulmonary and Critical Care Medicine
Johns Hopkins Hospital
Baltimore, Maryland

Gino Scalabrini
Johns Hopkins University School of Medicine
Baltimore, Maryland

Marcos Schechter, MD
Fellow, Infectious Diseases
Emory University
Atlanta, Georgia

David Scordino, MD
Instructor of Emergency Medicine
Johns Hopkins University, School of Medicine
Baltimore, Maryland

Michelle Sharp
Fellow, Pulmonary and Critical Care
Johns Hopkins University
Baltimore, Maryland

Zach Smith, MMS, PA-C
University of Maryland Medical Center
R. Adams Cowley Shock Trauma Center
Critical Care Resuscitation Unit
Baltimore, Maryland

Lisa Steiner MMS, PA-C
Sr. Physician Assistant
The Johns Hopkins University School of Medicine
  Baltimore, Maryland

Mark Tenforde, MD, MPH
Division of Allergy and Infectious Diseases
University of Washington School of Medicine
Seattle, Washington

Ximena Tobar MMS, PA-C
Sr. Physician Assistant
The Johns Hopkins University School of Medicine
  Baltimore, Maryland

Susan Tuddenham, MD, MPH
Fellow, Infectious Diseases
Johns Hopkins University, School of Medicine
Baltimore, Maryland

Vanessa Vasquez, MD
Emergency Physician
West Palm, Florida

Michael Vulfovich
Director of Medical Education
Department of Emergency Medicine
Metrowest Physicians
Framingham, Massachusetts

Deanna Wilson
Adolescent Health Program
Johns Hopkins University
Baltimore, Maryland

Raymond Young, MD
Fellow, Cardiovascular Medicine
Georgetown University
Washington, DC

Principals of Infectious Disease Management

Chapter 1

Laboratory Testing for Microbial Detection

Michael Arce

Laboratory Modalities

The approach to microbial detection in patients who present to the emergency department (ED) should be focused and should aim for clinically significant findings while minimizing the chances of a clinically deleterious false negative result. Judicious selection of laboratory tests, efficient sample collection, and laboratory reporting are all important considerations. In this chapter, general guidelines are provided for the initial evaluation of potential microbial infections in patients presenting to the ED. In some cases, the diagnosis will remain uncertain during the patient's stay, but diagnostic testing initiated in the ED may be beneficial for the inpatient or outpatient team and for the future care of the patient.

The methodology of point of care testing (POCT) differs from that of core laboratory testing. POCT is diagnostic testing performed at or near the site of clinical care delivery. It provides the advantage of rapid test results with the potential for faster patient treatment. When used appropriately, it typically has high sensitivity and, thus, is an effective screening tool in the ED. The disadvantage of POCT is its lower specificity. Some POCT is useful in the identification of certain specific organisms that cause infectious disease, including group A *Streptococcus* (rapid Strep test or RST), HIV (human immunodeficiency virus), *Influenzavirus A* and *B*, and *human respiratory syncytial virus* (RSV). Other POCT can also help assess for the likelihood of a non-specific microbe being present, such as the urine dipstick.

Reverse transcriptase (RT) polymerase chain reaction (PCR; RT-PCR) is one of the more well-developed molecular techniques to date and has a wide range of clinical applications: specific or broad-spectrum pathogen detection, evaluation of emerging novel infections, surveillance, early detection of bioterrorism agents, and antimicrobial resistance profiling. In regard to emergency care, PCR-based methods are often cost-effective with excellent sensitivity and specificity profiles, and they have a rapid turnaround time relative to traditional testing procedures.

Direct fluorescent antibody (DFA) testing is designed to specifically target antigens unique to the infecting organism but not present in the human host. This technique can be used to quickly determine if a subject has a specific viral, bacterial, or parasitic infection. These immunoassays are cost-effective, highly specific (99% in some cases), and, generally, moderately sensitive (84% in some cases). Because of this, DFA tests can be used for both screening and confirmation at a fraction of the turnaround time and cost of other forms of definitive microbial testing.

Viral Testing

The vast majority of viral infections affecting immunocompetent populations rarely pose significant morbidity or mortality risks. Therefore, with certain exceptions, there is little gained from viral testing initiated during an ED visit. Some exceptions include suspected cases of meningitis or encephalitis, respiratory infections of epidemiologic significance (ie, SARS), viral sexually transmitted diseases, and infectious mononucleosis (IM) in patients at risk for complications.

Certain viral respiratory infections like *Influenzavirus* and *SARS coronavirus* are on the forefront of public consciousness because these viruses have the potential to cause large-scale epidemics. Given the rise in concern about recent influenza pandemics, the CDC (Centers for Disease Control and Prevention) and other infectious disease governing bodies have established testing recommendations for patients with febrile respiratory illness.

Testing for *Influenzavirus* infections should be initiated with a screening test such as rapid antigen testing (RAT). A positive RAT is most likely to represent a truly positive patient during peak influenza season. Likewise, when influenza season has passed, negative RAT most likely represents a true negative patient, and confirmatory testing is not needed. However, due to the limited sensitivity of RAT, a negative *Influenzavirus* screen during peak flu season should be interpreted with caution, and a confirmatory test should be sent. The test of choice for diagnosing *Influenzavirus* infection is DFA. DFA is highly sensitive and specific when compared to a viral culture, and it is timely and cost-effective. Turnaround time typically is 24 to 48 hours.

The additional advantage of RT-PCR is its ability to type and subtype strains of *Influenzavirus* (eg, H1N1 or H5N1). A viral culture may be useful for public health surveillance but has no utility for ED care.

RSV infections can be diagnosed with reasonable accuracy based on clinical features during winter months. Laboratory confirmation should only be sent during treatment to confirm diagnosis but not necessarily used to guide a decision to treat. Nasopharyngeal washings followed by rapid antigen assays are generally diagnostic (sensitivity and specificity of 90%). PCR-based assays are a reasonable alternative to culture for confirming the rapid antigen detection assay results. Turnaround time is 24 to 48 hours.

The respiratory viral panel is a molecular assay that detects multiple viral pathogens. It is used to confirm negative screening tests (eg, rapid antigen assay). These panels typically detect *Influenzavirus A* and

B and RSV as well as adenovirus, rhinovirus, and parainfluenza virus species/subtypes. Turnaround time is less than 24 hours. IM testing is recommended in adolescents and adults with exam findings consistent with IM because monitoring for complications may be necessary. Complications are rare but include splenic rupture, hemolytic anemia, thrombocytopenia, aplastic anemia, thrombotic thrombocytopenic purpura, and disseminated intravascular coagulation. Heterophile antibody testing (ie, monospot) or ELISA (enzyme-linked immunosorbent assay) techniques are approximately 85% sensitive and approach 100% specificity. As a result, further confirmatory testing is generally not indicated.

Bacterial Testing

Bacterial sources of infection are far-reaching, affect all ages, and are the cause of significant morbidity and mortality around the globe. An important part of initiating care for these patients includes localizing the source of infection in order to gain source control and identifying the pathogen in order to provide appropriate treatment. Common sources for the spread of bacterial infection include cerebrospinal fluid (CSF), blood, urine, oropharyngeal, pulmonary, intra-abdominal, bone, and soft-tissue infections. In this chapter, testing for specific bacterial infections is organized by localization.

Suspected central nervous system (CNS) bacterial infections require special attention. Depending on a patient's clinical presentation, a screening head computed tomography (CT) may be warranted prior to obtaining CSF for analysis. Head CT is recommended for patients with alterations in mental status, papilledema (or other signs of pupillary reactions), or focal neurologic changes in order to assess for the likelihood of potential cerebral herniation if a lumbar puncture (LP) were performed. Analysis of CSF by way of lumbar puncture is the test of choice when evaluating a patient for a CNS infection. Some CSF findings are highly suggestive of bacterial meningitis, but there are a variety of deviations from the standard findings. It is important to note that CSF pleocytosis can result from noninfectious situations, including traumatic LP, seizure, or subarachnoid hemorrhage. A correction factor can be used to further clarify whether the measured white blood cell (WBC) elevations in sample CSF are the result of a traumatic LP or are truly representative of the WBC in the patient's CSF (Equation 1.1).

$$\text{True CSF WBC} = \text{Measured CSF WBC} - \frac{\text{Serum WBC} - \text{CSF RBC}}{\text{Serum RBC}} \qquad (1.1)$$

RBC = red blood cell

Gram stain can suggest a bacterial etiology (when positive) 24 hours earlier than culture results. However, CSF culture remains a gold standard for diagnosing and guiding treatment of CNS infections.

Direct bacterial antigen detection is available for rapid detection of the more concerning causes of bacterial CSF infection (e.g. *Streptococcus pneumoniae*, *Haemophilus influenzae* type B, group B *Streptococcus*, and *Neisseria meningitidis*). However, these tests have been shown to be of limited sensitivity, and they are not cost-effective. Moreover, they rarely change management because neonates, non-immunized individuals, and many patients suspected of having bacterial meningitis should receive antibiotic treatment regimens empirically for these pathogens when they are suspected.

Bacterial causes of pharyngitis can lead to significant morbidity in the acute phase of the illness, and long-term complications can result from pharyngeal streptococcal infections. A peritonsillar or retropharyngeal abscess can lead to upper airway obstruction or extension of the infection through fascial planes, potentially leading to CNS infection, mediastinitis, and even cervical osteomyelitis in the right circumstances.

The most widely recommended testing strategy for the detection of group A beta-hemolytic *Streptococcus* (GABHS) in pediatrics is an RST specific for *Streptococcus* antigen in order to screen for infection in patients presenting with symptoms consistent with strep infection, including scarlatiniform rash. Negative RSTs in pediatric patients should be followed by a throat culture given the risk of false negatives, but positive RSTs are reliable and are grounds for initiating treatment. Cultures are not useful 2–3 weeks post infection. Given a lower prevalence of *Streptococcus* in adults, a negative RST yields a sufficient negative predictive value to forgo throat culture. Cultures are not recommended for a test of cure after treatment because they may remain positive due to a low-level carriage state (ie, some patients are chronically colonized by GABHS without clinical consequence). RST has a turnaround time of 3 to 5 minutes.

In contrast, throat culture has a turnaround time of 24 to 48 hours, and an additional 24 hours is required for isolation and identification from contaminated specimens. For the evaluation of patients suspected of having poststreptococcal disease (ie, rheumatic fever or glomerulonephritis), streptozyme, antistreptolysin O (ASO), and anti-DNase B (antideoxyribonuclease B or ADB) titers are used to establish the presence of a preceding streptococcal infection.

Respiratory illness caused by bacteria is generally a clinical diagnosis that is supported by radiologic imaging (eg, chest x-ray, CT). However, certain pathogens, if not identified or if inadequately treated, pose greater risks to patients. Some examples include pulmonary abscesses, pulmonary tuberculosis, and *Legionella* infections. Obtaining diagnostic pulmonary secretions and subsequent culturing can be useful in cases of pulmonary infections that fail appropriate antibiotic management and in cases that are suspicious for *Mycobacterium* infections, especially pulmonary tuberculosis. Bacterial respiratory cultures have a turnaround time of 48 or more hours.

The evaluation of a symptomatic urinary tract infection (UTI) begins with urine collection. In stable patients who are able to cooperate with specimen collection, a midstream, clean catch urine sample is as accurate as a catheterized urine sample. A urine dipstick is a POCT that is fast and inexpensive. A negative urine dipstick in a patient with a low pretest probability can be used to rule out urine as a source of infection. However, a urine dipstick is not sensitive enough to rule out infection in symptomatic patients with higher pretest probabilities. Moreover, a urine dipstick can be subject to inaccuracies due to improper testing and handling practices. A urine dipstick positive for nitrate is 95% specific but only 45% sensitive for a UTI. A urine dipstick positive for leukocyte esterase is anywhere between 50% and 96% sensitive and 91% and 99% specific.

Microscopic urinalysis (UA) can be useful for differentiating between infection and colonization of the genitourinary (GU) tract. The presence of bacteria alone on microscopic UA is suggestive of colonization, which may or may not represent infection. If WBCs are also present, then infection is more likely. UA also helps to delineate a simple UTI from pyelonephritis. The presence of WBC casts is suggestive of an ascending infection (ie, pyelonephritis), and treatment for a complicated UTI should be administered. However, the accuracy of microscopy in diagnosing UTI is similar to that of a urine dipstick, so a negative test in a symptomatic patient with intermediate to high pretest probability is not enough to rule out infection. Urine culture can be used when microscopic UA or urine dipstick findings are negative in patients with intermediate to high pretest probability for a GU infection. Urine culture is also useful for close monitoring in patients who are not started on antibiotics or in patients with previous treatment failures. Urine culture is indicated in patients at risk for a complicated UTI.

The detection of bloodstream infections and serious local infections in the setting of systemic inflammatory response syndrome (SIRS) or sepsis requires blood culture analysis of two to three independently drawn blood samples. Multiple samples yield the greatest sensitivity for detection of a blood stream infection (BSI) and minimizes the misinterpretation of contaminated samples. Most true positive blood cultures become positive within 24 to 48 hours, and the pathogen responsible is typically isolated from a majority of samples. Routine microbial testing for gastrointestinal infection is generally not useful in the emergency setting.

Stool testing is time consuming, yields little value, and rarely influences management. Patients presenting with abdominal pain or symptoms consistent with colitis in the setting of a diarrheal illness should prompt consideration of microbial causes that have the potential for serious complications in the appropriate clinical setting. Detection of *Clostridium difficile* infection is often done by immunodiagnostic assays (*C. difficile* PCR). In adults, *C. difficile* PCR is reported as 88% sensitive and 96% specific. Cytotoxic culture remains the gold standard but is slow and labor intensive. ELISA toxin assays are also available. Sensitivities vary widely, ranging from 50% to 90%. *C. difficile* PCR has a turnaround time of 24 hours, and cytotoxic assays have turnaround times of 24 to 72 hours. Stool culture takes 96 hours to produce results.

Enterohemorrhagic *E. coli* (*E. coli* 0157:H7) requires a specialized stool culture that may be of use in patients who present with signs and symptoms of hemolytic uremic syndrome. Turnaround time is 48 to 72 hours, but additional time is needed for confirmation of a positive test.

Sexually Transmitted Infections

Sexually transmitted infections (STIs) are commonly seen and treated in the emergency setting. A variety of testing techniques have made ED testing more efficient. For example, *N. gonorrhea* and *Chlamydia* testing can be done by nucleic acid amplification testing (NAAT) from either urogenital or urine samples. Adding to the convenience of these methods is the availability of combination tests for the simultaneous detection of both pathogens. Culture continues to be the gold standard for diagnosis; in cases of suspected sexual abuse or rape, culture is highly recommended. Turnaround time for amplified nucleic acid testing is 24 to 72 hours. Turnaround times for cervical or urethral cultures are between 48 and 72 hours.

Herpes is generally a clinical diagnosis, but microbial testing can be warranted when isolation of *herpes simplex virus* (HSV) is required for patient management, such as in cases of disseminated disease or CNS infection. DFA detection is helpful in detecting HSV in typical skin lesions, and it provides rapid and specific identification of HSV infection. However, sample collection is somewhat labor-intensive.

HSV PCR is the most sensitive method for HSV detection and is particularly useful in the diagnosis of CNS infections due to the rapid turnaround time when compared to HSV culture, which can take up to two days.

In the past, HIV antibody screening was difficult to routinely perform during an ED visit because of the lengthy turnaround time. Recently, six POCTs for the presumptive diagnosis of HIV infection were approved for use in the United States. When compared to standard antibody screening, these POCTs have proven to be accurate screening tests with high sensitivity and specificity. HIV POCT is becoming more widely available in US EDs. A negative screening test is regarded as a true negative. Confirmation is only indicated for a positive screening test. Western blot assay remains the confirmatory test of choice for HIV infection in the setting of a positive POCT.

Treponema pallidum is commonly diagnosed by serologic testing as well as by IgG (immunoglobulin G) and IgM (immunoglobulin M) antibody detection. There are two types of serologic testing. Traditionally, nontreponemal tests (ie, rapid plasma reagin [RPR] or the venereal disease research laboratory [VDRL]) are used as screening tests and can be used to follow the response to treatment. Treponemal tests (TP-PA [treponema pallidum particle agglutination], FTA-ABS [fluorescent treponemal antibody-absorbed], and MHA-TP [microhemagglutination assay for antibodies to treponema pallidum]) are used for confirmation of a reactive nontreponemal test. In other words, when a VDRL or RPR screen for syphilis is positive (reactive), then confirmation testing with one of the direct treponemal tests is indicated.

Parasitic Infection

Parasite and vector-related infections cause a great deal of morbidity and mortality worldwide but rarely impact the United States on a large scale. However, there are a few notable infections. Malaria, babesiosis, Chagas disease, and leishmaniasis are parasitic infections that can be detected in peripheral blood samples. Testing for these parasites requires thick and thin smears, which are inspected for the level of parasitemia. The turnaround time for a positive smear is around 24 hours. If malaria is suspected, a STAT (signal transducer and activator of transcription) preliminary result should be ordered. STAT testing can result in less than 4 hours. Repeat samples should be sent during malaria treatment after 24, 48, and 72 hours to assess the effectiveness of therapy by trending the decline of parasitemia.

Borrelia burgdorferi is a tick-borne disease that is classically diagnosed clinically without laboratory testing. In some cases, testing can help if Lyme disease is suspected in at-risk patients. If laboratory testing is performed, an ELISA antibody screen is used for the detection of IgG or IgM antibodies. False negatives are common in the first one to two weeks of infection because it can take time to create a measurable concentration of antibodies against *B. burgdorferi*. If the ELISA is positive or inconclusive, a Western blot should be done to confirm infection. This two-tiered approach is recommended by the CDC to minimize false positive findings.

Fungal

Cultures are the most sensitive routine laboratory method for the detection of fungal infections. Fungal culture is indicated in patients who are immunocompromised, septic and receiving extensive treatment with broad-spectrum antibiotics, and, sometimes, victims of severe trauma. Fungal cultures are rarely sent from the ED but should be considered in patients who have a lack of response to appropriate antibacterial treatment. Cultures for yeast are incubated for seven days, whereas routine fungal cultures are incubated for up to four weeks.

Suggested Readings and References

1. Wolfson AB. *Harwood-Nuss' Clinical Practice of Emergency Medicine*. 5th ed. Philadelphia, PA: Lippincott Williams and Wilkins; 2010:869–935.
2. Marx JA, Hockberger R, Walls R. *Rosen's Emergency Medicine Concepts and Clinical Practice*. 7th ed. Philadelphia, PA: Mosby; 2010:1676–1848.
3. Roberts JR, Hedges JR. *Clinical Procedures in Emergency Medicine*. 5th ed. Philadelphia, PA: Saunders; 2010:1283–1298.

4. Slaven EM, Stone SC, Lopez FA. *Infectious Diseases: Emergency Department Diagnosis and Management.* New York: McGraw-Hill; 2007.

5. US Centers for Disease Control and Prevention. Clinical Description and Lab Diagnosis of Influenza. http://www.cdc.gov/flu/professionals. Accessed October 15, 2012.

6. National Institute of Allergy and Infectious Disease, Lyme Disease http://www.niaid.nih.gov/topics/lymedisease/research/pages/diagnostics.aspx Accessed April 18, 2015.

Chapter 2

Infection Control

Michael Vulfovich

Infection control is a field concerned with the scientific study of nosocomial-associated infections and the development of protocols and interventions to reduce rates of transmission. The Joint Commission for Accreditation of Hospitals has mandated that each hospital have an infection control program in order to be certified. This program is responsible for various activities, such as the analysis of the nosocomial infection outbreaks, monitoring antibiotic resistance patterns, creating awareness and education for health care workers regarding protocols, writing infection control policies, and overseeing the cleaning of equipment and the disposal of infectious waste. The CDC (Centers for Disease Control and Prevention) has taken a leadership role in the development of practice guidelines that aid in the creation of individual institutional protocols for infection control programs.

Within the Emergency Department (ED), multiple patients with a wide variety of potentially infectious and contagious diseases are in close proximity to other patients and in contact with health care providers caring for multiple patients concurrently. This can increase the risk of exposure and contamination for both patients and staff. In this setting, standardization and monitoring play an especially vital role in infection prevention and control. This chapter will provide a broad overview of isolation precautions and environmental cleaning.

Isolation Precautions

There are four major types of isolation precautions: standard, contact, droplet, and airborne. See Table 2.1. Standard precautions are applicable in the care of all patients, and the other categories expand on the foundation built by the standard precautions. In the ED, isolation precaution signs should be visibly posted in the patient's room with easily accessible supplies either inside or just outside the patient room.

Standard Precautions

These precautions were first issued in 1996 by the CDC and Hospital Infection Control Advisory Committee (HICPAC) and were updated in 2007. They should be utilized in the care of all patients and are especially critical when the health care worker may have mucous membrane or non-intact skin exposure to contaminated blood, body fluids, or secretions.

Hand Hygiene
The most important tenet of infection control is hand hygiene. See Box 2.1. It is not only the easiest and most cost-effective tenet but also the most commonly used method to reduce rates of nosocomial infection transmission. Observational studies have shown variability in adherence to handwashing policies with various factors shown to influence lack of adherence (see Box 2.1). There are numerous options for hand hygiene, and they offer variable levels of protection against microbial flora. The use of hand hygiene also has become a major focus for the "SAVE LIVES: Clean Your Hands" initiative of the WHO, and it is also one of the 2010 National Patient Safety Goals developed by JCAHO. The two main forms of hand hygiene used in the ED are soap and water or the use of an alcohol-containing antiseptic.

Plain soap and water offers no antimicrobial activity, but it may be effective against flora and spores that are loosely adherent to the skin, such as *Clostridium difficile* spores. For handwashing to be effective, however, it is important that health care providers utilize proper technique. After wetting hands with water, physicians should apply a small amount of plain soap and rub their hands together vigorously for 15 to 30 seconds. Spending less time rubbing hands together results in an incomplete reduction of hand contaminants. After thoroughly rubbing all areas of the hands (with particular attention paid to the fingernails), the hands should be rinsed with water and dried thoroughly using a disposable towel. That towel should then be used to turn off the faucet prior to discarding it. Proper hand drying is essential because wet hands have been described to increase the risk of cross-contamination.

The most common form of hand hygiene in the ED is waterless alcohol-containing antiseptics, which have excellent germicidal activity against gram positive and gram negative bacteria, including some multidrug-resistant pathogens like vancomycin-resistant enterococci (VRE), methicillin-resistant *Staphylococcus aureus* (MRSA), *Mycobacterium tuberculosis*, and various fungi. Alternative options include chlorhexidine, iodophors, chloroxynelol, hexachlorophene, quaternary ammonium compounds, and triclosan. To use any of the preceding, physicians should apply a small amount of the product to their hands and rub it into all areas of the hands with particular attention paid to the fingernails until the hands are dry. It is very important to note that these alcohol-containing antiseptics do not have any antimicrobial activity against spore-forming bacteria, such as *C. difficile* (for which soap and water should be used). If hands are visibly dirty, then wash with soap and water before using any of the previously mentioned germicidal agents. Alcohol-based hand disinfection is faster than the use of soap and water and has been

Table 2.1 Infection Prevention Precautions

Type of Isolation	Type of Patients	Recommendations
Standard	All patients Minimum level of infection prevention	1) hand hygiene; 2) use of personal protective equipment (eg, gloves, gowns, face masks), depending on the anticipated exposure; 3) respiratory hygiene and cough etiquette; 4) safe injection practices; and 5) safe handling of potentially contaminated equipment or surfaces in the patient environment
Contact	• Presence of stool incontinence (may include patients with norovirus, rotavirus, or Clostridium difficile), draining wounds, uncontrolled secretions, pressure ulcers, or presence of ostomy tubes and/or bags draining body fluids • Presence of generalized rash or exanthems • Patients with suspected infections/colonization with Multi drug resistant organization, such as VRE and MRSA	• Standard precautions plus gloves and gowns for any patient contact. Consider use of face mask. Place patients in private rooms or cohort patients. • Clean/disinfect the exam room accordingly. • Instruct patients with known or suspected infectious diarrhea to use a separate bathroom, if available; clean/disinfect the bathroom before it can be used again.
Droplet	• Respiratory viruses (eg, influenza, parainfluenza virus, adenovirus, respiratory syncytial virus, human metapneumovirus) • Bordetella pertusis • For first 24 hours of therapy: Neisseria meningitidis, group A streptococcus	Contact Precautions plus face mask for any close procedure or contact. Place the patient in an exam room with a closed door ASAP (prioritize patients who have excessive cough and sputum production); if an exam room is not available, the patient is provided a face mask and placed in a separate area as far from other patients as possible while awaiting care.
Airborne	For patients with any pathogen that can be transmitted by airborne route; these include, but are not limited to • Tuberculosis • Measles • Chickenpox (until lesions are crusted over) • Localized (in immunocompromised patient) or disseminated herpes zoster (until lesions are crusted over)	Place the patient immediately in an airborne infection isolation room (AIIR) • If an AIIR is not available, provide a face mask (eg, procedure or surgical mask) to the patient and place the patient immediately in an exam room with a closed door • Instruct the patient to keep the face mask on while in the exam room, if possible, and to change the mask if it becomes wet • Initiate protocol to transfer patient to a health care facility that has the recommended infection-control capacity to properly manage the patient • Wear a fit-tested N95 or higher level disposable respirator, if available, when caring for the patient; the respirator should be donned prior to room entry and removed after exiting room

Box 2.1 Indications for Hand Hygiene

Always perform hand hygiene in the following situations:

• Before touching a patient, even if gloves will be worn
• Before exiting the patient's care area after touching the patient or the patient's immediate environment
• After contact with blood, body fluids, or excretions, or wound dressings
• Prior to performing an aseptic task (eg, accessing a port, preparing an injection)
• If hands will be moving from a contaminated-body site to a clean-body site during patient care
• After glove removal

shown to improve health care provider compliance, which is the biggest barrier to infection control and is estimated to average only 40%.

Personal Protective Equipment

The CDC has recommended that all health care workers wear nonsterile gloves while caring for patients in order to reduce the risk of infection transmission between and among healthcare providers and patients. The use of gloves is especially important because handwashing and antiseptics may not destroy all contaminants and flora. Health care providers should also be aware that gloves do not offer complete protection against contamination. Confounding factors, such as the type of glove used and the presence of jewelry, may alter effectiveness. It is important to practice hand hygiene both before the application of gloves and after their removal. Sterile gloves need to be used for ED procedures, such as central line placement, lumbar puncture, and emergent transvenous pacing.

The use of other personal protective equipment—including gowns, shoe covers, face shields, masks, and goggles—is determined by institutional infection control protocols and depend on the setting and facility. The immediate disposal or disinfection of all personal protective equipment is mandated by the Occupational Safety and Health Administration (OSHA) in order to prevent the transmission of infectious materials from patient to patient.

Contact Precautions

Contact precautions are intended for patients who harbor organisms that are spread by direct or indirect contact with the patient or contaminated objects within their environment. These patients should be preferentially placed in private patient rooms or cohorted with patients who are infected with the same pathogen. Personnel should use nonsterile gloves and gowns at all times when administering care to these patients. The addition of gowns to the universal precautions has significantly reduced the rate of transmission of these organisms. Personal protective equipment should be put on prior to entering the patient's room and removed immediately after.

Multidrug-Resistant Organisms (MDRO)

As MDROs, including VRE and MRSA, become more prevalent, it is increasingly important to identify patients infected or colonized with MDROs and to utilize infection control isolation protocols. The transmission of MDRO's from one patient to another primarily occurs via the hands of health care workers. Both the Society for Healthcare Epidemiology of America and the Health care Infection Control Practices Advisory Committee of the CDC have separately published recommendations to prevent the transmission of MDRO's. These include the use of surveillance cultures to identify carriers of these infections. Patients should be placed under contact precautions, and disposable equipment should be used solely for that patient when possible. Shared nondisposable equipment should be thoroughly cleaned because these organisms can remain viable for prolonged periods outside the body.

Clostridium Difficile

C. difficile is a spore-forming, anaerobic, gram-positive bacillus that is now the most common cause of nosocomial diarrhea. It is a significant cause of morbidity and mortality in hospitalized patients. Health care institutions should use surveillance to track the rate of C. difficile infections in their facility. Infected patients should be cohorted or isolated in private rooms for at least the duration of the diarrhea. All personnel coming into contact with infected patients should use gloves and gowns for any patient contact. It is important to remember that alcohol-based hand antiseptic does not effectively remove C. difficile spores from the hands of health care workers, so vigorous hand washing for at least 30 seconds with soap and water is recommended. Any equipment used to examine these patients should either be dedicated to that patient alone or promptly. Rooms should be rigorously cleaned after patient discharge.

Droplet Precautions

Droplet precautions are applicable to patients with those organisms that cause respiratory illnesses with particles that are larger than 5 μm in size, which is sufficiently large to limit their time in the air. Organisms that require droplet precautions include *Bordetella pertussis, Haemophilus, influenzavirus*, adenovirus, rhinovirus, *Neisseria meningitidis*, and Group A Streptococci until the infected patient has been on antimicrobial therapy for 24 hours. A private room is preferable, and medical personnel should wear a mask for any contact within 6 feet of infected patients. In addition, any patient on droplet precautions being transported outside the room should wear a mask. If they are unable to tolerate a mask, they should adhere strictly to cough hygiene.

Influenza

Influenzavirus is a viral illness that is spread via large aerosolized particles. It is highly infectious. Especially during peak influenza season, certain practices should be enacted in addition to preventative vaccinations. These practices include screening and triage of symptomatic patients, implementation of respiratory hygiene, cough etiquette, hand hygiene, and minimization of elective visits. Patients thought to be infected should be kept under isolation precautions for seven days or from the onset of symptoms until 24 hours after the resolution of fever and respiratory symptoms, whichever is longer. Until the precautions can be lifted, all health care personnel should utilize universal precautions as well as face masks because this has been shown to significantly decrease influenza transmission.

Airborne Precautions

When particles are less than 5 μm in size, they can remain in the air for longer periods of time, prolonging the risk of exposure. Suspected or confirmed organisms that require airborne precautions include *Mycobacterium tuberculosis*, rubeola virus, varicella virus, and disseminated herpes zoster in any patient or localized herpes zoster in immunocompromised patients. Patients with these infections should be placed in negative pressure isolation rooms. Personnel should use appropriately sized certified respirators, such as the N95 or the Powered Air Purifying Respirator (PAPR) when entering infected patients' rooms.

Tuberculosis

Public health measures and effective chemotherapy have reduced the incidence and prevalence of tuberculosis in the United States. Tuberculosis (TB) is more prevalent in some populations (See Box 2.2), and latent infection is more likely to progress to active disease in others (Box 2.3). Health care personnel should be cognizant of patients with epidemiologic risk factors. TB is transmitted via inhalation of droplet nuclei (particles 1 to 5 μm in diameter are more likely to be produced during procedures, such as endotracheal intubation and aerosol treatments). All patients infected with tuberculosis should immediately be placed on airborne precautions, and these should be continued until the patient is on effective therapy, is improving clinically, and has three consecutive sputum samples from different days that are acid-fast bacilli negative.

Environmental Cleaning

Environmental cleaning, disinfection, and sterilization are the final steps in reducing infection transmission in the health care setting. Some infectious organisms have been shown to survive for months on

---

Box 2.2 Groups with a higher prevalence of TB infection include

- Foreign-born persons from areas with high TB prevalence (especially those who have arrived in the United States from endemic areas less than 5 years earlier) and individuals who travel frequently to such areas
- Homeless or marginally housed persons
- Residents and employees of congregate settings that are high-risk (eg, correctional facilities, long-term care facilities, and homeless shelters)
- The elderly (based on having been alive during a time of higher TB prevalence in the United States)
- Health care workers (HCWs) who serve patients at high risk in the United States
- HCWs, other professionals, and volunteers who travel abroad to work in health care facilities or with refugees in regions in which TB is endemic
- HCWs with unprotected exposure to a patient with TB disease before the identification and correct airborne precautions of the patient
- Certain populations who are medically underserved and who have low incomes
- Infants, children, and adolescents exposed to adults in high-risk categories

Box 2.3 Groups with a higher risk of progression to active TB include

- Those who have been infected with TB within the previous 2 years
- Infants and children younger than 4 years of age
- Persons with a history of untreated or inadequately treated TB disease, including those with fibrotic lesions on chest radiography suggestive of healed TB
- Persons with immunocompromising conditions, including
  - HIV infection
  - Hematologic malignancy
  - Cancer of the head, neck, and/or lung
  - Organ transplantation
  - Prolonged corticosteroid therapy
  - Treatment with other immunosuppressive agents, such as calcineurin inhibitors, cytotoxic chemotherapeutic agents, and tumor necrosis factor alpha (TNF-alpha) inhibitors
- Persons with other underlying medical conditions including
  - Silicosis
  - Diabetes mellitus
  - Chronic kidney disease
  - Gastrectomy or intestinal bypass
- Body weight 10% or more below ideal body weight

Box 2.4 Common Emergency Department Procedures

Peripheral IV Placement:
1. Wash hands with antiseptic soap
2. Wear gloves
3. Prep the skin with antiseptic solution—isopropyl alcohol or chlorhexidine

Central Line Placement:
1. Wash hands with antiseptic soap
2. Prep the skin with antiseptic solution—chlorhexidine or povidone-iodine solution
3. Maintain full barrier precautions—cap, face mask, gown, and sterile gloves for physician and full barrier drape for patient; all others in the room should also wear a cap, face mask, and avoid contaminating the sterile field
4. Re-prep skin with antiseptic solution
5. Use sterile materials from central line cart
6. When the procedure is complete, place sterile occlusive dressing on central line while still under sterile precautions

Lumbar Puncture:
1. Wash hands with antiseptic soap
2. Prep the skin with antiseptic solution—chlorhexidine or povidone-iodine solution
3. Use sterile gloves, face mask with eye protection, and local sterile drape; all others in the room should also wear cap, face mask, and avoid contaminating the sterile field
4. Make sure that you clean off the chlorhexidine or povidone-iodine solution from entry site to avoid possible meningeal irritation
5. Use sterile materials from lumbar puncture kit

Laceration Repair:
1. Administer tetanus immunization as recommended by guidelines
2. Thoroughly irrigate and explore laceration; anesthetize if necessary
3. Use gloves; nonsterile gloves are acceptable
3. Debride nonviable tissue
4. Consider prophylactic antibiotics based on wound size, location, and degree of contamination

countertops and other surfaces depending on environmental conditions. Proper cleaning begins with the removal of all foreign material from objects and with the removal of large, visible contaminants. The next step involves disinfection of the environment. Sterilization, or the complete eradication of pathogens, is the final step in environmental cleaning. Different levels of environmental cleaning exist, depending on the item or area being cleaned.

Common Procedures

In the ED, several procedures are commonly performed. Infection prevention should remain an important consideration during the performance of any of these procedures. See Box 2.4.

Suggested Readings and References

1. Edmond MB, Wenzel RP. Organization for infection control. In: Mandell GL, Bennett JE, Dolin R, eds. *Principles and Practice of Infectious Diseases*. 6th ed. Philadelphia, PA: Churchill Livingstone; 2005:3323.
2. UTD: General Principles of Infection Control.
3. Garner JS. Guideline for isolation precautions in hospitals: The Hospital Infection Control Practices Advisory Committee. *Infect Control Hosp Epidemiol*. 1996;17:53.
4. Siegel JD, Rhinehart E, Jackson M, et al. Healthcare Infection Control Practices Advisory Committee 2007 guideline for isolation precautions: Preventing transmission of infectious agents in healthcare settings. http://www.cdc.gov/ncidod/dhqp/gl_isolation.html Published June 2007. Accessed on December 06, 2011.
5. Pittet D, Allegranzi B, Sax H, et al. Evidence-based model for hand transmission during patient care and the role of improved practices. *Lancet Infect Dis*. 2006;6:641.
6. Boyce JM, Pittet D. Healthcare Infection Control Practices Advisory Committee, HICPAC/SHEA/APIC/IDSA Hand Hygiene Task Force. Guideline for Hand Hygiene in Health-Care Settings. Recommendations of the Healthcare Infection Control Practices Advisory Committee and the HICPAC/SHEA/APIC/IDSA Hand Hygiene Task Force. Society for Healthcare Epidemiology of America/Association for Professionals in Infection Control/Infectious Diseases Society of America. *MMWR Recomm Rep* 2002;51:1.
7. World Health Organization. SAVE LIVES: Clean Your Hands: WHO's global annual campaign. http://www.who.int/gpsc/5may/en/ Accessed on December 06, 2011).
8. http://www.patientsafety.gov/TIPS/Docs/TIPS_JanFeb10Poster.pdf
9. Merry AF, Miller TE, Findon G, Webster CS, Neiff SP. Touch contamination levels during anaesthetic procedures and their relationship to hand hygiene procedures. *Br J Anesthesiol*. 2001;87:291–294.
10. Kampf G, Kramer A. Epidemiologic background of hand hygiene and evaluation of the most important agents for scrubs and rubs. *Clin Microbiol Rev*. 2004;17:863–893.
11. Puzniak LA, Leet T, Mayfield J, et al. To gown or not to gown: the effect on acquisition of vancomycin resistant enterococci. *Clin Infect Dis*. 2002;35:18.
12. Srinivasan A, Song X, Ross T, et al. A prospective study to determine whether cover gowns in addition to gloves decrease nosocomial transmission of vancomucin resistant enterococci in an intensive care unit. *Infect Control Hosp Epidemiol*. 2002;23:424.
13. Muto CA, Jernigan JA, Ostrowsky BE, et al. SHEA guideline for preventing nosocomial transmission of multidrug-resistant strains of Staphylococcus aureus and enterococcus. *Infect Control Hosp Epidemiol*. 2003;24:362.
14. Kyne L, Hamel MB, Polavaram R, Kelly CP. Heath care costs and mortality associated with nosocomial diarrhea due to Clostridium difficile. *Clin Infect Dis*. 2002;34:346.
15. Cohen SH, Gerding DN, Jognson S, et al. Clinical practice guidelines for Clostridium difficile infection in adults: 2010 update by the Society for Healthcare Epidemiology of America (SHEA) and the Infectious Disease Society of America (IDSA). *Infect Control Hosp Epidemiol*. 2010;31:431.
16. Aiello AE, Murray GF, Perez V, et al. Mask use, hand hygiene, and seasonal influenza like illness among young adults: a randomized intervention trial. *J Infect Dis*. 2010;201:491.
17. Sepkowitz KA. How contagious is tuberculosis? Clin Infect Dis. 1996;23:954.
18. CDC. Guidelines for Environmental Infection Control in Health-Care Facilities. Recommendations of CDC and the Healthcare Infection Control Practices Advisory Committee (HICPAC). *MMWR Morb Mortal Wkly Rep* 2003;52(RR10):1–42.
19. Bolyard EA, Tablan OC, Williams WW, Pearson ML, Shapiro CN, Deitchmann SD. Guideline for infection control in healthcare personnel, 1998. Hospital Infection Control Practices Advisory Committee. *Infect Control Hosp Epidemiol*. 1998;19:407–463.
20. Bhalla A, Pultz NJ, Gries DM, et al. Acquisition of nosocomial pathogens on hands after contact with environmental surfaces near hospitalized patients. *Infect Control Hosp Epidemiol*. 2004;25:164–167.

Infectious Disease Mimics

Tyler Martinez

Summary Box

Disease Description: Infection is not the only etiology of the Systemic Inflammatory Response Syndrome (SIRS).*

The diseases that can mimic sepsis fall into four main categories: malignancy, autoimmunity, xenobiotic-related, and others—notably pulmonary embolus (PE).

Treatment: Therapy is based on the underlying disease process.

Other Key Issues: Always maintain a broad differential diagnosis for SIRS.

*See box 4.1 for a description of the SIRS criteria.

Disease Description

Malignancy

The initial manifestations of malignancy are often vague. They are often as ascribed to a viral syndrome in the early stages, so the underlying malignancy sometimes is not discovered until later in the course of the disease. Some of the most common complaints in those with underlying malignancy are weight loss (or possibly gain), anorexia or decreased oral intake, malaise, generalized fatigue, and night sweats. A mildly elevated temperature can also be seen. When these symptoms persist for weeks to months and/or gradually increase in severity, an infectious etiology becomes less likely, and other causative diseases should be considered. Especially in older patients, nonspecific constitutional symptoms are more likely to represent underlying malignancy, but these symptoms can be due to an undiagnosed primary malignancy in younger patients as well.

If malignancy is suspected in a patient with nonspecific constitutional symptoms, serum electrolytes can be used to screen for certain paraneoplastic syndromes. An abnormally low sodium level can suggest the syndrome of inappropriate antidiuretic hormone (SIADH) due to small-cell lung cancer, other small cell malignancies, and head or neck malignancies. An elevated calcium level can occur due to bone lysis in multiple myeloma and in certain bone metastases, such as those from primary breast, lung, and certain genitourinarycancers (eg, renal, cervical, uterine, and ovarian cancer). Of note, prostate cancer bone metastases are blastic rather than lytic and, thus, are less commonly associated with hypercalcemia. Elevated blood calcium can also result from any cancer that produces parathyroid hormone-related peptide (eg, breast cancer and certain types of lung cancer, including squamous cell lung cancer), which increases bone resorption. Any severe electrolyte disorder warrants admission, possibly to the intensive care unit (ICU), for medical management.

Complete blood count (CBC) abnormalities can be misleading. Because a highly elevated WBC is frequently associated with sepsis (especially in conjunction with fever, malaise, fatigue, anorexia, and sweating), providers can prematurely narrow their differential diagnosis to solely infectious processes when, in fact, these symptoms could be due to malignancy. Especially when the WBC is significantly elevated, approaching 100,000 or more, a diagnosis of acute myeloid leukemia (AML) should be considered. Typically, a leukocytosis of greater than 100,000 results from either AML or severe *Clostridium difficile* infection. A decrease in the other cell lines (eg, anemia and thrombocytopenia) is common when leukocytosis has been present for enough time; thus, decreases in these other cell lines can aid in differentiating hematologic malignancy from infection. Unfortunately, all of the preceding CBC findings can also be seen in the setting of infection or sepsis; and AML can present with leucopenia as well, making definitive diagnosis more difficult.

Increased production of any cell line can cause a complication known as hyperviscosity syndrome, which is the impedance of normal vascular blood flow due to the increase in intravascular viscosity that results from the increased concentration of hematologic cells. Hyperviscosity syndrome typically presents with the previously mentioned constitutional symptoms and then progresses to abdominal pain, altered mental status, and focal neurologic or peripheral findings due to thromboses. Treatment involves early consultation with a hematologist and IV (intravenous) hydration followed by plasmapheresis if the preceding interventions are unsuccessful.

Autoimmunity

The initial presentation of autoimmune diseases is similar to that of malignancy: fatigue, malaise, anorexia, weight changes, myalgias, arthralgias, night sweats, and/or low-grade temperature elevations of insidious onset. Autoimmune diseases that can be mistaken for infection include systemic lupus erythematosus (SLE), rheumatoid arthritis (RA), systemic scleroderma (SS), Takayasu arteritis (TA), granulomatosis with Polyangiitis (ie, Wegener's granulomatosis), Behcet's disease, polymyositis, dermatomyositis, ankylosing spondylitis, and polyarteritis nodosa (PAN), among others.

Most of the preceding diseases are more commonly seen in adults, although PAN, SLE, and juvenile idiopathic arthritis (formerly JRA or juvenile RA) can be considered in children with fever of unknown origin.

Differentiating systemic autoimmune diseases from infection or sepsis in the emergency department is difficult and often delayed, especially if the patient has no prior diagnosis. Laboratory testing often yields nonspecific findings, nearly all of which can also be seen in certain infections. Serum test results can include leukocytosis, anemia, thrombocytopenia, elevated inflammatory markers (ie, C-reactive protein and erythrocyte sedimentation rate). A urinalysis may reveal an increase in WBCs and/or red blood cells due to genitourinary involvement of the autoimmune disease, which can be confused with a genitourinary infection. Often, however, an infection of the genitourinary system will additionally yield bacteria, positive leukocyte esterase, and nitrite, which can aid in differentiating infection from an auto-immune process.

A chest radiograph can also yield overlapping findings, as many of the autoimmune diseases can present with pulmonary fibrosis, pneumonitis, pulmonary hemorrhage, and even acute respiratory distress syndrome (ARDS).

Many autoimmune diseases also have varying degrees of cardiovascular inflammation, including pericarditis, myocarditis, cardiac tamponade, and aortitis. Without a broad differential diagnosis, these cardiac manifestations can be erroneously ascribed to infectious causes, such as syphilis, bacterial endocarditis, septicemia, and streptococcal infection.

Unless there is a high index of suspicion, a patient with a mild fever, elevated inflammatory markers, and one or more other findings (eg, evidence of pericarditis on an EKG [electrocardiogram] or physical exam; infiltrate on chest radiograph; or warm, red, and swollen joint) can be admitted and covered for a presumed infectious process, delaying proper diagnosis until symptoms do not improve despite antibiotic treatment.

Conversely, there must also be a high index of suspicion for infection when an autoimmune process is suspected because systemic steroids are one of the most common treatments for acute rheumatologic flares, and systemic steroids given to a patient with a serious infection could result in major morbidity or mortality. Thus, early rheumatology consultation can be helpful when trying to delineate between infection and an autoimmune process regardless of which etiology is favored.

Xenobiotic-related

Many xenobiotics (chemicals in an organism that are not normally produced by or not normally present in that organism), either alone or in combination, are known to cause alterations in temperature, heart rate, blood pressure, respiratory rate, and mental status. These findings, as well as many other physical exam and laboratory findings, can lead to a clinical picture similar to that of sepsis. The astute clinician needs to be aware of the most common causes of xenobiotic-induced pseudosepsis because delays in appropriate treatment can be detrimental.

Serotonin Syndrome

Serotonin syndrome results from excess serotonin within the blood stream, most commonly due to combining serotonergic medications or due to increasing the dosage of a single agent. The most common medication combination resulting in serotonin syndrome is that of selective serotonin reuptake inhibitors (SSRI) and monoamine oxidase inhibitors (MAOI), but there are many other medications that have serotonin agonist properties (see Table 3.1).

The manifestations of serotonin syndrome exist along a clinical spectrum, ranging from mild to life-threatening. Thus, an accurate medication history, including recent medication or dosage changes, is crucial to the diagnosis of serotonin syndrome, especially if the symptoms are mild or atypical. Unfortunately, there is no specific diagnostic test for serotonin syndrome, so the diagnosis is purely clinical. Differentiating between serotonin syndrome and sepsis or infection without an accurate medical history can be quite difficult.

Table 3.1 Serotonergic Xenobiotics	
Amantadine	LSD (lysergic acid diethylamide)
Amitriptyline	MDMA
Amphetamine	Meperidine
Buspirone	Mescaline
Bromocriptine	Mirtazapine
Buproprion	Nortriptyline
Citalopram	Paroxetine
Clomipramine	Phenelzine
Desipramine	Selegiline
Dexfenfluramine	Sertraline
Doxepin	St. John's Wort
Fenfluramine	Tramadol
Fluoxetine	Trazodone
Fluvoxamine	Venlafaxine
Imipramine	

The classic triad of serotonin syndrome includes hyperthermia, muscle rigidity and hyperreflexia, and altered mental status. More broadly, this triad reflects the autonomic dysfunction, neuromuscular dysfunction, and cognitive dysfunction that can occur in serotonin syndrome. Signs and symptoms of autonomic dysfunction can include elevated temperature, tachycardia, hypertension, hypotension (less commonly), tachypnea, diaphoresis, flushed and dry skin, and dilated or unreactive pupils. Signs and symptoms of neuromuscular dysfunction include hyperreflexia, myoclonus, rigidity, nystagmus, opisthotonus, tremor, and Babinski sign. Signs and symptoms of cognitive dysfunction include confusion, altered mental status, agitation, seizures, insomnia, hallucinations, lethargy, and even coma.

Laboratory testing can yield some or all of the markers associated with sepsis, including elevated lactate, metabolic acidosis, and/or leukocytosis. Head CT (computed tomography), lumbar puncture, and drug levels are usually all within normal limits.

Treatment includes supportive management and discontinuation of the serotonin agonist. Patients usually improve within 24 hours but typically require admission for further monitoring, sometimes to the ICU. A trial of cyproheptadine (a serotonin antagonist) can be considered in more critically ill patients, but cyproheptadine, like many of the serotonergic xenobiotics that cause serotonin syndrome, has anticholinergic properties and thus must be used cautiously.

Salicylate Overdose

There are many common over-the-counter medications that contain salicylate. Both an acute overdose (more common in the young or those with mental health problems) and a chronic ingestion (more common in the elderly) of salicylates can mimic the signs, symptoms, and physiologic appearance of bacterial sepsis so closely that it can be nearly indistinguishable without a high index of suspicion or a good exposure history from the patient or a witness. However, a pseudosepsis picture is more likely to be seen in a large, acute ingestion.

Initial symptoms of salicylate poisoning include nausea and vomiting, diaphoresis, increased respiratory rate, and tinnitus or decreased hearing. Hyperthermia can be seen in significant ingestions secondary to the uncoupling of oxidative phosphorylation. Normal or even high glucose levels have been seen, but hypoglycemia is more common.

Salicylates cause a mixed metabolic picture, initially increasing a patient's respiratory drive and yielding a respiratory alkalosis. An acute ingestion can also cause excessive vomiting, which causes a superimposing metabolic alkalosis due to volume contraction. As toxicity progresses, salicylate induces an increase in lipolysis and uncouples oxidative phosphorylation. This results in increased anaerobic metabolism and lactate production, which yields an anion gap metabolic acidosis. Progressive toxicity also causes lethargy and obtundation, leading to decreased respiratory drive and a consequent respiratory acidosis. Thus, salicylate toxicity can progress from a combined respiratory and metabolic alkalosis initially to a combined respiratory and metabolic acidosis.

Hypotension with reduced systemic vascular resistance can also be seen in large salicylate ingestions. Multiorgan failure (eg, acute renal failure, encephalopathy, disseminated intravascular coagulation, ARDS, and cardiac dysrhythmias) can also be present and further cloud the clinical picture.

Definitive diagnosis is made with serial serum salicylate concentrations. Treatment for salicylate toxicity is immediate resuscitation with attention to airway, breathing, and circulation followed by reducing the body's overall salicylate burden by alkalinizing the urine. It is important to monitor electrolytes, especially potassium. If serious toxicity is evident or if standard measures do not appear to improve the patient's clinical status, emergent hemodialysis is indicated.

Pulmonary Embolism

PE is not normally thought of as a mimicker of sepsis, but, in the right setting, PE can mimic moderate infection. The most common complaint in someone with a PE is shortness of breath. Unexplained dyspnea almost always results in further evaluation for possible cardiac, pulmonary, or hematologic causes.

Patients with a PE will typically complain of shortness of breath, chest pain (pleuritic in nature), dyspnea with exertion, and cough. Less likely complaints include hemoptysis, syncope, chest pain, shortness of breath, mild fever (usually less than 102°F), or unilateral leg swelling. In addition to tachypnea and hypoxemia, objective findings include sinus tachycardia and an abnormal chest radiograph, most commonly demonstrating basilar atelectasis.

In the setting of an abnormal chest radiograph, tachycardia, tachypnea, hypoxia, hypocapnia, mildly elevated temperature, and cough, a provider without a broad differential could erroneously diagnose sepsis due to presumed pneumonia in the setting of two or more SIRS criteria.

PE should always remain on the differential for shortness of breath, especially if the patient has one or more risk factors for PE. These risk factors include age greater than 50, recent surgery requiring general anesthesia in the last four weeks, estrogen usage, pregnancy, recent long travel, active malignancy (specifically adenocarcinoma or brain cancer), and new-onset limb or body immobility for greater than 48 hours.

PE is diagnosed with either a CT angiography of the chest (usually PE protocol) or a ventilation/ perfusion scan. A CT scan can help differentiate an occult pneumonia from a PE, but this benefit must be weighed against the risks of increased radiation and the possibility of renal injury from IV contrast.

Treatment for a PE is with anticoagulation, typically either unfractionated heparin as an IV bolus and then drip, or with fractionated heparin like enoxaparin as a subcutaneous injection.

Suggested Readings and References

1. Birmes P et al. Serotonin syndrome: a brief overview. *Can Med Assoc J.* 2003;168:1439–1442.
2. Boyer EW, Shannon M. The serotonin syndrome. *New Engl J Med.* 2005;352:1112–1120.
3. Flombaum CD. Metabolic emergencies in the cancer patient. *Semin Oncol.* 2000;27:322–334.
4. Grill V, Martin TJ. Hypercalcemia of malignancy. *Rev Endocr Metab Disord.* 2000;1:253–263.
5. Kline JA et al. New diagnostic tests for pulmonary embolism. *Ann Emerg Med.* 2000;35:168–180.
6. Leatherman JW, Schmitz PG. Fever, hyperdynamic shock, and multiple-system organ failure: A pseudo-sepsis syndrome associated with chronic salicylate intoxication. *Chest* 1991;100:1391–1396.
7. Mundy GR et al. Hypercalcemia of malignancy. *Clinical Endocrine Oncology.* 2nd ed. Blackwell Publishing; 2009.
8. Salvarani C et al. Polymyalgia rheumatica and giant-cell arteritis. *New Engl J Med.* 2002;347:261–271.
9. Slobodin G et al. The emergency room in systemic rheumatic diseases. *Emerg Med J.* 2006;23:667–671.
10. Susec O et al. The clinical features of acute pulmonary embolism in ambulatory patients. *Acad Emerg Med.* 1997;4:891–897.
11. Williams F et al. Critical illness in systemic lupus erythematosus and the antiphospholipid syndrome. *Ann Rheum Dis.* 2002;61:414–421.

General Management of Severe Infection in Acute and Emergency Environments

Chapter 4

Sepsis

Kamna S. Balhara, Basem F. Khishfe, and Jamil D. Bayram

Summary Box

Disease Description: Sepsis is a clinical syndrome of systemic inflammation due to infection, which may be occult.

Organisms: Gram positive and negative bacteria, fungi, and viruses

Treatment: Airway, breathing, and circulation (ABCs) management
  Aggressive fluid resuscitation
  Early administration of broad-spectrum antibiotics: consider combination of vancomycin (loading dose 20–25 mg/kg IV, adjust for renal insufficiency) and antipseudomonal coverage (cefepime 2 g IV)
  Early goal-directed therapy and severe sepsis resuscitation bundle (see text)

Other Key Issues: Diagnosis can be challenging in pediatric and geriatric populations.

25

Disease Description

Sepsis is a clinical syndrome characterized by systemic inflammation due to infection.

Epidemiology

Sepsis affects approximately 750,000 Americans every year and carries a mortality rate as high as 28.6%. Sepsis affects people of all ages, but it is especially common and fatal in the elderly. Whereas over 60% of sepsis cases are cared for in advanced or intensive care units, it has been estimated that 500,000 patients with severe sepsis first present to the emergency department (ED). The early recognition and treatment of sepsis upon presentation to the ED is paramount for reducing morbidity and mortality.

Presenting Features and Complications

General Features: Fever, tachycardia, and tachypnea are usually present, along with other signs and symptoms of source-specific infection. Some septic patients may not look "ill." Patients that appear nontoxic are often described as having "cryptic" or "occult" sepsis. In more severe cases of sepsis, signs of inadequate perfusion may be present.

Cardiovascular Manifestations: Due to systemic inflammation and consequent vasodilation in early sepsis, patients frequently present with decreased systemic vascular resistance, reflex tachycardia, and normal or increased cardiac output. Although the exact causes of myocardial depression in sepsis remain unclear, decreased ejection fractions and increased end-diastolic volumes have been observed in adequately resuscitated survivors of sepsis, likely due to decreased contractility and impaired myocardial compliance. Under conditions of adequate volume resuscitation, the profound reduction in systemic vascular resistance leads to an increase in cardiac index that obscures myocardial dysfunction.

Pulmonary Manifestations: Sepsis is the most common condition associated with the development of acute respiratory distress syndrome (ARDS). In sepsis, microvascular insults result in increased alveolar capillary permeability, which predisposes patients to pulmonary edema and, eventually, acute lung injury and ARDS. The resultant ventilation/perfusion mismatch and right-to-left shunting of deoxygenated blood induces a compensatory tachypnea and hyperventilation, which produces the respiratory alkalosis often seen in sepsis patients.

Renal Manifestations: Severe sepsis can cause acute renal failure (ARF). ARF may result from pre-renal hypoperfusion, acute tubular necrosis secondary to renal hypoperfusion, or from glomerulonephritis or interstitial nephritis caused by certain pathogens or drugs used in treatment of sepsis.

Hematologic Manifestations: Neutrophilic leukocytosis is commonly produced by sepsis, although neutropenia may rarely be seen. Red cell production is decreased in sepsis, but anemia does not result unless infection is prolonged or unless sepsis is complicated by a hemolytic process. Anemia, reticulocytosis, decreased haptoglobin, and increased lactate dehydrogenase and/or indirect bilirubin can suggest a hemolytic process. Disseminated intravascular coagulopathy (DIC) may also occur in sepsis and can have thrombotic manifestations (microvascular occlusion leading to organ failure) and hemorrhagic manifestations (when platelets and clotting factors cannot be replenished at a rate high enough to match consumption).

Neurologic Manifestations: Neurologic manifestations of sepsis are usually nonfocal and may include disorientation, confusion, lethargy, and agitation.

Gastrointestinal Manifestations: Elevated bilirubin levels (especially indirect bilirubin) and jaundice may be present due to hepatocellular dysfunction as well as red blood cell (RBC) hemolysis. Stress gastric ulceration may occur but rarely causes significant bleeding.

Other Abnormalities: Hyperglycemia can occur. Hypoglycemia is less frequently seen. Adrenal insufficiency and venous thromboembolism may also be seen. A metabolic acidosis with elevated anion gap is seen due to lactic acid elevation, which results from poor tissue oxygenation (leading to increased anaerobic glycolysis) as well as poor hepatic clearance of lactate.

Diagnostic Considerations and Tests

Definitions: Sepsis was first defined in 1991 by the American College of Chest Physicians and the Society of Critical Care Medicine and today remains largely unchanged. It is defined as a source of infection plus the systemic inflammatory response syndrome (SIRS). Because sepsis is largely a clinical diagnosis, the source of infection may be either confirmed or suspected. SIRS is defined in Box 4.1.

As described in Table 4.1, sepsis can be described as a progression along a continuum from severe sepsis to septic shock to, finally, multiple organ dysfunction syndrome (MODS).

Diagnostic Tests: Diagnostic tests in suspected sepsis must be guided by the clinical picture. Initial tests should include a complete blood count, complete metabolic profile, urine analysis, urine and blood cultures, venous blood gas, and serum lactate. Other blood tests—such as prothrombin time, partial thromboplastin time, international normalized ratio, DIC panel, and arterial blood gas—should be

---

Box 4.1 Definition of SIRS

SIRS = 2 or more of the following:

- Temperature > 38°C (100.4°F) or < 36°C (96.8°F)
- Heart rate > 90 bpm
- Respiratory rate > 20 breaths per minute, or arterial carbon dioxide tension (PaCO$_2$) < 32 mm Hg
- Abnormal white blood cell count (> 12,000/μL or < 4,000/μL or > 10% bands)

---

considered as indicated. Further studies, such as chest radiograph, computed tomography of the abdomen, or lumbar puncture, should be performed as guided by clinical suspicion to identify a source of infection.

Lactate level, a product of anaerobic metabolism and a surrogate marker for global tissue hypoxia, plays an important role in the diagnosis, prognosis, and treatment of sepsis. A serum lactate value of greater than 4 mmol/L (36 mg/dL) is correlated with an increased severity of illness (severe sepsis) and a poor prognosis, regardless of hemodynamic status. Importantly, lactate clearance of 10% or greater in 2 hours has been described as an indication of adequate resuscitation.

Procalcitonin is under investigation as a sepsis marker, and some studies suggest that it may help differentiate SIRS from sepsis. Other biomarkers, such as interleukin 6 (IL-6) and C-reactive protein (CRP), are elevated in sepsis and have been proposed as potential diagnostic and prognostic markers but have not been shown to be specific.

Differential Diagnosis: Several medical conditions can mimic sepsis, such as gastrointestinal hemorrhage, pulmonary embolism, acute myocardial infarction, acute pancreatitis, and adrenal insufficiency.

Organisms

Bacteria (gram positive and negative) are most commonly associated with sepsis, although fungi, viruses, and parasites can cause sepsis. Infections in the lungs, urinary tract, abdomen, skin, brain, and other areas can cause bacteremia and lead to sepsis.

Treatment

The mainstays of sepsis treatment include aggressive intravenous fluid resuscitation, early administration of empiric antibiotics, and hemodynamic stabilization (with oxygen, vasopressors, blood transfusion, and/or inotropes as needed).

Severe Sepsis Bundles: Following the 2008 evidence-based recommendations, the Surviving Sepsis Campaign recommends the implementation of the Severe Sepsis Bundles, which are evidence-based "groups" of individual therapies whose goals must be completed in patients with severe sepsis, septic shock, and/or a lactate of greater than 4 mmol/L (36 mg/dL). These bundles have been designed to achieve a 25% reduction in mortality from severe sepsis or septic shock. There are two Severe Sepsis Bundles: Severe Sepsis Resuscitation Bundle and Severe Sepsis Management Bundle (see Box 4.2).

Early Goal-Directed Therapy (EGDT): EGDT has been advocated in the treatment of severe sepsis and septic shock to reduce mortality. It is outlined in Box 4.3.

Antibiotics: Broad-spectrum antibiotics need to be administered within 1 hour of the diagnosis of severe sepsis or septic shock. The choice of antimicrobials usually depends on the source of infection, allergies, and susceptibility patterns of pathogens in the community and the hospital. Given that there is very little margin for error in patients with severe sepsis and septic shock, the choice of antimicrobial

Table 4.1 Spectrum of Sepsis

Sepsis	SIRS + source of infection (confirmed or suspected)
Severe Sepsis	Sepsis + organ dysfunction, hypotension, or hypoperfusion (lactate ≥ 4 mmol/L, SBP < 90 mm Hg, or SBP drop > 40 mm Hg of normal)
Septic shock	Severe sepsis with hypotension despite adequate fluid resuscitation
MODS	Septic shock + evidence of ≥ 2 organs with dysfunction

MODS: multiple organ dysfunction syndrome.

Box 4.2 Specific Elements of the Severe Sepsis Bundles

Severe Sepsis Resuscitation Bundle (must be completed within 6 hours):

1. Measure serum lactate.
2. Obtain blood cultures prior to antibiotic administration (be cautious of unwarranted delays [> 45 minutes] in antibiotic administration).
3. Administer broad-spectrum antibiotics within 3 hours of ED admission (must be within 1 hour of diagnosis of severe sepsis or septic shock).
4. In the event of hypotension and/or a serum lactate > 4 mmol/L:
   • Deliver an initial minimum of 30 ml/kg of crystalloid* or an equivalent.
   • Apply vasopressors for hypotension not responding to initial fluid resuscitation to maintain a mean arterial pressure (MAP) > 65 mm Hg. Norepinephrine is first line.
5. In the event of persistent hypotension despite fluid resuscitation (ie, septic shock) and/or a lactate > 4 mmol/L:
   • Achieve a central venous pressure (CVP) of > 8 mm Hg.
   • Achieve a central venous oxygen saturation (ScvO2) > 70% or mixed venous oxygen saturation (SvO2) > 65%.
   • Achieve normalization of lactate.

Severe Sepsis Management Bundle (must be completed within 24 hours):

1. Intravenous corticosteroids (hydrocortisone 200 mg IV daily) are suggested in adult septic shock patients if adequate vasopressor therapy and fluid resuscitation fail to restore hemodynamic stability. Steroids may be tapered when vasopressors are no longer needed.
2. Maintain adequate glycemic control (≤180 mg/dL).
3. Prevent excessive inspiratory plateau pressures on mechanically ventilated patients (< 30 cm H2O).

* Although controversy exists regarding use of crystalloid vs colloid solutions, the current Surviving Sepsis Campaign advocates use of crystalloids, with addition of albumin if substantial amounts are needed.

therapy should be sufficiently broad to cover all likely bacterial pathogens in patients with no clear source of infection (see Box 4.4).

Additional treatment guidelines

• A higher target central venous pressure (CVP) of 12 to 15 mmHg is recommended in the presence of mechanical ventilation or preexisting decreased ventricular compliance.
• Norepinephrine is the first-line vasoactive agent. Some studies suggest that norepinephrine is superior to dopamine in sepsis.

Box 4.3 Early Goal-Directed Therapy

EGDT:

1. Supplemental oxygen and, if needed, endotracheal intubation and mechanical ventilation
2. Central venous and arterial catheterization
3. Check central venous pressure (CVP): If CVP < 8 mm Hg, give crystalloid/colloid fluids until CVP is 8–12 mm Hg.
4. Check mean arterial pressure (MAP): If MAP < 65 mm Hg after CVP goal is achieved, give vasoactive agents until MAP is ≥65 and ≤90 mm Hg.
5. Check central venous oxygen saturation (ScvO2):
   • If ScvO2 < 70% after CVP and MAP goals are achieved, evaluate the hematocrit level and, if needed, transfuse packed RBCs until hematocrit ≥ 30%.
   • If ScvO2 < 70% with CVP, MAP, and hematocrit goals achieved, start inotropic agents until ScvO2 ≥ 70%.
6. When all goals are achieved (CVP, MAP, hematocrit, and ScvO2), admit patient.

Box 4.4 Empiric Antibiotics in Adults with Sepsis and Septic Shock with No Clear Source of Infection

Accepted antibiotic regimens (covers *Pseudomonas*):

- Vancomycin* plus antipseudomonal cephalosporin (eg, cefepime 2 g IV q8 hours
- Vancomycin* plus beta-lactamase inhibitor (eg, piperacillin-tazobactam 4.5 g IV q6 hours)
- Vancomycin* plus carbapenem (eg, meropenem 1–2 g IV q8 hours)

If true penicillin allergy:

- Consult infectious diseases service
- Consider vancomycin* plus aminoglycoside (eg, tobramycin**) plus monobactam (eg, aztreonam 2 g IV q8 hours) or antipseudomonal fluoroquinolone (eg, ciprofloxacin 400 mg IV q8 hours)

Other tips:

- Consider adding double antibiotic coverage for *Pseudomonas* (eg, adding an aminoglycoside) as part of the regimen ONLY if there is very high clinical suspicion for *Pseudomonas*.
- Consider adding metronidazole (500 mg q8 hours) as part of the regimen if there is high suspicion for intra-abdominal infection.
- Use linezolid (600 mg q12 hours) instead of vancomycin if there is a true vancomycin allergy.
- Consult the infectious disease service for patients with suspected fungal sepsis.

* Vancomycin: loading dose 20–25 mg/kg, followed by 15–20 mg/kg q8–12 hours; loading dose for those in renal insufficiency should be adjusted accordingly and redosed by level.
** Tobramycin: 5 mg/kg IV daily only in select patients (stable renal function, stable volume status, not pregnant, creatinine clearance > 60 ml/min, not burned); redose by level in patients at risk for nephrotoxicity.
Note: all antibiotics mentioned, with the exception of linezolid and metronidazole, will require dose adjustment in renal insufficiency.

- Use epinephrine or vasopressin as the alternative agent in septic shock when blood pressure is poorly responsive to norepinephrine.
- Dopamine may be considered as an alternative to norepinephrine in patients at low risk for tachyarrhythmias.
- Dobutamine is the preferred inotropic agent.
- The urine output goal is 0.5 ml/kg per hour or higher.
- In patients with suspected catheter-related infection, at least 2 sets of blood cultures should be obtained with at least 1 set percutaneously and 1 set from any vascular device placed > 48 hours prior.
- Avoid bicarbonate therapy when treating hypoperfusion-induced lactic acidemia in patients with a pH of 7.15 or greater.
- Consider stress ulcer prophylaxis with proton pump inhibitors, especially if the patient is mechanically ventilated, coagulopathic, or in acute renal failure.
- Consider recombinant activated protein C in patients with severe sepsis and a high risk of death.

For newborns and infants in the first 6 to 8 weeks of life, give IV ampicillin and gentamicin or ampicillin and cefotaxime. For older infants and children, give a third-generation cephalosporin or beta-lactamase inhibitor. Consider adding vancomycin if methicillin-resistant Staphylococcus aureus is suspected.

Other Key Issues

Pediatric Considerations: Neonates are at the highest risk for mortality from sepsis. Almost half of neonatal deaths are caused by sepsis. Symptoms maybe subtle in neonates and infants; activity level, sleeping pattern, appetite, and urine output should be evaluated.

Geriatric Considerations: In the elderly, altered mental status may be the only presenting symptom of sepsis.

Suggested Readings and References

1. Dellinger RP, Levy MM, Carlet JM, et al. Surviving sepsis campaign: International guidelines for management of severe sepsis and septic shock 2008. *Crit Care Med.* 2008;36:296–327.

2. Rivers E, Nguyen B, Havstad S, et al. Early goal-directed therapy in the treatment of severe sepsis and septic shock. *N Engl J Med.* 2001;345:1368–1377.

3. Angus DC, Linde-Zwirble WT, Lidicker J, et al. Epidemiology of severe sepsis in the United States: analysis of incidence, outcome, and associated costs of care. *Crit Care Med.* 2001;29(7):1303–1310.

4. Wang HE, Shapiro NI, Angus DC, et al. National estimates of severe sepsis in United States emergency departments. *Crit Care Med.* 2007;25:1928–1936.

5. Parrillo JE. Pathogenetic mechanisms of septic shock. *N Engl J Med* 1993;328:1471–1477.

6. Levy MM, Fink MP, Marshall JC, et al. 2001 SCCM/ESICM/ACCP/ATS/SIS International Sepsis Definitions Conference. *Crit Care Med.* 2003;31:1250–1256.

7. Winters BD, Eberlein M, Leung J, et al. Long-term mortality and quality of life in sepsis: a systematic review. *Crit Care Med.* 2010;38:1276–1283.

8. Marshall JC, Cook DJ, Christou NV, et al. Multiple Organ Dysfunction Score: a reliable descriptor of a complex clinical outcome. *Crit Care Med.* 1995;23:1638–1652.

9. Ventetuolo CE, Levy MM. Biomarkers: diagnosis and risk assessment in sepsis. *Clin Chest Med.* 2008;29:591–603.

10. Tang BMP, Eslik GD, Craig JC, et al. Accuracy of procalcitonin for sepsis diagnosis in critically ill patients: systematic review and meta-analysis. *Lancet Infect Dis.* 2007;7:210–217.

11. Nguyen HB, Rivers EP, Knoblich BP, et al. Early lactate clearance is associated with improved outcome in severe sepsis and septic shock. *Crit Care Med.* 2004;32:1637–1642.

12. Hotchkiss RS and Karl IE. The pathophysiology and treatment of sepsis. *N Engl J Med.* 2003;348:138–150.

13. Remick DG. Pathophysiology of sepsis. *Am J Pathol.* 2007;170:1435–1444.

14. Kumar A, Roberts D, Wood KE, et al. Duration of hypotension prior to initiation of effective antimicrobial therapy is the critical determinant of survival in human septic shock. *Crit Care Med.* 2006;34:1589–1596.

15. NICE-SUGAR Study Investigators, Finfer S, Chittock DR, et al. Intensive versus conventional glucose control in critically ill patients. *N Engl J Med.* 2009;360:1283–1297.

Central Nervous System Infections

Chapter 5

Bacterial Meningitis

Mary P. Chang

Summary Box

Disease Description: Bacterial infection causing inflammation of the meninges.

Organisms: Group B *Streptococcus, Escherichia coli, Listeria monocytogenes, Streptococcus pneumoniae, Neisseria meningitidis, Haemophilus influenzae* type b.

Treatment: Antibiotics should be given early. Standard empiric antibiotic therapy is vancomycin 15 to 20 mg/kg IV q8 to 12 hours with ceftriaxone 2 g IV q12 hours.

Other Key Issues: Early recognition is key to reducing morbidity and mortality. If the patient is critically ill and suspicion for meningitis is high, give antibiotics immediately followed by diagnostic workup. Give dexamethasone prior to antibiotics for bacterial meningitis.

Disease Description

Meningitis is inflammation of the meninges, the lining around the brain and spinal cord.

Epidemiology

In the United States, between 2003 and 2007, there were about 4,100 cases of bacterial meningitis, resulting in 500 deaths.

Per the Centers for Disease Control and Prevention (CDC), there are several risk factors for bacterial meningitis. These include age, community setting, immunosuppression, individuals working with meningitis-causing pathogens (ie, microbiologists), and travel to certain regions (see Table 5.1). Younger patients are at higher risk for bacterial meningitis overall. However, certain meningitis pathogens have a predilection for certain age groups (see table 5.1). People living in more crowded conditions, such as college students and military personnel, are also at a higher risk of infection and are encouraged to get the meningococcal vaccine. People who live in the "meningitis belt" in sub-Saharan Africa are at higher risk of meningococcal meningitis during the dry season.

Presenting Features

Per the World Health Organization (WHO), meningitis is defined as having a temperature of greater than 38°C; headache; and either altered sensorium, neck stiffness, or another meningeal sign. Patients will typically present with a fever, stiff neck, and severe, nonfocal headache. Fever is the most common symptom of meningitis with a sensitivity of 85%. Altered mental status can be seen if the patient presents at an advanced stage. If a patient also has a rash, meningococcal or pneumococcal meningitis should be high on the differential diagnosis. A 1999 JAMA review of 10 meningitis studies calculated that less than two-thirds of infected patients in these studies presented with the triad of fever, headache, and neck pain. The study also concluded that low risk patients who did not have any of the typical triad symptoms (fever, headache, or neck pain) on physical exam were not likely to have meningitis (sensitivity 99%–100%).

Typical Disease Course

Bacterial meningitis often begins as a sinusitis or from a recently implanted device, which via direct or hematogenous spread penetrates the blood brain barrier. Bacterial meningitis can also be transmitted through inhalation of infected respiratory secretions or through the exchange of throat secretions, which subsequently seed the bloodstream. Once the organism passes through the blood brain barrier, it can irritate the meninges, cause cerebral edema, and increase intracranial pressure. Symptoms typically develop three to seven days after exposure.

Complications

Neurologic complications include cerebral edema, seizures, altered mental status, hydrocephalus, and brain herniation secondary to elevated intracranial pressure. Brain swelling can cause obtundation, posturing, cranial nerve VI palsy, and Cushing's triad of hypertension, bradycardia, and irregular breathing. Papilledema is not frequently seen because symptoms develop quickly. In patients with untreated bacteremia, their disease can progress to septic shock and death.

Diagnostic Tests

To confirm a diagnosis of bacterial meningitis, cerebrospinal fluid (CSF) and blood cultures should be obtained. The opening pressure of a lumbar puncture in the setting of bacterial meningitis can range from 20 to 50 cm H_2O. The fluid generally has a cloudy appearance. The white blood cell (WBC) count typically is elevated and ranges from 1000 to 5000 cells/mm with a neutrophilic predominance (80%–95%). CSF glucose concentration is generally low at less than 40 mg/dL. The CSF protein concentration is usually elevated, ranging from 100 to 500. An initial CSF gram stain should be sent to quickly

Table 5.1 Pathogens That Cause Meningitis by Specific Age Group	
Age Group	Causes
Newborns	Group B Streptococcus, Escherichia coli, Listeria monocytogenes
Infants and Children	Streptococcus pneumoniae, Neisseria meningitidis, Haemophilus influenzae type b
Adolescents and Young Adults	Neisseria meningitidis, Streptococcus pneumoniae
Older Adults	Streptococcus pneumoniae, Neisseria meningitidis, Listeria monocytogenes

characterize the class of organism, and a CSF culture should be sent to identify the specific organism and its antibiotic susceptibilities. If CSF collection occurs within four hours of antibiotic administration, the gram stain and culture may still yield a positive result. Even outside this window, the diagnosis of bacterial meningitis can still be supported by a suggestive WBC count, glucose level, and protein level in the CSF. Latex agglutination tests can detect certain bacterial antigens, but the sensitivity for the most common meningeal pathogens ranges from 50% to 100%. Per the Infectious Diseases Society of America (IDSA) 2004 guidelines, agglutination testing can be useful in patients who have been pretreated with antibiotics (Level 3b recommendation).

Before performing a lumbar puncture, a possible brain mass should always be considered because brain herniation is a possible complication of a lumbar puncture in this subset of patients. Herniation in these cases results from the acute decrease in spinal column CSF pressure (due to the direct removal of CSF) relative to the increased intracranial pressure, which remains unchanged during an LP if there is a brain lesion obstructing communication with the spinal column CSF. This pressure differential results in brain herniation from the high pressure intracranial space toward the low pressure spinal column. A study published in the *New England Journal of Medicine* in 2001 reviewed 235 cases of suspected meningitis patients who had a CT (computed tomography) head scan before lumbar puncture. They discovered that those with an abnormal CT head scan had the following characteristics: age ≤ 60 years; immunocompromised state; a history of central nervous system disease; a history of seizure within one week of presentation; and neurologic abnormalities, such as altered level of consciousness, an inability to answer two consecutive questions correctly or to follow two consecutive commands, or aphasia. The patients who did not have any of these criteria and had a normal CT scan had a negative predictive value of 97%. Correspondingly, the current IDSA guidelines recommend that the following adult patient populations undergo CT head prior to lumbar puncture: immunocompromised patients or patients with papilledema, altered consciousness, a focal neurologic deficit, or a history of CNS disease (mass, stroke, or focal infection). (Class 2b level of evidence)

Treatment

First-line recommendations

The treatment of bacterial meningitis depends on the age group. Empiric antibiotics can be administered until culture narrows the pathogen.

- Neonates: Ampicillin (150 mg/kg IV q8 hours) with cefotaxime (100–150 mg/kg IV q8–12 hours) or an aminoglycoside to cover for *Streptococcus agalactiae, Escherichia coli, Listeria monocytogenes*, and *Klebsiella*. Ceftriaxone should be avoided in this population to avoid the risk of hyperbilirubinemia.
- Ages 1 month to 23 months: Vancomycin 15 mg/kg IV q6 hours and ceftriaxone 75 to 100 mg/kg IV q12 to 24 hours
- Ages 2 years to 50 years: Vancomycin 15 to 20 mg/kg IV q8–12 hours (up to 2 g) with a third-generation cephalosporin to cover for organisms such as *S. pneumoniae, Neisseria meningitidis, Haemophilus influenzae*, and *E. coli*.
- Age > 50 years old: Vancomycin (30–45 mg/kg IV q8–12 hours), ampicillin (1–2 g IV q4 hours), and a third-generation cephalosporin to cover for *S. pneumoniae, N. meningitides*, aerobic gram-negative bacilli, and *L. monocytogenes*.
- Patients with a recent penetrating head injury or CSF shunt should receive cefepime (2 g IV q12 hours) in addition to vancomycin for added *Pseudomonas* coverage.
- Pregnant patients: Ampicillin 2 g IV q4 hours (add to therapy for *Listeria* coverage)
- Immunocompromised patients: Vancomycin 15 mg/kg q8 hours with ampicillin 2 g IV q4 hours and ceftriaxone 2 g IV q12 hours.

If pneumococcal meningitis is suspected and antibiotics are to be given, consider giving dexamethasone (0.15 mg/kg IV q6 hours for 2–4 days) 10 minutes before antibiotics. Experimental animal studies have shown that the inflammatory response from treating bacterial meningitis with antibiotics can increase morbidity and mortality. The anti-inflammatory property of dexamethasone mitigates the surge in inflammatory marker release. Per IDSA guidelines, giving dexamethasone in neonates is a class 1c recommendation. For infants and children who have *H. influenza* type b meningitis, administering dexamethasone is a class 1a recommendation. However, it is difficult to know what organism is causing bacterial meningitis in the emergency department without having culture results. More studies are needed before a formal recommendation can be given because the current data does not show a clear benefit in this population. In adults, dexamethasone administration benefited those with pneumococcal meningitis and those with a Glasgow Comas Scale score ≤ 11. The recommendations for dexamethasone administration in adults is to give it in pneumococcal meningitis (Class 1a) and all meningitis patients (Class 3b). If an adult patient has already received antibiotics, they should not receive dexamethasone (Class 1a).

Early treatment of suspected bacterial meningitis is critical given its rapidly progressive course and high mortality. There have been no studies that indicate when antibiotics need to be given, but several studies show a worse outcome when there are more organisms seen in collected CSF samples prior to antibiotic administration.

Second and third line recommendations

- Beta-lactam allergy: Vancomycin 15 to 20 mg/kg IV q8 to 12 hours plus Moxifloxacin—400 mg IV q24 hours, addition of trimethoprim-sulfamethoxazole 5 mg/kg IV q6 to 12 hours if *Listeria* coverage is needed
- Multiple drug allergy patients: fluoroquinolones
- Vancomycin-resistant history: linezolid 600 mg IV/PO q12 hours

Other Key Issues

It is important for emergency physicians to recognize potential bacterial meningitis early. They are usually the providers that patients present to first. Lumbar puncture will aid in definitive diagnosis, but, if this procedure is delayed and suspicion is high, antibiotics should be given first. Meningitis is a treatable condition, and early intervention will have a great impact on reducing morbidity and mortality.

Suggested Readings and References

1. Thigpen MC, Whitney CG, Messonnier NE, et al. Emerging infections programs network: bacterial meningitis in the United States, 1998-2007 external Web Site icon. *N Engl J Med.* 2011;364:2016–2025.
2. *Bacterial meningitis.* http://www.cdc.gov/meningitis/bacterial.html#reference. Accessed August 31, 2013.
3. Attia J, Hatala R, Cook DJ, Wong JG. The rational clinical examination: does this adult patient have acute meningitis? *JAMA* 1999;282:175–181.
4. Immunization surveillance, assessment and monitoring. http://www.who.int/immunization_monitoring/diseases/meningitis_surveillance/en/. Accessed September 4, 2013.
5. Swartz M. Acute bacterial meningitis. In: Gourbach SL, Barlett JG, Blacklow NR, eds. *Infectious Diseases.* 2nd ed. Philadelphia, Pa: WB Saunders; 1998:1377–1381.
6. Carpenter RR, Petersdorf RG. The clinical spectrum of bacterial meningitis. *Am J Med.* 1962;33:262–275.
7. Tan JS, Salata RA. *Expert Guide to Infectious Diseases.*
8. Tunkel AR, Hartman BJ, Kaplan SL, et al. Practice guidelines for the management of bacterial meningitis. *Clin Infect Dis.* 2004;39:1267–1284.
9. Gray LD, Fedorko DP. Laboratory diagnosis of bacterial meningitis. *Clin Microbiol Rev.* 1992;5:130–145.
10. Gulian J-M, Gonard V, Dalmasso C, Palix C: Bilirubin displacement by ceftriaxone in neonates: evaluation by determination of "free" bilirubin and erythrocyte-bound bilirubin *J Antimicrob Chemother.* 1987;19:823–829.
11. Tunkel AR. *Bacterial Meningitis.* Philadelphia, Pa: Lippincott Williams & Wilkins; 2001.
12. American Academy of Pediatrics. Pneumococcal infections. In: Pickering LK, ed. *Red Book: 2003 Report of the Committee on Infectious Diseases.* 26th ed. Elk Grove Village, Ill: American Academy of Pediatrics; 2003:490–500.
13. Hasbun R, Abrahams J, Jekel J, Quagliarello VJ. Computed tomography of the head before lumbar puncture in adults with suspected meningitis. *N Engl J Med.* 2001;345:1727–1733.
14. Feldman WE, Ginsburg CM, McCracken GH Jr, et al. Relation of concentrations of Haemophilus influenzae type b in cerebrospinal fluid to late sequelae of patients with meningitis. *J Pediatr.* 1982;100:209–212.
15. Michael B, Menezes BF, Cunniffe J, et al. Effect of delayed lumbar punctures on the diagnosis of acute bacterial meningitis in adults. *Emerg Med J.* 2010;27:433–438.
16. Tunkel AR, Hartman BJ, Kaplan SL, et al. Practice guidelines for the management of bacterial meningitis. *Clin Infect Dis.* 2004;39:1267–1284.

Chapter 6

Aseptic Meningitis

Michelle Sharp

Summary Box

Disease Description: Acute meningeal inflammation, fever, and headache with no organisms in the cerebral spinal fluid.[1-3]

Organisms (if caused by organisms): Viruses (enteroviruses being most common), fungi, atypical bacteria, or parasites.[3]

Treatment: Supportive care.

Other Key Issues: Additional causes include drug-induced aseptic meningitis (eg, nonsteroidal anti-inflammatory drugs and antibiotics), chemical meningitis from the rupture of an epidermoid cyst or malignancy, and immune diseases, such as lupus.[1,3]

Disease Description

Aseptic meningitis is defined as acute meningeal inflammation, fever, and headache in the absence of detectable organisms in the cerebral spinal fluid (CSF).[1-3] Often, encephalitis (inflammation of the brain) and meningitis overlap. In contrast to the mental status changes typical of encephalitis, however, aseptic meningitis characteristically presents as a headache without alteration of mentation or personality.[2]

Epidemiology

With all causes combined, it is estimated that at least 75,000 individuals develop aseptic meningitis yearly.[3,4] It is very difficult to fully delineate the epidemiology of the disease because milder cases may not present to medical personnel. Of the identified cases, approximately 70% to 85% are caused by enteroviruses.[3,4] During 2003, outbreaks in the Western United States were commonly caused by echovirus 30, whereas in the Eastern United States, echovirus 9 was common.[5] Aseptic meningitis secondary to viruses develop more frequently in the summer and fall.[3]

Diagnosis

Aseptic meningitis is defined by several basic criteria: acute onset with signs and symptoms of meningeal involvement (fever, headache, and stiff neck), CSF abnormalities with the absence of bacteria in the CSF, short and benign course of illness, lack of local parameningeal infection or systemic disease (which might present like meningitis), and lack of a community epidemic disease of which meningitis is a feature.[6,7]

The differentiation between bacterial and viral meningitis has been an ongoing clinical dilemma because the clinical presentation of each is similar, yet the mortality and treatment of each is quite disparate. The diagnosis usually pivots on CSF analysis. In viral meningitis, the typical findings in the CSF include a normal glucose, an elevated WBC count (generally < 1000) with a lymphocytic pleocytosis, and an elevated protein.[4,8] The CSF analysis may vary with other causes of aseptic meningitis; however, no bacteria are seen on the gram stain. Of note, the CSF of viral meningitis and partially treated bacterial meningitis can have similar features.

The diagnostic accuracy and rapidity for viral meningitis has improved with the development of reverse transcriptase polymerase chain reaction assay (RT-PCR). RT-PCR has been shown to decrease both the length of hospital stay and the amount of antibiotic use in patients with aseptic meningitis.[9] The analysis of CSF with RT-PCR for viruses has replaced cell culture in the diagnosis of viral meningitis. Additional viral testing options include antibodies in the CSF, oropharyngeal secretions, and serum.

Disease Course

In viral meningitis, the host is typically infected with a virus by respiratory droplets, by fecal-oral transmission, or by a vector, such as a mosquito. The incubation period is approximately four to six days, during which time viremia occurs and results in dissemination to the meninges.[3,5] It is important to note that the clinical course of the disease varies based on the host immune response and the viral source. The onset of viral symptoms generally includes headache and nuchal rigidity. Fever typically accompanies symptoms in enterovirus infections; it typically ranges from 38°C to 40°C and lasts for up to five days.[3] The fever has been described as being biphasic, presenting first before the development of neck stiffness and then reoccurring along with meningeal symptoms.[5] Other symptoms noted are pharyngitis, nausea, vomiting, diarrhea, and photophobia.[3,5]

Some patients may have recurrent aseptic meningitis (Mollaret meningitis).[4] Herpes simplex virus type 2 (HSV-2) is typically the culprit in recurrent episodes.[4] Other less common causes of Mollaret meningitis are HSV type 1 (HSV-1), Epstein-Barr virus, intracranial epidermoid or dermoid cysts, and systemic lupus erythematosus.[3,4] In Mollaret meningitis, one can often see large mononuclear cells, which resemble endothelial cells.[3,4] Reye's syndrome can also be a complication if the fever is treated with aspirin.

Organisms

Multiple organisms have been implicated in aseptic meningitis. In cases where an etiology is able to be identified, enteroviruses are the most common cause (eg, coxsackievirus, echovirus, and poliovirus) followed by HSV-2 and varicella zoster virus.[1,2] However, cases of HSV-1, Epstein-Barr virus, and para-influenza virus as well as tick-borne encephalitis virus have also been identified.[2] Other sources to be considered include partially treated bacterial meningitis, *Mycobacterium tuberculosis*, *Treponema pallidum*, atypical bacteria (eg, *Mycoplasma pneumoniae* and *Chlamydia pneumoniae*), and parasites (eg, *Strongyloides stercoralis* and *Acanthamoeba* species).[3]

This chapter predominantly focuses on the enteroviruses that cause the majority of identified cases of aseptic meningitis.

The enteroviruses are members of the *Picornaviridae* family and thus are non-enveloped viruses with positive-sense, single-stranded, and linear RNA.[10] The main virus groups referred to as the enteroviruses are poliovirus, coxsackievirus A, coxsackievirus B, and echoviruses.[1,10] There are multiple serotypes of each group. Humans are the primary host organisms for enteroviruses. Enteroviruses have the ability to infect hosts in acids with a pH as low as 3.0, allowing them to replicate in the GI (gastrointestinal) tract.[11]

The viral cycle of enteroviruses include adsorption, penetration/uncoating, synthesis of virus-specific protein and RNA, and assembly followed by release from the host cell.[11] In adsorption, there are cell surface receptors (ICAM-1, CD54, DAF, CD55, VLA-2, and CD155) that enteroviruses bind in order to enter cells.[11] The virus creates a pore in the host cell membrane, and the viral RNA travels into the cytoplasm.[11] Viral protein synthesis then occurs at the host's rough endoplasmic reticulum, and viral RNA synthesis occurs at the host's smooth endoplasmic reticulum. The virus is then assembled and released from the host cell.

Treatment

Aseptic meningitis is typically self-limited, and, therefore, treatment is supportive. Most patients require treatment with antibiotics until CSF is obtained to rule out bacterial meningitis.

Other Key Issues to Consider

Aseptic meningitis has been described in association with systemic diseases, such as adult-onset Still's disease, and has been shown to improve with prednisone 60 mg daily.[12] Multiple drugs have been described in association with aseptic meningitis. Among these are amoxicillin, ibuprofen, and lamotrigine. Malignancy-induced aseptic meningitis has been observed with CNS tumors and in leukemia. Mechanical sources of aseptic meningitis have also been described, such as with epidermoid cyst rupture.

Suggested Readings and References

1. Robbins SL, Coltran RS. *Pathologic Basis of Disease.* 7th ed. Philadelphia, Pa: Saunders; 2004.
2. Kupila L, Vuorinen T, Vainionpaa R, Hukkanen V, Marttila RJ, Kotilainen P. Etiology of aseptic meningitis and encephalitis in an adult population. *Neurology* 2006;66:75–80.
3. Cherry JD, Bronstein DE. Aseptic meningitis and viral meningitis. In: Feigin RD, Cherry JD, Demmler-Harrison GJ, Kaplan SL, eds. *Feigin and Cherry's Textbook of Pediatric Infectious Diseases.* 6th ed. Philadelphia, Pa: Saunders Elsevier; 2009:494–503.
4. Sawyer M, Rotbart, HA. Aseptic and viral meningitis. Clinical syndromes and cardinal features of infectious diseases: Approach to diagnosis and initial management. In: Long SS, Pickering LK, Prober CG, eds. *Principles and Practice of Pediatric Infectious Disease.* 3rd ed. London, United Kingdom: Churchill Livingstone; 2007:305–309.
5. Centers for Disease Control and Prevention. Outbreaks of aseptic meningitis associated with echoviruses 9 and 30 and preliminary surveillance reports on enterovirus activity—United States, 2003. *MMWR Morb Mortal Wkly Rep.* 2003;52:761–764.
6. Saslaw S, Wooley CF, Anderson GR. Meningitis syndrome: report of eleven cases with cerebrospinal fluid isolation of enterovirus. *Arch Intern Med.* 1960;150:69–75.
7. Wallgren A. Une nouvelle maladie infectieuse du systeme nerveux central? Acta Paediatr Scand. 1925;4:158–182.
8. Kumar, R. Aseptic meningitis: diagnosis and management. *Indian J Pediatr.* 2005;72:57–63.
9. Stellrecht KA, Harding I, Woron AM, Lepow ML, Venezia RA. The impact of an enteroviral RT-PCR assay on the diagnosis of aseptic meningitis and patient management. *J Clin Virol.* 2002;25(suppl 1):S19–26.
10. Goering RV, Dockrell HM, Zuckerman M, Chiodini PL, Riott IM, eds. *Goering: Mims' Medical Microbiology.* 5th ed. Philadelphia, Pa: Saunders; 2012. Accessed via MD Consults.com on October 28, 2012.
11. Palacios G, Casas I, Trallero G. Human enteroviruses. In: Cohen J, Opal SM, Powderly WG, Calandra T, eds. *Infectious Diseases.* 3rd ed. St. Louis, Mo: Mosby Elsevier; 2010:1528–1538.
12. Akkara Veetil BM, Yee AH, Warrington KJ, Aksamit AJ Jr, Mason TG. Aseptic meningitis in adult onset Still's disease. *Rheumatol Int.* 2010;32:4031–4034. doi: 10.1007/s00296-010-1529-8. Epub 2010 May 22.

6. Lee BE, Davies HD. Aseptic meningitis. *Curr Opin Infect Dis.* 2007;20:272–277.

8. Wittmann A, Wooten GF. Amoxicillin-induced aseptic meningitis. *Neurology.* 2001;57:1734.

9. Rodriguez SC, Olguin AM, Miralles CP, Viladrich PF. Characteristics of meningitis caused by Ibuprofen: report of 2 cases with recurrent episodes and review of the literature. *Medicine (Baltimore).* 2006;85:214–220.

10. Dubos F, Moulin F, Gajdos V, et al. Serum procalcitonin and other biologic markers to distinguish between bacterial and aseptic meningitis. *J Pediatr.* 2006;149:72–76.

11. Yang S, Rothman RE. PCR-based diagnostics for infectious diseases: uses, limitations, and future applications in acute-care settings. *Lancet. Infect Dis.* 2004;4:337–348.

Chapter 7

Encephalitis

Tyler Martinez

Summary Box

Disease Description: Inflammation of the brain parenchyma, typically due to a viral infection.

Organisms:
 Most Common: Herpes simplex virus 1 (HSV-1)
 Common: HSV-2, Varicella Zoster Virus (VZV), and West Nile virus (WNV).
 Less common: Protozoans, helminthes, fungi, *Listeria, measles virus, mumps virus, rubella virus, Cytomegalovirus* (CMV), *human immunodeficiency virus 1* (HIV-1), HIV-2, *Borrelia burgdorferi, Rickettsia rickettsii, Colorado tick fever virus, rabies virus, Eastern equine encephalitis virus* (EEE), *Western equine encephalitis virus* (WEE), and *Saint Louis encephalitis virus* (SLEV).

Treatment:
 Parenteral: Acyclovir 10 mg/kg q8 hours
 Oral: no adequate oral substitute

Other Key Issues: Question the patient about foreign travel, immunocompromised state, and potential exposures.

Disease Description

Epidemiology

The incidence of viral encephalitis varies both regionally and yearly. WNV and other arthropod-borne viruses (eg, EEE, WEE, SLEV) vary seasonally with mosquito populations. WNV has only been monitored since an initial outbreak in 1999 in New York. Since that time, it has spread to almost every state in the United States. Additionally, WNV can be seen in Asia, Africa, and Europe. SLEV is seen predominantly in the Midwestern and Southern regions of the United States. EEE is seen in the Atlantic and Gulf Coast regions, and WEE is seen in the Western half of the United States as well as South America. While HSV was classically the most common cause of encephalitis, WNV has since emerged as the most common cause in the United States. WNV cases are likely greatly underreported because most cases are asymptomatic or present with only a mild febrile illness.

HSV, occurring in 1 to 4 per 1,000,000 in the United States, is the other major cause of encephalitis. HSV-1 accounts for approximately 90% of these HSV infections. The remaining are caused by HSV-2. HSV-1 is typically seen in adults and older children, whereas HSV-2 is usually seen in neonates due to perinatal transmission.

Presenting Features

Encephalitis has been described as meningitis with focal neurologic findings. However, this more aptly describes meningoencephalitis (an inflammation of both the meninges and the brain parenchyma), which is a more common presentation than pure encephalitis. Pure encephalitis (ie, without a superimposed meningitic component) will lack the signs and symptoms of meningeal irritation (eg, stiff neck and photophobia). New-onset seizures, cognitive deficits, new psychiatric symptoms, lethargy/coma, cranial nerve abnormalities, or movement disorders should alert the clinician to possible encephalitis. Fever is usually present but can be absent up to 30% of the time.

Diagnostic Considerations

It is always important to rule out other causes of altered mental status and/or fever. Urinary tract infections or pneumonia in the young or elderly can cause altered mental status. A patient's medication list should be inspected because drug–drug interactions can result in toxic levels of medications, which can lead to states that mimic encephalitis. Occult trauma should also be investigated if there is any clinical concern. Subarachnoid hemorrhage should also be considered. Previously undetected malignancy with metastases can also result in an altered mental status, new neurologic findings, and even fever.

Typical Disease Course

Patients with encephalitis are typically ill-appearing from the onset. However, their presentation can range from a mild alteration in mental status to fulminant septic shock and coma requiring airway protection and hemodynamic support. The morbidity of HSV encephalitis depends upon the patient's neurologic condition at the time of acyclovir administration. Of those with HSV encephalitis who are treated with acyclovir, mortality is approximately 30%. Moreover, 30% of those who survive will have permanent neurologic deficits. Untreated HSV encephalitis has a mortality of 70% to 100%. Rabies encephalitis is generally fatal. EEE has morbidity/mortality figures similar to HSV. Of those hospitalized with WNV, there is approximately a 15% mortality.

Complications

The most concerning complication of encephalitis is the development of life-threatening cerebral edema with resultant brainstem compression and herniation.

Diagnostic Tests

Neuroimaging (CT or MRI) will typically occur as an initial test for any patient suspected of having encephalitis. In addition to evaluating for the potential for cerebral edema and brain herniation, neuroimaging can also survey for abnormalities in distributions that are suggestive of certain infecting agents. Classic findings for HSV encephalitis, for example, are located in the temporal lobe. WNV infections tend to affect the basal ganglia, thalamus, brainstem, cerebellum, and spinal cord. Most other causes of encephalitis will show various nonspecific findings.

Evaluation for encephalitis in any patient in the emergency department requires a lumbar puncture for cerebral spinal fluid (CSF) analysis, provided there isn't a risk of herniation based on imaging or exam findings. In addition to the standard CSF labs sent for suspected CSF infection (ie, cell counts, gram stain, bacterial culture, glucose, and protein), HSV polymerase chain reaction (PCR) should also be sent if there is concern for encephalitis. PCR is much more sensitive and specific for HSV-1, HSV-2, and enteroviruses. If there is concern for influenza, parainfluenza, measles, or mumps, a viral culture should be sent because there are PCR tests available for these organisms. Culture for HSV and enteroviruses is low yield and not routinely performed. If there is any concern for rarer causes of encephalitis (eg, EEE, WEE, SLEV, or *Listeria*, etc.), it is recommended that one to three extra tubes of CSF be obtained and stored for possible testing in the future.

Diagnosis of WNV is best accomplished by analyzing both the serum and CSF for specific immunoglobulin M (IgM) antibodies against WNV.

Organisms

Approximately only 20% to 40% of people infected with WNV will develop symptoms. Incubation period is anywhere from 2 to 14 days. WNV is transmitted via mosquitos and thus typically peaks in the warm months, although it can occur year round in more temperate climates.

HSV encephalitis can occur at any time of year. The mechanism by which the virus gains access to the central nervous system (CNS) is poorly understood. It is thought that reactivation of dormant HSV or contact with someone who is actively excreting HSV can lead to HSV encephalitis in susceptible hosts. Once there is CNS penetration, transport to the brain occurs via retrograde axonal flow. Approximately one-third of cases of HSV encephalitis is due to a primary infection. Two-thirds of cases result from reactivation of a latent virus. HSV-2 encephalitis in neonates is almost always the result of vertical transmission during a vaginal birth in the setting of an active herpes infection. The actual mechanism by which the virus gains access to the CNS is still debated.

Other causes of encephalitis include *rabies virus*, HIV, CMV, *Borrelia burgdorferi*, *Rickettsia rickettsii*, and *Colorado tick fever virus*.

Treatment
Empiric treatment for presumed viral encephalitis is the antiviral acyclovir at 10 mg/kg every 8 hours for 21 days. Empiric broad-spectrum antibiotics are typically also given to cover for possible bacterial meningitis until CSF studies result. Corticosteroids have been suggested for the acute treatment of viral encephalitis. If there are signs of elevated intracranial pressure (ICP), neurosurgical consultation should be obtained for possible decompressive craniotomy. Whether craniotomy or steroids has a positive impact on overall outcome has not been determined, but these interventions are postulated to help limit secondary brain damage while the patient responds to antiviral therapy. In the setting of increased ICP, standard indications for the treatment of elevated intracranial pressure (ie, hyperventilation, steroids, mannitol, hypertonic saline, and elevation of the head of the bed) should also be considered.

Suggested Readings and References

1. Whitley RJ. Herpes simplex encephalitis: adolescents and adults. *Antiviral Res.* 2006;71:141–148.
2. Whitley RJ, Gnann JW. Viral encephalitis: familiar infections and emerging pathogens. *Lancet.* 2002;359:507–513.
3. Kupila L et al. Etiology of aseptic meningitis and encephalitis in an adult population. *Neurology.* 2006;66:75–80.
4. Adamo MA, Deshaies EM. Emergency decompressive craniectomy for fulminating infectious encephalitis. *J Neurosurg.* 2008;108:174–176.
5. Fitch MT et al. Emergency department management of meningitis and encephalitis. *Infect Dis Clin North Am.* 2008;22:1.
6. Benson PC, Swadron SP. Empiric acyclovir in infrequently initiated in the emergency department to patients ultimately diagnosed with encephalitis. *Ann Emerg Med.* 2006;47:1100–1105.
7. Petropoulou KA et al. West Nile virus meningoencephalitis: MR imaging findings. *Am J Neuroradiol.* 2005;26:1986–1995.
8. Granerod J et al. Causes of encephalitis and differences in their clinical presentations in England: a multicenter, population-based prospective study. *Lancet. Infect Dis.* 2010;10:835–844.

Chapter 8

Brain Abscess

Sneha A. Chinai

Summary Box

Disease Description: A brain abscess is a life-threatening infection within the brain that originates as cerebritis and evolves into an encapsulated collection of purulent material.

Organisms: Recovered organisms are primarily bacterial (aerobic, anaerobic, or mixed flora) with fungi and parasitic infections seen less frequently.

Treatment:
  Oral antibiotics: not recommended
  Parenteral: dependent on the source of infection (see Table 8.1)
  Surgical drainage

Other Key Issues: This diagnosis requires neurosurgical consultation for management and inpatient admission.

Table 8.1 Suggested Drug Choices and Scheduled Regimens[a]

Condition	Antibiotic	Additional Antibiotic
Postoperative	Vancomycin (15 to 20 mg per kilogram per dose every 8 to 12 hours)	Either Ceftazadime 2 g IV every eight hours or ceftazadime 2 grams and IV every eight hours or meropenem 2 g IV every eight hours
Post traumatic	Vancomycin (15 to 20 mg per kilogram per dose every 8 to 12 hours)	Ceftriaxone 2 g every 12 hours or cefotaxime 2 g every four to six hours
Oral (including dental) or sinus source	Metronidazole 15 mg per kilogram	Ceftriaxone 2 g every 12 hours or cefotaxime 2 g every four to six hours

[a]In the case of a positive blood culture in the presence of endocarditis, use therapy for endocarditis. Adapted from Alvis Miranda H et al.[16]

Disease Description

A brain abscess is an infection within the brain that begins as cerebritis and becomes an encapsulated collection of purulent material, usually within two weeks. The incidence of brain abscess is estimated to be up to 2% in the general population although higher incidences are seen in developing countries. Epidemiologically, brain abscesses are seen more frequently in immunocompromised patients.

Studies conducted a few decades ago reported mortalities ranging from 20% to 50%. Despite medical advances over the past two decades (eg, broad-spectrum antibiotics, advanced radiographic imaging, and newer capabilities for tissue sampling), a brain abscess remains a life-threatening condition. Recent studies report a mortality rate of 5% to 20%. Moreover, even with proper treatment, 30% to 60% of patients suffer neurological sequelae, such as hemiparesis, cranial nerve palsies, hydrocephalus, seizure disorders, visual defects, and memory deficits.

Routes of Infection

There are two general methods of inoculation: direct spread from a contiguous infectious site and hematogenous spread (see Table 8.2). Direct spread accounts for 25–50% of cases and generally presents as a single brain abscess. Common sources for direct spread include odontogenic infections and sinusitis, particularly frontal and ethmoid sinus infections. A smaller percentage of cases are the result of ear infections, including otitis media and mastoiditis. Foreign bodies, especially in the setting of traumatic injuries, can create a nidus of infection. Less commonly, bacteremia can result in abscess formation. When the etiology of the brain abscess is bacteremia, multiple abscesses are generally seen in the middle cerebral artery distribution. Additionally, invasive neurosurgical procedures may

Table 8.2 Summary of BA Sources Characteristics[a]

Source	Frequency %	Probable Focus	Comments
Spread from pericranial contiguous focus	25 to 50	Paranasal sinuses, middle ear, or dental infection	Dental infections, ethmoid, or frontal sinusitis usually spreads to the frontal lobe
			Subacute/chronic otitis media or mastoiditis preferentially spreads to the inferior temporal lobe and cerebellum
			Generally causes a solitary BA
Hematogenous spread	15 to 30	Lung abscess or empyema, bacterial endocarditis, skin infections, intra-abdominal (including pelvic)	Many are multifocal and are located in the distribution of the middle cerebral artery
Direct inoculation	8 to 19		Mainly due to traumatic brain injury or neurosurgical procedures

Abbreviation: BA, brain abscess.
[a]Adapted from Alvis Miranda H et al.[16]

be complicated by direct inoculation, leading to abscess formation. There is no identifiable source of infection in 20% to 40% of cases.

Presentation

The signs and symptoms of a brain abscess are influenced by the location and size of the infection, the causative pathogen, and the patient's immune status and medical comorbidities (see Table 8.3). Brain abscesses are most frequently located in the frontal or temporal lobes; followed by the parietal lobes; cerebellum; and, least frequently, the occipital lobe. Headache is the most common occurring in 70–90% of patients. Patients typically present with a constant headache on the side of the infection, and the headache is generally not relieved by anti-inflammatory medications. Neck pain is seen more often in patients with occipital lobe infections or in patients who have abscesses that have ruptured into the ventricles. Vomiting can be associated with an elevated intracranial pressure due to obstructive hydrocephalus. Diffuse and local cerebral edema or mass effect with midline shift can also result in altered mental status or neurological deficits. Approximately 25% of patients will present with seizures, and this may be the first sign of an underlying brain abscess.

Fever is unreliable and is seen in only 50% of patients on initial presentation. Focal neurologic deficits are found in approximately 50% of patients and are dependent upon the location of the abscess. Frontal abscesses are associated with lethargy, contralateral hemiparesis, and primitive reflexes. Primitive reflexes are suppressed by the frontal lobe after infancy but can reappear when not properly inhibited due to frontal lobe damage. There are a number of primitive reflexes that may be elicited on exam, such as the moro reflex, the tonic neck reflex, the walking reflex, and the sucking reflex. Patients with temporal abscesses may present with aphasia, contralateral facial weakness, and homonymous superior quadrantanopia. Parietal infections may result in homonymous inferior quadrantopia and impaired position sense. Patients with cerebellar involvement may have nystagus, ataxia, and tremors on exam. Multiple cranial nerve palsies, dysphagia, and contralateral hemiparesis are found with brainstem lesions. In cases of elevated intracranial pressure, there may be papilledema or cranial nerve palsies, particularly in cranial nerves III and VI.

Diagnostic Tests

The appearance of a brain abscess on imaging will be dependent in its stage (see Table 8.4). The most easily accessible test for brain abscesses is computed tomography (CT) of the head with intravenous contrast. Early infection identified within the first one to two weeks is associated with edema and poorly demarcated borders on CT. Hydrocephalus and other associated intracranial infections may also be seen. After two to three weeks, a vascularized fibrotic capsule with central necrosis can be visualized. Magnetic resonance imaging (MRI) of the head with gadolinium contrast is more sensitive for defining both abscess and cerebral edema, distinguishing early cerebritis, and illuminating brainstem lesions. MRI of the head with diffusion-weighted imaging can help further distinguish brain abscesses from neoplastic lesions. The best modality for the accurate identification of the causative organism is culturing a

Table 8.3 Common Presenting Signs and Symptoms in BA[a]	
Signs/Symptom	Frequency (%)
Fever	54.5 to 60
Headache	72 to 92.8
Hemiparesis/cranial nerve	14.5
Hemiparesis	20.2
No neurological deficit	39.8
Meningismus	52.2
Altered level of consciousness	10 to 100
Seizure	21 to 25.3
Nausea/vomiting	31 to 40
Papilledema	4.1 to 50
GCS, at admission	
3 to 8	10.3
9 to 12	28.0
13 to 15	61.7

Abbreviations: BA, brain abscess; GCS, Glasgow coma scale.
[a]Adapted from Alvis Miranda H et al.[16]

specimen obtained by CT-guided aspiration or by neurosurgical intervention. In cases of hematogenous spread, blood cultures may be useful. Serology can be utilized in the diagnosis of brain abscesses caused by *Toxoplasma gondii* (anti-toxoplasma immunoglobulin antibody in blood) and neurocysticercosis (anti-cysticercal antibodies in cerebrospinal fluid). Lumbar puncture is contraindicated in the setting of a neurological deficit or papilledema due to the risk of herniation.

Organisms

The microbiology of brain abscesses will vary based on the source of infection and the immune status of the host. The causative pathogens are primarily bacterial and can involve anaerobic organisms, aerobic organisms, or mixed bacterial infections. Fungi and parasitic infections are also possible in immunocompromised hosts. Sinus and dental infections tend to be mixed flora and most commonly cause brain abscesses in the frontal lobes. Bacterial flora may include *Streptococcus, Bacteroides, Fusobacterium, Haemophilus*, and *Enterbacter* species. Ear infections are also generally mixed flora infections and, due to geographic proximity, tend to spread to the temporal lobes or cerebellum. Causative organisms include *Streptococcus, Enterobacter*, and *Pseudomonas* species. Neurosurgical procedure-related infections are associated with *Staphylococcus, Streptococcus*, and *Pseudomonas* species. Posttraumatic abscesses in the setting of retained foreign body, such as bullet fragments, typically result in infections with *Staphylococcus, Streptococcus*, and *Enterobacter* species. The organisms found in cases of hematologic spread will be influenced by the original source of infection. The pulmonary, genitourinary, and cardiac systems are frequent sources. In these cases, bacteremia is often caused by *Streptococcus, Klebsiella, Actinomyces, Enterobacter*, and *Pseudomonas* species. *Toxoplasma gondii, Listeria monocytogenes, Nocardia, Aspergillus, Cryptococcus*, and *Coccidiodes* are often found in immunocompromised patients. *Taenia solium* causes cysticercosis, which is highly prevalent in Mexico. *Entamoeba, Schistosoma*, and *Salmonella* may also be considerations in immigrant patients (see Table 8.5).

Treatment

Brain abscesses continue to be a serious and potentially fatal problem despite medical advances in imaging, culture techniques, antibiotics, and neurosurgery. Neurosurgical consultation is mandatory in all patients with suspected brain abscesses. Select cases may be medically managed with intravenous antibiotics and steroids, especially if there is a small abscess (less than 2.5 cm), the organism has been isolated for directed therapy, and the patient has good neurologic status at the time of presentation.

The majority of patients undergo either needle aspiration or surgical excision. This is critical for obtaining a specimen for culture to direct accurate and specific therapy. Needle aspiration is more commonly utilized and has a lower mortality rate than surgical excision. It is performed through a Burr hole using CT or ultrasound guidance. Surgical excision is best used for abscesses that are related to foreign bodies, fungal brain abscesses, multiloculated abscesses, failure to diagnose on previous image-guided aspiration, or worsening clinical condition or radiological appearance following 1 to 2 weeks of medical management.

Repeat imaging is required for any change in mental status. Empiric antibiotic selections are guided by the most likely source of infection and are adjusted for renal function (see Table 8.5). First-generation cephalosporins, aminoglycosides, erythromycin, clindamycin, or tetracyclines should not be used in the

Table 8.4 Stages of Brain Abscess Formation[a]		
Stage	Time	Characteristics
Early cerebritis	1 to 4 days	This stage is typified by neutrophil accumulation, tissue necrosis, and edema. Microglial cells and astrocytes are activated.
Late cerebritis	4–10 days	This phase is associated with a predominant macrophage and lymphocyte infiltrate.
Early capsule formation	11–14 days	Associated with the formation of well-vascularized abscess wall. This wall is crucially sequestering the lesion, maintaining the integrity of the brain function, and limiting the expansion of the infective process.
Late capsule formation	> 14 days	At 3 to 4 weeks, the abscess capsule becomes thick and is amenable to excision.

[a]Adapted from Alvis Miranda H et al.[16]

Table 8.5 Pathogens Related to Clinical Scenario

Paranasal sinusitis	Microaerophilic and anaerobic streptococci, *Haemophilus* sp., *Bacteroides* sp. (nonfragilis), and *Fusobacterium* sp.
Otitis media and mastoiditis	*Bacteroides* sp. (including B *Bacteroides fragilis*), streptococci, *Pseudomas aeruginosa*, and *Enterobacteriaceae Morganella morganii*
Dental infections	Streptococci and gram-negative bacilli: *B. fragilis*
Endocarditis	*Viridans streptococci* or *S. aureus*
Cyanotic congenital heart disease	Streptococci
	Anaerobic: *Bacteroides, Prevotella melaninogenica. Propionibacterium, Fusobacterium, Actinomyces*
Pyogenic lung infection	*Streptococcus* sp., *Actinomyces* sp., and *Fusobacterium* sp
Urinary sepsis	Enterobacteriaceae and Pseudomonacaea
Penetrating head trauma or neurosurgical procedures	*S. aureus*
Immigrants	Parasites: *Taenia, Entamoeba, Schistosoma, Paragonimus, Echinococcus*
Immunocompromised T-cell dysfunction	*Toxoplasma gondii*
	Nocardia asteroides
	Cryptococcus neoformans
	Mycobacteria
	Listeria monocytogenes
	Primary CNS lymphoma
	(EBV associated)
	Progressive multifocal leukoencephalopathy
	(JC virus)
Neutropenia	*Asperigillis* sp.
	Candida sp.
	Mucoraceae
	Enterobacteriaceae
	Pseudomonas aeruginosa

Abbreviations: CNS, central nervous system; EBV, Epstein-Barr virus; JC, John Cunningham.
[a]Adapted from Alvis Miranda H et al.[16]

setting of intracranial infection because of poor blood-brain barrier penetration. Once culture and serology sensitivities have resulted, antibiotic selection can be narrowed. Antibiotics are continued for 4 to 8 weeks based on clinical response and the extent of disease. Glucocorticoids are recommended for patients with signs of significant mass effect from the abscess or edema resulting in increased intracranial pressures and potential brain herniation particularly in the setting of depressed mental status. Select patients may require antiseizure prophylaxis.

Other Key Issues

This diagnosis requires neurosurgical consultation for management and inpatient admission.

Suggested Readings and References

1. Osenbach RK, Loftus CM. Diagnosis and management of brain abscess. *Neurosurg Clin N Am.* 1992;3:403–420.
2. Heilpern KL, Lorber B. Focal intracranial infections. *Infect Dis Clin N Am.* 1996;10:879.
3. Ratnaike TE, Das S, Gregson BA, Mendelow AD. A review of brain abscess surgical treatment—78 years: aspiration versus excision. *World Neurosurg.* 2011;76:431.
4. Chun CH, Johnson JD, Hofstetter M, Raff MJ. Brain abscess: a study of 45 consecutive cases. *Medicine (Baltimore).* 1986;65:415–431.
5. Schliamser SE, Bäckman K, Norrby SR. Intracranial abscesses in adults: an analysis of 54 consecutive cases. *Scand J Infect Dis.* 1988;20:1–9.
6. Ng PY, Seow WT, Ong PL. Brain abscesses: review of 30 cases treated with surgery. *Aust N Z J Surg.* 1995;65:664–666.

7. Yang SY, Zhao CS. Review of 140 patients with brain abscess. *Surg Neurol*. 1993;39:290–296.

8. Nielsen H, Gyldensted C, Harmsen A. Cerebral abscess. Aetiology and pathogenesis, symptoms, diagnosis and treatment. A review of 200 cases from 1935–1976. *Acta Neurol Scand*. 1982;65:609–622.

9. Seydoux C, Francioli P. Bacterial brain abscesses: factors influencing mortality and sequelae. *Clin Infect Dis*. 1992;15:394–401.

10. Tattevin P, Bruneel F, Clair B, et al. Bacterial brain abscesses: a retrospective study of 94 patients admitted to an intensive care unit (1980 to 1999). Am J Med. 2003;115:143–146.

11. Brook I. Aerobic and anaerobic bacteriology of intracranial abscesses. Pediatr Neurol. 1992;8:210–214.

12. Arlotti M, Grossi P, Pea F, et al. Consensus document on controversial issues for the treatment of infections of the central nervous system: bacterial brain abscesses. *Int J Infect Dis*. 2010;14(suppl 4):S79–S82.

13. Cavuşoglu H, Kaya RA, Türkmenoglu ON, et al. Brain abscess: analysis of results in a series of 51 patients with a combined surgical and medical approach during an 11-year period. *Neurosurg Focus*. 2008;24:E9.

14. Lakshmi V, Rao RR, Dinakar I. Bacteriology of brain abscess—observations on 50 cases. *J Med Microbiol*. 1993;38:187–190.

15. Mathisen GE, Johnson JP. Brain abscess. *Clin Infect Dis*. 1997;25:763–779.

16. Alvis Miranda H, Castellar-Leones SM, Elzain MA, Moscote-Salazar LR. Brain abscess: current management. *J Neurosci Rural Pract*. 2013;4(suppl 1):S67–S81. doi: 10.4103/0976-3147.116472.

Chapter 9

Epidural Abscess

David Mabey

Summary Box

Disease Description: An epidural abscess is a collection of pus that has accumulated between the dura and the calvarium or spine. It is rare but can lead to severe neurologic dysfunction or death.

Diagnostic tests: Magnetic resonance imaging (MRI), blood culture, erythrocyte sedimentation rate (ESR), and C-reactive protein (CRP)

Organisms:
  Often polymicrobial
  Staphylococcus and *Streptococcus* are common causes.

Treatment:
  Surgical drainage
  Initial antibiotics include IV vancomycin, metronidazole, and third- or fourth-generation
    cephalosporins.

Disease Description

Epidural abscess is a rare but potentially devastating infection of the central nervous system (CNS) that can result in neurological deficits, permanent neurological injury, sepsis, or even death. Early diagnosis is key to minimizing complications. Treatment requires prolonged hospitalization, surgical treatment in most cases, and long-term antibiotics. There are two main subsets of epidural abscess: spinal epidural abscess (SEA) and intracranial epidural abscess (ICEA).

Epidemiology and Pathogenesis

SEA occurs in 0.2 to 2 of every 10,000 admitted patients each year. It is more prevalent in patients 30 to 60 years of age, and it presents in males more often than in females. Infection occurs via two known mechanisms: contiguous spread (about one-third of infections) and hematogenous spread (about half of infections). The remaining causes of epidural abscesses are unknown. The enlarging accumulation of pus in SEA causes CNS damage via mechanical compression and local inflammation, including vascular thrombophlebitis.

In SEA, the outcome is largely determined by the degree of neurological deficit prior to the initiation of treatment. Almost half of SEA cases result in lasting neurological deficits. Paralysis is seen in almost 15% of cases. Local or systemic invasion leads to infections, such as vertebral osteomyelitis, endocarditis, and psoas muscle abscess.

SEA is more common in the posterior aspect of the epidural space and more commonly occurs in the thoracolumbar spine, which has more infection-prone fat. The abscess typically traverses three to four vertebral levels, but there are known cases of abscesses that traverse the entire spine.

ICEA is rarer than SEA, accounting for only 10% of epidural abscesses. ICEA is more prevalent in younger patients (7–20 years old). Frontal sinusitis is the source of ICEA in 60% to 90% of cases.

Presenting Features

Back pain is the most common presentation of SEA, along with spinal tenderness. It is present in 70% to 90% of patients with SEA. Fever occurs in about half of patients, and neurological deficits are present in about one-third of patients. The presence of paresthesias, radicular pain, and meningismus can also be seen and aid in diagnosis. Bowel or bladder dysfunction is a late sign. There are four stages of dysfunction in SEA:

1. Back pain at the level of the spine affected by the abscess
2. Nerve-root pain radiating from the involved spinal area
3. Motor weakness, sensory deficits, and bowel or bladder dysfunction
4. Paralysis

ICEA is associated with sinus infection and will often have purulent nasal or aural discharge as well as scalp swelling. Other findings include fever, nausea, vomiting, confusion, agitation, seizures, hemiparesis, and cranial neuropathies. Mass effect due to ICEA can cause confusion, cranial nerve compression, or herniation. Local or systemic inflammation can also cause direct damage.

Diagnostic Considerations

Risk factors for SEA include intravenous drug use, diabetes mellitus, malignancy, immunocompromised state, recent spinal procedure or instrumentation, spinal trauma, and local or systemic infection. The classic triad of fever, back pain, and neurological deficit is rarely present.

Risk factors for ICEA include frontal sinus infection, posttraumatic infection, and recent intracranial, transnasal, or transmastoid surgical procedure. Patient history often includes recent CNS procedure, known or suspected infection (ie, osteomyelitis or sinusitis), comorbidities, immunodeficiency, and trauma.

Differential Diagnosis

The differential diagnosis to consider when SEA is suspected includes intervertebral disk disease (including discitis), degenerative bone disease, vertebral osteomyelitis, and muscle strain. The differential diagnosis for suspected ICEA includes meningitis, sinusitis, migraine, intracranial tumor, and other intracranial abscesses.

Diagnostic Tests

The gold standard for both SEA and ICEA is MRI; gadolinium enhancement aids diagnosis. In ICEA, gadolinium will show a thickened dural surface, which can help differentiate ICEA from sterile collections. In SEA, gadolinium can help highlight subtle osteomyelitis or discitis.

Standard computed tomography (CT) is unreliable for SEA, but CT myelogram is a viable option if MRI is unavailable. CT is an effective screening tool for ICEA and will show a low-attenuation, extra-axial mass. Radiographs may show vertebral body abnormalities but are neither sensitive nor specific for SEA and ICEA. Extension of a SEA is difficult to determine by exam alone, so imaging of the entire spine is often required to fully characterize the abscess.

Laboratory Evaluation

Leukocytosis is present in about two-thirds of SEA. ESR is very sensitive for SEA; although not as sensitive as ESR, CRP is potentially useful. Neither the presence nor the magnitude of abnormality for ESR, CRP, or leukocyte count is specific. Lumbar puncture should not be done routinely, as it carries the risk of meningitis or subdural extension of the infection if the needle passes through the abscess. In addition, CSF cultures are positive in only 25% of SEA cases. Blood cultures are positive in approximately 60% SEA cases. Culture of the abscess, either from image-guided drainage or surgical drainage, is required to accurately select antibiotic therapy.

Organisms

Staphylococcus and *Streptococcus* species are common causes of SEA, especially in infections associated with injection-drug use and skin infections. *S. aureus* alone accounts for 50% to 66% of cases of SEA. Methicillin-resistant *S. aureus* (MRSA) now accounts for up to 40% of the *Staphylococcus* infections seen in SEA. Injection-drug use should raise concern for *Pseudomonas* spp (multiple species). Enteric organisms should be considered in SEA when there are distant infections, such as urinary tract infections. Immunosuppression should raise concern for mycobacterial or fungal organisms. Medical comorbidities increase the likelihood of polymicrobial infections.

ICEA is often polymicrobial and associated with the organisms that cause sinusitis. The most common microorganisms include *Staphylococcus, Streptococcus, Haemophilus*, and anaerobes.

Treatment

Neurosurgeons should be involved as early as possible. Initial antibiotics should be chosen to treat *Staphylococcus* (including MRSA) and *Streptococcus* species as well as gram negative and anaerobic organisms. A reasonable regimen is vancomycin, metronidazole, and a third- or fourth-generation cephalosporin.

In the stable patient, antibiotics should be withheld until culture data can be obtained. If surgical treatment is not readily available, biopsy is often performed to obtain samples for culture before starting antibiotics. In the majority of cases, treatment requires surgical drainage, although nonsurgical treatment is a possibility in the patient without neurological deficits and with a microorganism identified by culture. Long-term antibiotics are required and should be guided by abscess cultures. Most recommendations are for at least 2 weeks of parenteral therapy followed by at least 4 weeks of oral antibiotics.

Disposition

Consult neurosurgery for disposition. Except in rare cases, patients with SEA and ICEA will require admission.

Suggested Readings and References

1. Pradilla G, Ardila G, Hsu W, Rigamonti D. Epidural abscesses of the CNS. *Lancet Neurol.* 2009;8:292–300.
2. Darouiche R. Spinal epidural abscess. *N Engl J Med.* 2006;355:2012–2020.
3. Davis DP, Wold RM, Patel RJ, et al. The clinical presentation and impact of diagnostic delays on emergency department patients with spinal epidural abscess. *J Emerg Med.* 2004;26:285–291.
4. Reihsaus E, Waldbaur H, Seeling W. Spinal epidural abscess: a meta-analysis of 915 patients. *Neurosurg Rev.* 2000;232:175–204.
5. Heran NS, Steinbok P, Cochrane DD. Conservative neurosurgical management of intracranial epidural abscesses in children. *Neurosurgery.* 2003;53:893–898.
6. Zimmerer S, Conen A, Muller AA, et al. Spinal epidural abscess: aetiology, predisponent factors and clinical outcomes in a 4-year prospective study. *Eur Spine J.* 2011;20:2228–2234.

Ear, Nose, and Throat Infections

Chapter 10

Pharyngitis, Tonsillitis, and Peritonsillar Abscess

Gabrielle Jacquet

Summary Box

Disease Description: Pharyngitis typically presents with sore throat, fever, and pharyngeal inflammation. More serious cases may progress to peritonsillar abscess (PTA).

Organisms:
  Viruses (see following)
  Bacteria: Group A β-Hemolytic Streptococci (GABHS), *Mycoplasma pneumoniae*

Treatment:
  For all cases: supportive care with antipyretics, analgesics, and fluids
  For GABHS:
    Oral First Line: Penicillin VK 500 mg po 3 to times daily for 10 days
    Second Line: Azithromycin: 500 mg po daily × 5 days or clindamycin 600 mg po BID (twice a day)
    Parenteral: single dose of benzathine penicillin
    G 1.2 million units IM (intramuscular)

Other Key Issues: The carotid arteries and trachea are important nearby structures. Antibiotics are not appropriate in all cases. HIV (human immunodeficiency virus) infection can initially present with pharyngitis.

Disease Description

Epidemiology

Age: For pharyngitis, the highest burden of disease is in children and young adults. Approximately 50% of cases are diagnosed in patients between 5 and 24 years of age. Peritonsillar abscess (PTA) primarily develops in young adults.

Season: In temperate climates, most cases occur in the winter and early spring.

Presenting Features: Infection/inflammation of the throat that primarily affects the palatine tonsils are considered tonsillitis, whereas infections involving the posterior pharynx are considered pharyngitis. Tonsillitis and pharyngitis often occur together.

Viral Pharyngitis/Tonsillitis: Fever, odynophagia, and petechial or vesicular lesions on the soft palate and tonsils are often seen with associated cough, rhinorrhea, and congestion. Cases typically lack tonsillar exudates and cervical lymphadenopathy, except in the setting of mononucleosis, influenza, and acute retroviral syndrome (also known as acute HIV syndrome).

Bacterial Pharyngitis/Tonsillitis: Cases often present with acute-onset fever, sore throat, and odynophagia. Patients often have tonsillar erythema, exudates, and tender anterior cervical adenopathy. Cough, conjunctivitis, and rhinorrhea are typically lacking.

Peritonsillar Abscess: Patients often complain of fever, sore throat, odynophagia, trismus, dysphagia, and a muffled "hot potato" voice. Patients may appear ill and have an infected tonsil that is displaced medially, causing the uvula to be deflected to the opposite side.

Diagnostic Considerations

The differential includes infectious mononucleosis, retropharyngeal abscess, neoplasm, and internal carotid artery aneurysm.

Typical Disease Course

Pharyngitis: Most cases are due to common viral infections and are benign and self-limited.

PTA: Often considered a suppurative complication of tonsillitis, but other theories suggest an obstruction of the Weber glands (salivary glands in the superior tonsil) leading to a polymicrobial abscess formation that extends into the space between the palatine tonsil and its capsule.

Complications

Complications of pharyngitis may include peritonsillar abscess, parapharyngeal abscess, lymphadenitis, sinusitis, otitis media, mastoiditis, necrotizing fasciitis, and toxic shock syndrome.

Complications of GABHS include the following:

Scarlet fever

Acute rheumatic fever (rare in the United States)

Rheumatic heart disease (primarily in developing countries)

Acute glomerulonephritis

Lemierre's syndrome (thrombophlebitis and septic emboli)

Diagnostic Tests

For pharyngitis/tonsillitis due to GABHS

Centor criteria (used to determine whether testing is indicated):

(1) tonsillar exudates

(2) tender anterior cervical adenopathy

(3) absence of cough

(4) fever

For patients with 0 to 1 criteria: No antibiotic therapy recommended.

For patients with 2+ criteria: Test

For patients with 3+ criteria: Test or treat empirically (mixed evidence)

Rapid antigen-detection test (RADT): recommended for use by the Infectious Disease Society of America, the Committee on Infectious Diseases of the American Academy of Pediatrics, and the American Heart Association for confirmation of GABHS infection.

A negative RADT result should be confirmed by blood-agar plate culture for all children. *Culture is not recommended in the adult population.*

Multiplex PCR (polymerase chain reaction) can be used for detection of *Corynebacterium diphtheriae* but is not performed in the clinical setting.

For PTA: IV (intravenous) contrast-enhanced computed tomography of the neck is the gold standard. However, ultrasound is increasingly used to diagnose and treat PTA.

Organisms

Viral Pharyngitis: rhinoviruses (20%), *Coronavirus* spp. (>5%), adenoviruses (5%), herpes simplex viruses (4%), parainfluenza viruses (2%), influenza viruses (2%), coxsackievirus A (< 1%), Epstein-Barr virus (< 1%), *Cytomegalovirus* spp. (< 1%), and HIV (< 1%).

Bacterial Pharyngitis: GABHS (15%–30%), Group C β-Hemolytic Streptococci (5%), *Neisseria gonorrhea* (< 1%), *C. diphtheria* (< 1%), *Arcanobacterium hemolyticum* (< 1%), *M. pneumoniae* (< 1%), and *Chlamydia Pneumoniae* (< 1%).

PTA: typically polymicrobial; *GABHS* are the most commonly identified organisms.

Treatment

First Line Recommendations

For all cases: supportive care with antipyretics, analgesics, and fluids.

For GABHS Pharyngitis/Tonsillitis:

Supportive care PLUS

Antibiotics:

ORAL: Penicillin VK 500 mg po 3 to 4 times daily for 10 days or Amoxicillin 500mg to 875 mg po q12 hours or 250 to 500 po q8 hours for 10 days

PARENTERAL: 1 dose of benzathine penicillin G 1.2 million units IM

Alternative: Azithromycin: 500 mg po daily × 5 days or clindamycin

600 mg po BID or 600 mg to 900 mg IV every 8 hours

A single dose of 10 mg po dexamethasone reduces severe pharyngeal pain, especially in patients with an identified bacterial pathogen; but dexamethasone should not be considered in routine cases.

For Peritonsillar Abscess:

Supportive care and antibiotics listed above PLUS fine needle aspiration (FNA) with an 18- to 20-gauge needle or incision and drainage (I&D). There is no difference in outcome when comparing FNA with I&D. More than 90% of patients will be treated effectively after a single FNA. Use ultrasound guidance if available. Otolaryngology should be consulted if the emergency medicine physician is unable to drain the abscess and/or in cases of airway compromise.

Other Key Issues to Consider

Local Anatomy: Weber glands (a group of mucous salivary glands superior to the tonsil in the soft palate) have been implicated in the formation of PTA. It is important to consider their proximity to the trachea and to the carotid artery when performing FNA.

Antibiotic Therapy: Despite the much lower prevalence of GABHS infection (for which antibiotics is indicated), a staggering 49% to 57% of children and 64% of adults evaluated for pharyngitis receive an antibiotic prescription.

Consider HIV: Up to 90% of primary infections with HIV-1 are associated with acute retroviral syndrome, which includes pharyngitis 2 to 4 weeks after exposure.

Suggested Readings and References

1. Barksdale A. Neck and upper airway disorders. In: Cline DM, Ma OJ, Cydulka RK, Meckler GD, Handel DA, Thomas SH, eds. *Tintinalli's Emergency Medicine Manual.* 7th ed. New York, NY: McGraw-Hill Medical; 2012:Chapter 153. http://www.accessemergencymedicine.com/content.aspx?aID=56279797. Accessed October 19, 2012.

2. Bisno AL, Gerber MA, Gwaltney JM Jr, et al. Practice guidelines for the diagnosis and management of group A streptococcal pharyngitis. *Clin Infect Dis.* 2002;35:113–125.

3. Caserta MT, Flores AR. Pharyngitis. In: Mandell GL, Bennett JE, Dolin R, eds. *Mandell, Douglas, and Bennett's Principles and Practice of Infectious Diseases.* 7th ed. Philadelphia, Pa: Mosby; 2010.

4. Centor RM, Witherspoon JM, Dalton HP, et al. The diagnosis of strep throat in adults in the emergency room. *Med Decis Making.* 1981;1:239.

5. Johnson RF, Stewart MG, Wright CG: An evidence-based review of the treatment of Peritonsillar abscess. *Otolaryngol Head Neck Surg.* 2003;128:332–343.

6. Linder JA, Bates DW, Lee GM, et al. Antibiotic treatment of children with sore throat. *JAMA*. 2005;294:2315–2322.

7. Nash DR, Harman J, Wald ER, et al. Antibiotic prescribing by primary care physicians for children with upper respiratory tract infections. *Arch Pediatr Adolesc Med*. 2002;156:1114–1119.

8. Oxenius A, Price DA, Easterbrook PJ, et al: Early highly active antiretroviral therapy for acute HIV-1 infection preserves immune function of CD8+ and CD4+ T lymphocytes. *Proc Natl Acad Sci* 2000;97:3382–3387.

9. Shah RN, Cannon TY, Shores CG. Infections and Disorders of the Neck and Upper Airway. In: Tintinalli JE, Kelen GD, Stapczynski JS, eds. *Tintinalli's Emergency Medicine: A Comprehensive Study Guide*. 7th ed. New York: McGraw-Hill Education; 2011:Chapter 241. http://www.accessemergencymedicine.com/content.aspx?aID=6388487. Accessed October 19, 2012.

10. Shirley WP, Woolley AL, Wiatrak BJ. Pharyngitis and adenotonsillar disease. In: Flint PW, Haughey BH, Lund VJ, et al., eds. *Cummings Otolaryngology—Head and Neck Surgery*. 5th ed. Philadelphia, Pa: Mosby; 2010.

11. Steinman MA, Gonzales R, Linder JA, et al. Changing use of antibiotics in community-based outpatient practice, 1991–1999. *Ann Intern Med*. 2003;138:525–533.

12. Wing A, Villa-Roel C, Yeh B, et al: Effectiveness of corticosteroid treatment in acute pharyngitis: a systematic review of the literature. *Acad Emerg Med*. 2010;17:476–483.

Chapter 11

Otitis Externa, Otitis Media, and Mastoiditis

Susan Peterson and Staci Reintjes

Summary Box

Disease Description:
Otitis Externa: Infection of external auditory canal
Otitis Media: Infection of the middle ear
Mastoiditis: Infection of the mastoid bone

Organisms:
Otitis Externa: *Pseudomonas, Staphylococcus aureus, S. epidermidis,* and *Streptococcus*
Otitis Media: *S. pneumoniae, Haemophilus influenza,* and *Moraxella catarrhalis*
Mastoiditis: *S. pneumoniae, S. pyogenes, S. aureus, H. influenzae,* and *M. catarrhalis*

Treatment:
First line:
Otitis Externa: Neomycin-polymyxin B and hydrocortisone otic solution
Otitis Media: In healthy adults, observation without antibiotics for 3 days; if no resolution, consider high dose Amoxicillin 1 g PO TID (three times a day) for 7 days, or Levofloxacin 750 mg PO daily for 5 days, or Moxifloxacin 400 mg PO daily for 7 days. In children, high-dose amoxicillin (80–90 mg/kg per day in two divided doses) for 5 to 10 days as the treatment of first choice in most patients.
Mastoiditis: Ceftriaxone s 50 to 100 mg/kg per dose IM (intramuscularly) or intravenous (IV)† daily for 3 doses; and vancomycin 2 g/day IV divided either as 500 mg every 6 hours or 1 g every 12 hours.

Second line:
Otitis Externa: Ciprofloxacin 0.3%/dexamethesone 0.1% otic solution
Otitis Media: Amoxicillin/clavulanic acid 2000/125 mg PO BID (twice a day) for 7 days can be used. IV antibiotics should be reserved for those with serious complications.
Mastoiditis: Cefotaxime 1 to 2 g IV or IM every 8 hours and possible surgical drainage

Otitis Externa

Disease Description

Otitis Externa accounted for 8.1 of every 1000 doctor's visits in 2007, 20% of which were emergency department visits. The incidence of otitis externa is highest in children; less than 5% of cases occur in patients older than 20 years.[1] Patients typically present with inflammation of the auricle, external auditory canal, or outer tympanic membrane (TM). This causes otalgia, aural fullness, pruritus, discharge, and hearing loss. Severe infections may cause cranial nerve palsies, fever, and severe pain.[2] Symptoms are typically exacerbated by warm and humid climates, by swimming and frequent hair washing (most commonly in a bath tub), and by insertion of foreign bodies, such as hearing aids or cotton swabs. Excessive purulent discharge may point toward an occult or obstructing foreign body as the etiology.

Complications include TM rupture, osteomyelitis of the temporal bone, or malignant otitis externa (infection of the auditory canal extending to the temporal bone), which require more aggressive interventions. Otitis externa can become chronic if it persists for more than 3 weeks. The differential diagnosis includes otitis media with TM rupture, herpes zoster oticus (ie, Ramsay Hunt syndrome), eczema, cholesteatoma, abscess, and squamous cell carcinoma.

Infection typically occurs via penetration of the epithelial barrier. Excess cerumen traps water and bacteria in the external canal, creating a focus for bacteria to invade the epithelial lining. This is particularly notable in patients who swim frequently or who have foreign bodies in the canal, such as ear plugs or hearing aids. The result is the creation of a warm, moist, and alkaline environment, which is ideal for bacterial replication and invasive infection.

Physical Exam

With true acute otitis externa (AOE), the ear canal will be erythematous and edematous with cellular debris and purulent discharge. The pathognomonic finding is pain induced by pinna or tragus manipulation. Ideally, the ear canal should be cleaned out properly to ensure that the TM is intact and free of vesicles indicative of Ramsay Hunt syndrome. Spores and hyphae may be seen with fungal infections. Conductive hearing loss may also be present.

Organisms

The primary organisms that cause otitis externa are *S. epidermidis, S. aureus*, and *P. aeruginosa*. In one case review, *Pseudomonas* was found to cause 38% of infections in diabetics. *Pseudomonas* was also found to generally cause more severe symptoms, including fever. Candidal infections are seen in 2% to 10% of patients, and they typically occur after treatment for a bacterial otitis externa.[3]

Treatment

Initial treatment involves effectively cleaning the external canal of debris to improve the effectiveness of topical drops. If assessment of the canal is limited by edema, the patient may require specialty referral to an otolaryngologist for cleaning and a wick.[4] First line therapy includes topical acidic agents and antibiotic drops. First line therapy is Cortisporin (neomycin, polymyxin B, and hydrocortisone), four drops TID for 7 to 10 days. Second line therapy is Ciprodex (ciprofloxacin and dexamethasone), four drops BID for 7 to 10 days. Ciprodex is more expensive and carries a higher risk of pseudomonal resistance. Alternative options include tobramycin, gentamicin, or ofloxacin otic drops. **Ciprofloxacin, as well as tobramycin and gentamicin, are severely ototoxic and should be avoided if there is any concern for TM rupture.** Fungal AOE should be treated with aggressive cleaning of the external canal as well as topical astringents, such as VoSol HC (acetic acid, propylene glycol, and hydrocortisone), 4 to 6 drops TID for 10 days. Alternatively, clotrimazole solution can be administered 3 to 4 drops TID for 7 days.

Oral antibiotics should be considered for recurrent infections, those resistant to topical therapy, severe disease, extension beyond the external auditory canal, diabetics, or immunocompromised patients. Ciprofloxacin 750 mg PO BID is considered first line, as it is the only oral drug that has been shown to be effective against resistant pseudomonal strains. If *S. aureus* is suspected, then oral cephalexin or dicloxacillin can be used. For malignant otitis externa (MOE), IV antibiotics are required. An antipseudomonal beta-lactam is first line due to the increased resistance of *Pseudomonas* against fluoroquinolone monotherapy. Appropriate antibiotic choices for MOE include piperacillin/tazobactam 4.5 g IV every 6 hours; cefepime 2 g IV every 8 hours; and, for those with penicillin allergy, aztreonam 2 g IV every 8 hours.

Otitis Media

Disease Description

Acute otitis media (AOM) is the most common infection in childhood, and there are more than four million visits per year among patients older than 15 years.[5] Patients typically present with otalgia, otorrhea, fever, irritability, anorexia, and hearing loss. Otalgia is generally worse in adults than children. Patients may have purulent drainage from the ear in the setting of TM rupture. Otitis media often results from abnormal function of the Eustachian tube, causing a relative negative pressure in the middle ear. In children, this is commonly due to abnormal patency; whereas in adults, it is more commonly secondary to obstruction, such as with allergic rhinitis or an upper respiratory infection. Acute illness is self-limited in some patients. However, in others, the disease progresses to TM rupture. A minority of patients can have a persistent indolent effusion refractory to antibiotic treatment. Although pain is the most common complication of otitis media, hearing loss and mastoiditis are the most serious complications.

Physical Exam

Clinical diagnosis is made with visualization of the TM using an otoscope and may require the removal of cerumen with curettage or irrigation. Diagnostic criteria include having acute ear pain along with physical exam findings of an ear effusion or signs of inflammation. An effusion is identified by TM bulging, otorrhea, decreased mobility of the TM on insufflation with a pneumatoscope, or an air fluid level or air bubbles behind the TM. Inflammation is identified by erythema of the TM, pus appreciated behind the TM, or otalgia. Imaging is typically of no value in the diagnosis of AOM unless more invasive disease is suspected. If drainage is present, swabs can be taken for culture, which may be helpful in refractory cases.

Organisms

Otitis media is typically caused by bacteria that colonize the nasopharynx and enter the middle ear via the Eustachian tube. Eustachian tube dysfunction causes obstruction, entrapping bacteria and serous fluid. The two most common organisms causing AOM are *S. pneumoniae* (40%–50% of cases) and *H. influenza* (30%–40% of cases). *M. catarrhalis* causes 10% to 15% of cases, and *S. aureus* and *S. pyogenes* are only present in 2% of cultures.[5]

Treatment

Many cases of otitis media resolve spontaneously within 3 days without intervention. Among children, 19% of pneumococcal and 50% of *H. influenza* cases resolve clinically and have sterile aspirates of the middle ear without antibiotic treatment.[6] Observation without antibiotics is a safe first choice for healthy adults with mild or ambiguous signs of AOM and reliable follow-up. If there is no improvement, first line oral therapy for AOM is high dose amoxicillin 1 g PO TID for 7 days. Levofloxacin 750 mg PO daily for 5 days or Moxifloxacin 400 mg PO daily for 7 days can be used in patients allergic to penicillin. For AOM infection that fails to resolve or for patients with more severe infections, high dose amoxicillin/clavulanic acid 2000/125 mg PO BID for 7 days can be used. IV antibiotics should be reserved for those with serious complications. Cerebral abscesses should be treated with vancomycin plus ceftriaxone and metronidazole. Meningitis and acute mastoiditis should be treated with vancomycin and ceftriaxone. Patients with chronic mastoiditis should also have pseudomonal coverage and piperacillin/tazobactam can be added.

In children, the American Association of Pediatrics issued some revised guidelines in 2013 regarding the diagnosis and treatment of acute otitis media. Some of the key statements included the following:

1) Children can be diagnosed with acute otitis media when they present with moderate to severe bulging of the tympanic membrane or new onset otorrhea not to acute otitis media externa.

2) Children may be diagnosed with acute otitis media when they present with mild bulging of the tympanic membrane and recent onset of pain within 48 hours or intense erythema of the tympanic membrane.

3) Children without a middle ear effusion as demonstrated by pneumatic otoscopy and/or tympanometry likely do not have acute otitis media.

Mastoiditis

Disease Description

Although the current rate of surgical mastoiditis is extremely low, occurring in only 0.004% of cases, it was a significant cause of mortality prior to the advent of antibiotic therapy.[7] Patients with mastoiditis present with pain, swelling, and erythema over the mastoid bone, posterior to the ear. Fever, irritability, otalgia, and hearing loss are also often present. The diagnosis can often be made clinically, but CT scan is often used for confirmation. Patients typically develop progressive posterior auricular pain with erythema, swelling, and fever during or after the treatment of otitis media. Infection can be serious and may lead to sepsis, sigmoid sinus thrombosis, and intracranial abscess if not treated appropriately. More common complications include chronic infection, resistant bacteria, and mild hearing loss.

Organisms

The mastoid bone is an extension of the middle ear cleft. Typically, bacteria from otitis media extend past the mucosa into the mastoid air cells and cause osteitis with erosion of bone and cortex. The mastoid is lined with respiratory epithelium that swells when infection is present. This causes occlusion of the antrum, essentially entrapping the bacteria. The most common causative organisms include S. pneumoniae, S. pyogenes, S. aureus, H. Influenzae, and M. catarrhalis.[7]

Treatment

Mild mastoiditis may be treated on an outpatient bases, but the majority of cases are moderate to severe and require intravenous antibiotics. Antibiotics may decrease the swelling of the epithelium, allowing for spontaneous drainage of fluid from the antrum. If this cannot be accomplished with antibiotic therapy, such as vancomycin and ceftriaxone, surgical drainage of the fluid in the mastoid air cells may be required. Recent studies advocate for broad antibiotic coverage until culture data is available, as there have been recent increases in antibiotic resistant bacteria.[8]

Suggested Readings and References

1. CDC. Estimated burden of acute otitis externa—United States, 2003–2007. *MMWR Morb Mortal Wkly Rep.* 2011;60:605–609.

2. Walton L. Otitis externa. *BMJ.* 2012;344:e3623.

3. Roland PS, Stroman DW. Microbiology of acute otitis externa. *Laryngoscope.* Jul 2002;112(7Pt1):1166–1177.

4. Kaushik V, Saeed SR. Interventions for acute otitis externa. *Cochrane Database Syst Rev.* 2010;1:CD004740.

5. Culpepper L, Froom J, Bartelds AI, et al. Acute otitis media in adults: a report from the international primary care network. *J Am Board Fam Pract.* 1993;6:333–339.

6. Howie VM, Ploussard JH. The "in vivo sensitity test"—bacteriology of middle ear exudates, durine antimicrobial therapy in otitis media. *Pediatrics* 1969; 44:940. And Kaleida PH, Casselbrant ML, Rockette HE, et al. Amoxicillin or myringotom or both for acute otitis media: results of a randomized clinicaltrial. *Pediatrics* 1991;87:466.

7. Nussinovitch M, Yoeli R, Elishkevitz K, Varsano I (2004). "Acute mastoiditis in children: epidemiologic, clinical, microbiologic, and therapeutic aspects over past years." *Clin Pediatr (Phila)* 43:261–267.

8. Roddy MG, Glazier SS, Agrawal D. Pediatric mastoiditis in the pneumococcal conjugate vaccine era: symptom duration guides empiric antimicrobial therapy. *Pediatr Emerg Care.* Nov 2007;23(11):779–784.

Chapter 12

Rhinosinusitis

Staci Reintjes and Susie Peterson

Summary Box

Disease Description: Inflammation of the nasal passages and paranasal sinuses, commonly caused by allergies or viral infection and less frequently by bacterial or fungal infections.

Organisms:
  Most Common:
    Viral: Rhinovirus, Parainfluenza, Influenza
    Bacterial: *S. pneumoniae, H. influenzae, M. catarrhalis, S. aureus, P. aeruginosa,* anaerobes
    Fungal: *Rhizopus* spp. (multiple species), *Mucor* spp. (causative agents of mucormycosis), *Aspergillus* spp.

Treatment: Only after diagnosis of bacterial sinusitis
    First line: Amoxicillin/Clavulanate 875/125 mg PO TID for 7 days
    Second Line: doxycycline 100 mg BID for 7 days
    Levofloxacin 500 mg BID for 14 days

Key Facts: History and physical exam are more specific than imaging. Consider avoiding antibiotics if symptoms are of short duration and are consistent with viral sinusitis. Evaluate for severe complications in immunocompromised patients.

Disease Description

Sinusitis occurs after the development of rhinitis (inflammation of the nasal passages). Rhinitis is most commonly caused by allergens, but it also can result from an infectious or autoimmune process. For rhinitis to progress to rhinosinusitis (RS), there must be obstruction of the ostiomeatal complex within the medial meatus, which is the draining center for the maxillary, anterior ethmoid, and frontal sinuses. Drainage can be obstructed by progression of edema and inflammation from rhinitis, or patients can be predisposed to bouts of RS due to a nasal polyp that partially obstructs drainage chronically. Other factors that increase the likelihood of progression include smoking, dental infection, and frequent swimming.

The initial clinical presentation of RS parallels the symptoms of a viral upper respiratory tract infection. The progression of symptoms and length of disease is key to making the diagnosis of bacterial RS. Only 0.5% to 2.0% of patients with viral rhinosinusitis will develop acute bacterial sinusitis.[1] The diagnosis of bacterial RS can be made clinically if the patient has either two major symptoms or one major symptom and two minor symptoms for more than 7 to 10 days. Major symptoms include facial pain, purulent nasal discharge, fever > 39°C, nasal congestion, and hyposmia/anosmia. Minor symptoms include headache, cough, fatigue, halitosis, dental pain, or ear pain.

The most common differential diagnosis for RS is viral or allergic disease that has not progressed to true bacterial sinusitis. Other diseases that mimic RS include intranasal cocaine use, vasomotor rhinitis, basilar skull fracture resulting in CSF (cerebrospinal fluid) rhinorrhea, foreign body in the nasal passage, migraine, and tension headaches, or dental disease. Disease course is classified based on the timing from the onset of symptoms. Acute RS resolves in less than 4 weeks, subacute RS lasts 4 to 12 weeks, and chronic RS is diagnosed if there are more than 12 weeks of persistent symptoms.

Complications arising from sinusitis cause extensive morbidity if not recognized early. The most common complication is periorbital cellulitis arising from ethmoidal sinusitis. Other less common yet significant complications include meningitis, osteomyelitis, brain abscess, and cavernous sinus thrombosis. A complication specific to frontal sinusitis is Pott's puffy tumor, which is characterized by a subperiosteal abscess and osteomyelitis of the frontal bone due to direct extension of bacteria from the inflamed frontal sinus. Other complications may arise from sinusitis in immunocompromised populations, including diabetics and the elderly. These patients are at risk for developing fungal sinusitis, presenting with thick brown or black nasal discharge. Complications include mycetomas (ie, fungal infections characterized by swelling and draining sinuses that secrete granules), commonly from *Aspergillus* infection as well as ischemic bone necrosis, resulting in perforation with resultant fungemia. Fungal infection can then rapidly spread to the orbit, skin, and brain, potentially resulting in coma or death.

Diagnostic Tests

History and physical exam are by far the most sensitive and specific ways to accurately diagnose RS. Pain with leaning forward may be more reliable in diagnosing sinusitis than percussion or transillumination. An otoscope can be used to perform bedside anterior rhinoscopy. Findings suggestive of RS include mucosal edema, narrowing of the medial meatus, turbinate hypertrophy, and the presence of mucopurulent discharge. Radiographic imaging, including plain film and computed tomography (CT), have little role in making the diagnosis. Classic RS findings, such as air-fluid levels, mucosal thickening, and sinus opacification, are rarely seen on x-ray. However, they may be seen frequently on CT in patients with only simple viral rhinitis. This may lead to an increased number of patients being treated unnecessarily with antibiotics. CT is useful in diagnosing serious complications associated with sinusitis and should be considered for high-risk cases. Both nasal cultures and sinus aspiration have little utility in the emergency department assessment of RS.

Organisms

The most common causative organisms are viral, most frequently from strains of rhinovirus, followed by parainfluenza, and influenza. Viral RS will generally last less than 7 to 10 days; therefore, antibiotic treatment may not be indicated during this time period. Bacterial causes of RS include *Streptococcus pneumoniae*, followed closely by *Haemophilis influenza*. Less common bacterial sources include *Moraxella catarrhalis*, *Staphylococcus aureus*, and anaerobic organisms. *Pseudomonas aeruginosa* is common in patients with cystic fibrosis and HIV. Fungal causes of RS include *Rhizopus*, *Rhizomucor*, *Mucor*, and *Aspergillus* species. Fungal sinusitis is typically seen in immunocompromised, diabetic, and elderly patients and can present as an acute, subacute, or chronic infectious process.

Treatment

Adjunctive therapies to relieve nasal obstruction include anticongestants and medications that decrease mucosal edema as well as increase clearance of congestion. To decrease edema, alpha-adrenergic agonists, such as oxymetazoline 0.05% nasal spray, are recommended in viral RS, but they are only to be used for 3 days due to the risk of rebound vasodilation. Intranasal steroids have been found to be helpful only in patients with allergic rhinitis and should be reserved for this group alone. Guaifenesin is an expectorant (ie, increases the volume and decreases the viscosity of respiratory secretions), which promotes mucus clearance. Intranasal saline irrigation yields similar results via dilutional effects. Oral decongestants, oral steroids, and antihistamines are generally not found to be beneficial. Current first line therapy is to help alleviate bothersome symptoms.

Many clinical studies, based on symptoms alone and not sinus aspiration, indicate 40% to 60% of bacterial cases of sinusitis may resolve spontaneously within the first week without antibiotic treatment.[2] Patients at higher risk for a bacterial source are those with high fever, purulent discharge, and face pain for more than 3 days or those who present with worsening symptoms after 5 days of a viral upper respiratory infection that was initially improving. The Infectious Disease Society of America (IDSA) guidelines for 2012 recommend withholding antibiotics for 3 days after onset of symptoms in patients with mild to moderate symptoms. Antibiotics should be initiated after 3 days of symptoms if there is no improvement.

Antibiotic treatment for RS is dynamic. Current first line therapy includes amoxicillin/clavulanate at 875/125 mg PO BID or the higher dose of 2000/125 mg PO BID if resistance is likely. People at risk for resistant bacteria include the elderly, children less than 2 years old or in day care, prior antibiotic treatment in the past month, hospitalization in the past 5 days, immunocompromised patients, patients with other comorbidities, or those living in communities where S. pneumoniae penicillin resistance is more than 10%. Second line therapy includes doxycycline 100 mg PO BID, moxifloxacin 400 mg PO QD, and levofloxacin 500 mg PO QD. It is currently recommended that antibiotics be given for 7 days in adults and 10 to 14 days in children. Per current IDSA guidelines, trimethoprim/sulfamethoxazole, cephalosporins, and macrolides are no longer recommended due to their resistance patterns.

Treatment failure should be considered in patients who do not improve within 3 to 5 days of initiating antibiotics. Alternative regimens include increasing the amoxicillin/clavulanic acid dose to 2000/125 mg PO BID as well as changing to levofloxacin 500 mg daily or moxifloxacin 400 mg daily. Hospitalization should be considered for those with severe infection manifested by high fever, orbital edema, severe headache, meningeal signs, or visual symptoms. Patients admitted for acute severe sinusitis should be treated with an intravenous respiratory fluoroquinolone, such as moxifloxacin or levofloxacin, intravenous ampicillin/sulbactam at 1.5 to 3.0 g every 6 hours, ceftriaxone 1 to 2 g IV every 24 hours, or cefotaxime 2 g IV every 6 hours. Otolaryngology consultation should be considered for admitted patients as well as those at risk for fungal infection, nosocomial infection, and those with possible granulomatous disease. Surgery usually plays no role in the management of acute bacterial sinusitis, but urgent otolaryngology consultation should be part of the management of sinus and extra-sinus fungal disease.

Further Reading

1. Fokkens W, Lund V, Mullol J. EP3OS 2007: European position paper on rhinosinusitis and nasal polyps 2007: a summary for otorhinolaryngologists. *Rhinology*. 2007;45:97–101.
2. Falagas ME, Giannopoulou KP, Vardakas KZ, et al. Comparison of antibiotics with placebo for treatment of acute sinusitis: a meta-analysis of randomized controlled trials. *Lancet Infect Dis*. 2008;8:543–552.

Chapter 13

Odontogenic Infections

Gabrielle Jacquet and Lawrence Page

Summary Box

Disease Description: Odontogenic infections typically arise from infected teeth or from dental extraction. They may spread into the parapharyngeal and retropharyngeal spaces, involving the airway and mediastinum.

Organisms: Typically polymicrobial, including aerobes and anaerobes

Treatment:
> **Oral** (for local/mild infections): Amoxicillin/clavulanic acid, clindamycin, cefuroxime, or levofloxacin
> **Parenteral** (for deeper infections): IV (intravenous) ampicillin/sulbactam, piperacillin/tazobactam, imipenem/cilastatin, or ertapenem

Other Key Issues: Airway management is critical, as odontogenic infections can compromise airways via mass effect.

Disease Description

Epidemiology

Odontogenic infections often arise from dental caries (usually the mandibular teeth) or from dental extraction. Acute necrotizing ulcerative gingivitis (ANUG) is more common in immunocompromised patients (see following).

Presenting Features

Pulp infection: Localized dental tenderness

Dental abscesses: Neck mass, trismus, fever, leukocytes, dysphagia, and dyspnea

Ludwig's Angina (a rapidly progressing infection of the bilateral submental, sublingual, and submandibular spaces that may progress rapidly, causing airway compromise): tense, brawny, and elevated floor of the mouth

Necrotizing Infections: Patients are toxic and ill-appearing with subcutaneous crepitus and systemic signs, such as fever, tachycardia, hypotension, and confusion.

ANUG: Sudden onset of pain in the gingiva, exacerbated by chewing. On exam, the gingiva is marginated, punched-out, and eroded. Often, a superficial grayish pseudomembrane is seen along with a characteristic halitosis and altered taste sensation. Fever, malaise, and regional lymphadenopathy are typically present as well.

Diagnostic Considerations

A patient with any sign of airway involvement should not be sent to computed tomography (CT) scan before their airway is secured.

Typical Disease Course

Odontogenic infections can develop from 1 day to up to 3 weeks after the onset of odontalgia, and they may occur despite oral antibiotics. These infections may spread into the fascial planes, causing Ludwig's Angina.

Complications

Complications include the following: abscess, facial or orbital cellulitis, intracranial invasion (eg, cavernous sinus thrombosis), Ludwig's angina, Lemierre syndrome (ie, suppurative jugular thrombophlebitis), carotid artery erosion, descending necrotizing mediastinitis (mortality rate 25%–40%), airway compromise, hematogenous dissemination to distant organs, intraoral or dentocutaneous fistula formation, and cardiovascular disease.

Diagnostic Tests

A contrast-enhanced CT scan of the neck can help detect involvement of fascial planes as well as deep tissue spaces; such imaging should be considered, except in small, uncomplicated, and superficial dental abscesses.

Organisms

Dental infections are typically polymicrobial, including aerobes and anaerobes. *S. viridans* is identified most frequently. Common anaerobes include *Peptostreptococcus, Prevotella,* and *Bacteroides.*

ANUG is caused by *Prevotella intermedia, Fusobacterium* spp. (multiple species), *Tannerella forsythensis, Treponema denticola,* and other oral spirochetes.

Treatment

Antibiotics are *not* a substitute for definitive airway management. In addition, many cases of odontogenic infection will require surgical drainage, either at the bedside in the emergency department or in the operating room. Prior to performing incision and drainage, consider using a nerve block to obtain anesthesia to the affected area of the face. Patients with necrotizing infections need emergent surgery with wide local debridement. Penicillin has fallen out of favor due to emerging resistant bacteria.

First line Recommendations

Aerobic and anaerobic coverage:

Oral (for mild infections): Amoxicillin/clavulanic acid, clindamycin, cefuroxime, or levofloxacin

Parenteral (for deep neck infections): Ampicillin-sulbactam, piperacillin/tazobactam, imipenem/cilastatin, or ertapenem

For ANUG: Local debridement and lavage with oxidizing agents, chlorhexidine mouthwash, and the following oral antibiotics: metronidazole 500 mg PO or IV q8 hours *OR* amoxicillin/clavulanic acid 500 mg PO q8 hours *OR* ampicillin/sulbactam 1.5 g to 3 g IV q6 hours *OR* clindamycin, 450 mg PO q6 hours *OR* 600 mg IV q6 to q8 hours

Other Key Issues

When diagnosing a patient with ANUG, consider evaluating for sources of immunosuppression.

Suggested Readings and References

1. Christian JM. Odontogenic infections. In: Flint PW, Haughey BH, Lund VJ, et al., eds. *Cummings Otolaryngology—Head and Neck Surgery*. 5th ed. Philadelphia, Pa: Mosby; 2010.
2. Chow AW. Infections of the oral cavity, neck and head. In: Mandell GL, Bennett JE, Dolin R, eds. *Mandell, Douglas, and Bennett's Principles and Practice of Infectious Diseases*. 7th ed. Philadelphia, Pa: Mosby; 2010.
3. Gilbert DN, Moellering RC, Eliopoulos GM, HF Chambers, MS Saag, eds. *The Sanford Guide to Antimicrobial Therapy*. Sperryville, VA: Antimicrobial Therapy Inc.; 2010.
4. Rautemaa R, Lauhio A, Cullinan MP, et al. Oral infections and systemic disease—an emerging problem in medicine. *Clin Microbiol Infect*. 2007;13:1041–1047.
5. Shah RN, Cannon TY, Shores CG. Infections and disorders of the neck and upper airway. In: Tintinalli JE, Kelen GD, Stapczynski JS, eds. *Tintinalli's Emergency Medicine: A Comprehensive Study Guide*. 7th ed. New York, NY: McGraw-Hill Medical; 2011:Chapter 241. http://www.accessemergencymedicine.com/content.aspx?aID=6388487. Accessed October 19, 2012.
6. Shinn DL. Vincent's disease and its treatment. *Excerpta Medica*. 1977:307–308.

Chapter 14

Deep Space Infections of the Head and Neck

Gabrielle Jacquet

Summary Box

Disease Description: Infections in and around the airway, including the epiglottis, the parotid gland, and the retropharyngeal and parapharyngeal spaces

Organisms: Typically polymicrobial (most commonly *Streptococcus viridans* and *Streptococcus pyogenes*), including anaerobes (eg, *Bacteroides* and *Peptostreptococcus*)

Treatment:
  Parenteral: Clindamycin 600 mg to 900 mg IV (intravenous) *OR* ampicillin/sulbactam 3 g IV

Other Key Issues: These infections can extend into the airway and mediastinum, and their extent can be difficult to appreciate without imaging.

Disease Description

Epidemiology

In adults, deep space infections most commonly result from trauma, irradiation, surgical procedures, and human or animal bites. In children, they more commonly result from cervical adenitis and thyroiditis caused by bacteria or viruses.

Retropharyngeal abscesses (RPA) are most common in children 3 to 5 years old. The incidence of epiglottitis has significantly decreased in the pediatric population due to widespread vaccination against *Haemophilus influenza* type B, although cases due to other causative organisms (eg, *S. pneumoniae, S. pyogenes, Staphylococcus aureus,* and *Moraxella catarrhalis*) or due to lack of vaccination still occur. Cases can also be seen in adults (mean age 46 years). Due to the increasing size of the unvaccinated population, we may anticipate seeing more cases of epiglottitis due to *H. influenzae* type B. Parotitis affects primarily the elderly, the malnourished, the dehydrated, and postoperative patients.

Presenting Features

RPA commonly presents with sore throat (76%), fever (65%), torticollis (37%), dysphagia, neck pain, muffled "hot potato" voice, cervical lymphadenopathy, and respiratory distress. Cranial nerve IX, X, and XII deficits may also be seen. Epiglottitis symptoms classically include the triad of drooling, dysphagia, and distress but may include inspiratory stridor. Parotitis is recognized by a sudden firm, erythematous swelling of the preauricular and postauricular areas. This swelling extends to the angle of the mandible, which is often palpated as a blunted angle of the mandible on physical exam. Parotitis is often accompanied by exquisite local pain and tenderness. Signs of systemic toxicity include high fevers and chills.

Diagnostic Considerations

These infections can extend into airway and mediastinum, and their extent can be difficult to appreciate without imaging.

Typical Disease Course

Whereas epiglottitis presents rapidly and often compromises the airway, RPA generally progresses more slowly. However, RPA often requires surgical intervention for definitive treatment. Parotitis also typically requires surgical drainage, generally quite early. Spontaneous drainage is rare.

Complications

RPA can be complicated by upper airway asphyxia due to mass effect from the abscess, aspiration after sudden rupture of the abscess, and extension of the infection into the mediastinum (more common in adults). Airway obstruction and asphyxia can also occur in epiglottitis. Parotitis can yield massive neck swelling and secondary respiratory obstruction, septicemia, and osteomyelitis of the adjacent facial bones.

Diagnostic Tests

Deep Space Infection: Physical examination alone can misidentify the involved space and the number of involved spaces in 70% of cases. Contrast-enhanced computed tomography (CT) is a critical component in the evaluation of patients with suspected deep space infection.

Epiglottitis: Lateral plain radiograph of the neck may demonstrate a thickened epiglottis, which is often characterized as like a "thumb print" in appearance. Careful direct laryngoscopy may assist in diagnosis. CT of the neck is not needed to confirm the diagnosis. Patients should not be sent to the CT scanner without taking adequate airway precautions.

Organisms

RPA is usually polymicrobial, including anaerobes. *S. viridans* and *S. pyogenes* are the most commonly identified pathogens. Most isolated *Staphylococcus* species produce β-lactamase. The most commonly isolated anaerobes are *Bacteroides* and *Peptostreptococcus.*

Most cases of epiglottitis are caused by *Streptococcus* species, viruses, and fungi. Approximately 25% of cases are caused by *H. influenzae* type B.

Staphylococcus is the predominant isolate in parotitis, but *Enterobacteriaceae,* other gram-negative bacilli, and anaerobes have also been reported.

Treatment

Immediate airway management and otolaryngology consultation are required. Consider awake intubation. Most patients will require surgical intervention via transoral or transcervical incision and drainage in addition to IV fluid resuscitation and close observation.

First line antibiotic recommendations:

RPA: clindamycin 600 mg to 900 mg IV *OR* cefoxitin 2 g IV

Epiglottitis: ceftriaxone 2 g IV

Parotitis: an antistaphylococcal agent, such as nafcillin 2 g IV q4 hours *OR* vancomycin 1 g IV q12 hours AND metronidazole 0.5 g IV q6 hours *OR* clindamycin 600 mg IV q6 hours, plus early surgical drainage and decompression of the gland

Second line recommendations:

RPA: piperacillin-tazobactam *OR* ampicillin-sulbactam IV

Epiglottitis: clindamycin 600 mg to 900 mg IV *OR* ampicillin/sulbactam 3 g IV *OR* cefotaxime IV

Suggested Readings and References

1. Barksdale A. Neck and upper airway disorders. In: Cline DM, Ma OJ, Cydulka RK, Meckler GD, Handel DA, Thomas SH, eds. *Tintinalli's Emergency Medicine Manual*. 7th ed. New York, NY: McGraw-Hill Medical; 2012:Chapter 153. http://www.accessemergencymedicine.com/content.aspx?aID=56279797. Accessed October 19, 2012.

2. Fattahi TT, Lyu PE, Van Sickels JE. Management of acute suppurative parotitis. *J Oral Maxillofac Surg*. 2002;60:446–448.

3. Gilbert DN, RC Moellering Jr, GM Eliopoulos, HF Chambers, MS Saag, eds. *The Sanford Guide to Antimicrobial Therapy*. Sperryville, VA: Antimicrobial Therapy Inc.; 2010.

4. Herzon FS, Martin AD. Medical and surgical treatment of peritonsillar, retropharyngeal, and parapharyngeal abscesses. *Curr Infect Dis Rep*. 2006;8:196–202.

5. Shah RN, Cannon TY, Shores CG. Infections and disorders of the neck and upper airway. In: Tintinalli JE, Kelen GD, Stapczynski JS, eds. *Tintinalli's Emergency Medicine: A Comprehensive Study Guide*. 7th ed. New York, NY: McGraw-Hill Medical; 2011:Chapter 241. http://www.accessemergencymedicine.com/content.aspx?aID=6388487. Accessed October 19, 2012.

6. Shirley WP, Woolley AL, Wiatrak BJ. Pharyngitis and adenotonsillar disease. In Flint PW, Haughey BH, Lund VJ, et al., eds. *Cummings Otolaryngology—Head and Neck Surgery*. 5th ed. Philadelphia, PA: Mosby: 2010.

Ocular Infections

Periocular Infections

M. DeAugustinas, A Kiely

Conjunctivitis

Summary Box

Disease Description: Inflammation of the conjunctiva (inner lining of the eyelid and the ocular surface covering the sclera). More severe infections are notable for purulent discharge, membrane formation and scarring, and can lead to corneal change.

Organisms:
   Viral: Adenoviruses (most common) and Herpesviruses: Herpes simplex virus (HSV), Varicella Zoster virus (VZV), Epstein-Barr virus (EBV)
   Bacterial: *S. aureus, Streptococcus* spp. (multiple species), *H. influenza, C. trachomatis, Moraxella* spp.; *less commonly, N. Gonorrhea, P. aeruginosa*

Treatment:
   Viral: artificial tears, cold compresses, and hand hygiene
   Bacterial: broad spectrum topical antibiotic drop (Polymyxin B/ trimethoprim or a second generation fluoroquinolone) or ointment (erythromycin or ophthalmic bacitracin), 1 drop or ½ inch ribbon four times a day (QID) for 5 to 7 days
   Contact lens wearers: topical fourth or fifth generation fluoroquinolone (eg, moxifloxacin, besifloxacin) 1 drop (gtt) QID for 5 to 7 days*
   Severe bacterial (*N. Gonorrhea*): Ceftriaxone 1 g IV/IM single dose

Other Key Issues: Severe bacterial or Herpesvirus infections, as well as cases affecting vision (see following), warrant prompt ophthalmology consultation.

   *Drop concentration standardized to 1 gtt dosing.

Disease Description

Conjunctivitis refers to inflammation of the conjunctival lining, which covers the inner surface of the eyelids as well as the sclera. Presenting features include ocular surface injection due to hyperemia (often with tearing), mucoid or purulent discharge (rarely hemorrhagic), conjunctival follicles (discrete lymphoid nodules), papillae (nodules with vascular cores), membrane or pseudomembrane formation (fibrinous exudates), and associated keratitis (inflammation of the cornea). If conjunctivitis lasts beyond 4 weeks, it is termed "chronic."

Etiologies can be microbial (typically viral or bacterial—see "Organisms" following) or immune mediated (not discussed here). Beyond follicular conjunctivitis ("Pink Eye"), which is seen with many viruses, adenoviruses can additionally produce two distinct clinical syndromes: pharyngoconjunctival fever and epidemic keratoconjunctivitis. Pharyngoconjunctival fever presents with fever, headache, pharyngitis, preauricular lymphadenitis, and conjunctivitis. Epidemic keratoconjunctivitis includes chemosis (swelling of the conjunctiva); petechial hemorrhages; pseudo or true membrane* formation in fornices; and, ultimately, corneal erosions and subepithelial infiltrates.

Bacterial conjunctivitis is characterized by purulent discharge and can be categorized based on the severity and speed of onset. Mild to moderate disease arises over days to weeks, moderate to severe disease arises over hours to days, and severe or hyperacute disease arises in less than 24 hours. Hyperacute conjunctivitis results from sexual transmission of *Neisseria* spp., typically via genital-ocular spread. Rapid diagnosis is critical in such cases because hyperacute conjunctivitis can cause corneal infiltrates and corneal melting (in which proteases and collagenases from the infecting agent dissolve corneal stroma), leading to perforation in 15% to 40% of affected patients.

Other unique symptom constellations due to bacterial infections include trachoma and Parinaud's oculoglandular syndrome (POS). In trachoma, a severe follicular reaction to *C. trachomatis* leads to entropion (turning in of the eyelids so that the eye lashes rub against the ocular surface) and trichiasis (eyelashes that grow toward the eye, touching the cornea or conjunctiva), which induce conjunctival and corneal scarring. Trachoma is easily spread in ocular and nasal secretions via direct personal contact, flies, and shared laundry, such as towels and bedsheets. Spread tends to occur in communities with poor sanitation. POS is typically unilateral and is recognizable by its follicular, granulomatous conjunctival lesions as well as tender, ipsilateral preauricular and submandibular lymphadenopathy. Cat scratch fever (Bartonellosis) due to *B. henselae* is the most common etiology, but POS is actually an unusual feature of cat scratch fever. Additionally, POS is commonly the result of tularemia (*F. tularensis*) and sporotrichosis (*S. schenckii*). It occasionally presents in tuberculosis, syphilis, and coccidiodomycosis (*C. immitis*). Rarer etiologic agents also exist.

Diagnostic Tests

Diagnostic testing is not always indicated initially, although it can be useful for determining whether a patient is contagious and should be isolated in an inpatient setting or should take time away from work or school. Initial testing can be done with a forniceal swab (taken from the pocket between bulbar and palpebral conjunctiva) sent for viral, bacterial, and fungal culture. Given the wide range of species responsible for POS, the lab should be notified when there is suspicion for POS so that all of the proper stains and cultures can be performed.

Gram stain and cultures should always be performed in immunocompromised hosts such as neonates and immunocompromised adults, in severely purulent infections, and in those unresponsive to initial therapy.

Organisms

Infectious etiologies are most often viral and bacterial but can also be fungal or parasitic. The most common viruses include adenoviruses and the Herpesviruses HSV and VZV. Epstein Barr virus (associated with mononucleosis) is seen rarely. *Molluscum contagiosum*, measles virus, rubella virus, enterovirus, and coxsackie virus (acute hemorrhagic conjunctivitis) are seen even less often. In industrialized nations, HSV is a prominent cause of conjunctivitis; 40% to 80% of adults carry HSV-1, which is known to cause orofacial and ocular infections. Primary ocular HSV presents as a unilateral conjunctivitis,

---

* The exudate of a true membrane undergoes vascular invasion and is firmly adherent to the conjunctiva, resulting in tearing and bleeding of the conjunctival epithelium on removal. A pseudomembrane is a loosely adherent exudate that does not integrate into the conjunctival epithelium and does not undergo vascular invasion. Thus, it can be removed without bleeding and without disrupting the conjunctival epithelium.

sometimes in the setting of periocular/lid vesicles. These patients may also develop HSV keratitis, so patients with conjunctivitis and pain, foreign body sensation, photophobia, or vision changes should undergo careful slit lamp examination with fluorescein. Adenoviruses are transmitted by close contact with ocular or respiratory secretions, fomites, and even contaminated swimming pools. Different serotypes produce different syndromes. All serotypes continue shedding 10 to 14 days after the onset of symptoms.

Bacterial causes of conjunctivitis are also numerous. Mild to moderate bacterial disease that arises over days to weeks is typically caused by S. aureus, Moraxella, or Pseudomonas. Moderate to severe disease arising over hours to days is generally caused by H. influenza (often young children; can occasionally lead to preseptal cellulitis) or S. pneumonia. Severe, hyperacute (< 24 hours) disease is caused by N. gonorrhoreae or N. meningitides. Other causes include C. trachomatis and B. henselae, as previously discussed.

Treatment

Viral conjunctivitis is typically self-limited, so it can usually be managed with careful hand hygiene and lubrication of the eye with artificial tears. Within ophthalmology, some providers may recommend mild topical steroids to hasten recovery, but this should never be attempted before thorough slit lamp examination by an eye care provider. It should also be noted that topical steroids prolong virus shedding.

For suspected bacterial conjunctivitis, empiric therapy begins with broad-spectrum antibiotic eye drops (fluoroquinolone, polymyxin, or aminoglycoside) or ointment (macrolide, bacitracin) QID for 5 to 7 days; our practice favors moxifloxacin drops QID.

All drops are dosed 1 gtt per affected eye; all ointment is dosed as a ½ inch ribbon per affected eye.

Drops or ointment are supplemented with oral antibiotics in cases associated with pharyngitis and in children with H. influenza infection. For gonococcal conjunctivitis, systemic ceftriaxone is recommended for both adults and children (including neonates) due to the increasing prevalence of penicillin-resistant N. gonorrhoeae. If the cornea is not involved and the patient is extremely reliable, next day referral to an ophthalmologist in addition to management with IM ceftriaxone is sufficient. Otherwise, admission for IV therapy is advised. Copious, repeated irrigation is also advised to remove inflammatory mediators and debris that can contribute to corneal melting.

Other Key Issues

As a rule of thumb, the presence of purulent discharge, membrane formation, or bleeding in the fornices as well as vision loss or other symptoms of corneal or intraocular involvement—such as persistent foreign body sensation, severe pain, or photophobia—requires prompt ophthalmology consultation. Patients with a known history of HSV eye disease or immune compromise should also be referred.

Suggested Readings and References

1. American Academy of Ophthalmology Cornea/External Disease Panel. Preferred Practice Pattern® Guidelines. Conjunctivitis PPP 2013. San Francisco, CA: American Academy of Ophthalmology; 2013. www.aao.org/ppp.
2. Basic and clinical science course (BCSC) Section 8: External disease and cornea. San Francisco, CA: American Academy of Ophthalmology; 2011.
3. Centers for Disease Control and Prevention. Conjunctivitis (pink eye) for clinicians. 2014. http://www.cdc.gov/conjunctivitis/clinical.html Accessed August 9, 2014.

Canaliculitis

Summary Box

Disease Description: Inflammation of the lacrimal drainage apparatus marked by swelling, dilation, and erythema at or nasal to the punctum (orifice forming the entrance to the lacrimal ducts).

Organisms: Actinomyces israelii is most common

Treatment: Augmentin 875 mg q12 hours for 7 to 14 days

Other Key Issues: Canaliculotomy may need to be performed by an ophthalmologist for definitive long-term management.

Disease Description

Canaliculitis refers to inflammation of the lacrimal drainage apparatus in the eyelids. Presentation consists of often painful inflammation, persistent tearing, and occasionally follicular conjunctivitis at the medial canthus. Swelling, dilation, and erythema can often be seen at the punctum.

Diagnostic Tests

The canaliculus may be "milked" by applying pressure to the canaliculus with a cotton tip applicator; this is both therapeutic and diagnostic. If purulent material is expressed using this technique, the diagnosis is confirmed. Culture of purulent material should be obtained.

Organisms

The most common pathogen is *Actinomyces israelii*, a gram-positive rod.

Treatment

Treatment can often be lengthy and requires several steps. Initial conservative management involves digital massage (milking) of the canaliculus, removal of foreign matter, warm compresses, and topical antibiotic therapy.

Broad-spectrum oral antibiotics (Augmentin 875 mg PO q12 hours for 7 to 14 days) should initially be used prior to culture sensitivity results. More aggressive therapy is often necessary, especially with the formation of dacryoliths (lacrimal calculi), which are most common in *Actinomyces* infections. Dacryoliths can block the canaliculi, resulting in obstruction and secondary infection. Additionally, they can harbor the organism responsible for the infection, making them a nidus for persistent infection without proper treatment. Thus, surgical management is frequently required. Curettage through the punctum can be attempted, but canaliculotomy by an ophthalmologist is often necessary for removal of all concretions.

Other Key Issues

An ophthalmologist should rule out obstruction as a cause of canaliculitis.

Dacryocystitis

Summary Box

Disease Description: Inflammation of the lacrimal sac, usually due to obstruction. Dacryocystitis presents with edema, erythema, and distension of the lacrimal sac.

Organisms: Gram-positives in immunocompetent, gram-negatives in immunocompromised and diabetic individuals

Treatment: Oral First line: Augmentin 875 mg PO (oral administration) q12 hours for 7 to 14 days
   Parenteral: Ceftriaxone 1 g/day

Other Key Issues: Dacryocystitis may lead to orbital cellulitis, necessitating hospitalization and parenteral treatment. Consider referral, especially in pediatric patients, to rule out obstruction.

Disease Description

Dacryocystitis is inflammation of the lacrimal sac. The most common etiology is nasolacrimal duct obstruction, which causes chronic retention and stasis of tears and mucus in the nasolacrimal duct, followed by secondary infection. Patients with dacryocystitis typically present with edema, erythema, and distension of the lacrimal sac, which creates a red, tender mass inferomedially to the medial canthus. The punctum and canaliculus are normal, in contrast to canaliculitis. The pain patients experience is highly variable and ranges from absent to severe.

Diagnostic Tests

If a pyocele or mucocele is near the skin, aspiration can be performed and sent for culture.

Organism

The majority of infections are caused by gram-positive bacteria. Gram-negative bacteria should be suspected in patients who are immunocompromised, diabetic, or exposed to atypical organisms (eg, health care workers, nursing care centers).

Treatment

Oral antibiotics (eg, Augmentin 875 mg PO q12 hours) are effective in the majority of cases, although parenteral antibiotics (eg, ceftriaxone 1 g/day) should be considered in severe cases involving cellulitis or orbital inflammation.

Antibiotic therapy should be attempted before progressing to surgical management. If an abscess in the lacrimal sac involves adjacent tissues, management should include incision and drainage (I&D). After I&D, packing should be placed, and the wound should be allowed to heal by secondary intention.

Referral to an ophthalmologist is recommended regardless of initial therapy, as total nasolacrimal duct obstructions may require surgical intervention to prevent recurrence of infection, persistent tearing, and fistula formation.

Other Key Issues

Dacryocystitis may develop into chronic conjunctivitis or spread into adjoining structures, leading to orbital or facial cellulitis.

Approximately 50% of infants will have obstruction of the nasolacrimal duct at birth. This obstruction resolves spontaneously in the vast majority of infants within 6 weeks, and only 5% of full-term infants have clinically evident obstruction at 4 weeks of age (estimates range from 2% to 6%). Within 1 year of life, 90% of congenital nasolacrimal duct obstructions will clear spontaneously. Pediatric presentation is similar to that of adult nasolacrimal duct obstruction and involves unilateral or (in one-third of cases) bilateral tearing and mucoid discharge at the punctum. Active inflammation due to secondary infection may be present and should be treated with antibiotic therapy just as in adults. These pediatric patients should be referred to an ophthalmologist for follow-up and definitive management.

Suggested Readings and References

4. Basic and clinical science course (BCSC) Section 7: Orbit, eyelids, and lacrimal system. San Francisco, CA: American Academy of Ophthalmology; 2011.
5. Basic and clinical science course (BCSC) Section 8: External disease and cornea. San Francisco, CA: American Academy of Ophthalmology; 2011.
6. Tasman W, et al. *Foundations of Clinical Ophthalmology.* Volume 4. Philadelphia, PA: Harper & Row Publishers, Inc.; 2006:chapter 4.

Infectious Keratitis

M. DeAugustinas, A Kiely

Summary Box

Disease Description: Corneal opacity or ulceration with eye pain, foreign body sensation, redness, discharge, blurred vision, and/or photophobia.

Most Common Organisms:
  Viral: Herpes simplex virus
  Bacterial: Gram-positive cocci (*S. aureus, S. epidermidis, S. pneumoniae*) and gram-negative rods (*P. aeruginosa, Moraxella* spp.)
  Other: Fungal (*Aspergillus* spp., *C. albicans*), parasitic (*Acanthamoeba*)

Treatment:
  Viral first line: Valacyclovir 1 g PO TID for 7 days
  Bacterial first line: Fluoroquinolone drops (eg, moxifloxacin, ciprofloxacin, ofloxacin) 1 drops q30 minutes while awake, awaken 4 and 6 hours after retiring and instill 1 gtt. For severe or centrally located infiltrates, a loading dose (1 drop q5 to 15 minutes for 30 to 60 minutes) and around-the-clock initial therapy is advised.
  Patient will require reexamination by an ophthalmologist every 1 to 2 days to determine further dosing and duration.
  Other: Organism specific—consult ophthalmology

Other Key Issues: Same day ophthalmology consult/referral is mandatory, as more aggressive infections can cause corneal perforation.

Disease Description

Epidemiology

Keratitis is an inflammation of the cornea, which can result from a variety of causes and can lead to corneal opacification or ulceration. The annual incidence of infectious keratitis in the United States is approximately 11 per 100,000 per year. The majority of these cases occur in patients with corneal risk factors, such as contact lens wearers (relative risk of six) and those with a history of eye trauma or surgery, ocular surface disease, ocular anatomic abnormalities, systemic infection, or immune compromise.

The most common cause of infectious keratitis is herpes simplex virus type 1 (HSV-1). Approximately 20% of trigeminal nerve-distribution HSV or Varicella zoster (VZV) reactivations will involve the eye, for a total of more than 48,000 cases annually. However, the most common organisms identified by culture in cases of microbial keratitis are bacteria, with 25,000 to 30,000 cases of bacterial keratitis diagnosed each year in the United States.

Specific exposures are associated with particular infectious etiologies (see Table 16.1 for risk factors predisposing patients to bacterial keratitis). Soft or extended-wear contact lens use is a risk factor for *Pseudomonas aeruginosa* and other bacterial infections. Fresh-water swimming, bathing, or hot-tub use while wearing contact lenses can lead to parasitic *Acanthamoeba* infection, and trauma with plant matter is a known source of fungal infection.

Finally, noninfectious corneal infiltrates related to trauma, collagen vascular disease, autoimmune inflammation, vasculitis, or atopy (which predisposes to HSV keratitis) must be considered in any differential diagnosis of corneal inflammation.

Presenting Features

Infectious keratitis may present with eye pain, foreign body sensation, redness, mucopurulent discharge, blurred vision, and/or photophobia. Corneal opacity or ulceration is characteristic. Most patients will describe risk factors (like those previously mentioned) that correlate temporally with symptom onset, but detailed inquiry may be required to elicit relevant history for indolent infections (eg, fungal keratitis).

Diagnostic Considerations

Diagnosis and management of microbial keratitis requires consulting an ophthalmologist because keratitis has the potential to cause severe vision loss. Given the risk of a perforating injury, diagnostic procedures that involve manipulation of the cornea should be performed by an ophthalmologist.

Table 16.1 Risk Factors Predisposing Patients to Bacterial Keratitis

Extrinsic Factors	*Corneal Epithelial Abnormalities*
Use of contact lenses	Neurotrophic keratopathy (eg, trigeminal neuropathy)
Overnight wear	Recurrent erosion of the cornea
Overwear	Corneal abrasion or epithelial defect
Inadequate disinfection	Viral keratitis
Contamination of storage case	Corneal epithelial edema
Ineffective/contaminated solution	*Systemic Conditions*
Storage/rinsing in tap water	Diabetes mellitus
Sharing of lenses	Malnourishment
Trauma	Chronic assisted ventilation
Prior ocular or eyelid surgery	Connective tissue disease
Loose corneal sutures	Dermatologic/mucous membrane disorders
Medication-related immunosuppression	Immunocompromised status
Substance abuse (crack cocaine)	Atopic dermatitis
Abuse of topical anesthetic drops	Blepharoconjunctivitis
Ocular Surface disease	Gonococcal conjunctivitis
Tear-film deficiencies	Vitamin A deficiency
Abnormal eyelid anatomy and function	Neurologic lesion (damage to 5th and/or 7th cranial nerves)
Misdirection of eyelashes	Graft-versus-host disease
Adjacent infection/inflammation	Diphtheria

Typical Disease Course

The progression of infectious keratitis varies with the infecting organism but can be quite rapid. Prompt diagnosis and intervention, including prompt consultation with ophthalmology, is key to prevent vision loss and even loss of the eye. Examples of organisms capable of rapid tissue destruction are *Pseudomonas* spp., *Streptococcus pneumonia*, and *Neisseria gonorrheae*, which have the ability to invade intact cornea. Central or paracentral lesions affecting the visual axis are treated aggressively regardless of the organism to minimize corneal scarring.

Complications

Infectious keratitis can lead to visual compromise in a number of ways. The most common is corneal scarring, which can impair vision by obstructing the visual axis or by inducing irregular astigmatism. Untreated keratitis produces ulcers that can progress to corneal melting, in which proteases and collagenases from the infecting agent dissolve corneal stroma. If untreated, corneal melting can lead to corneal perforation and endophthalmitis (see Chapter 17: "Endophthalmitis"). Even in cases that do not progress to endophthalmitis, chronic intraocular inflammation can cause anatomic changes that affect vision.

Diagnostic Tests

Physical examination, including accurate visual acuity measurement, external examination, and slit lamp exam are essential. Intraocular pressure can safely be measured with a tonometer if no significant corneal thinning is noted on slit lamp exam, but this may also be deferred to ophthalmology if consultation is prompt. Pain and photophobia may limit examination; once corneal sensation has been assessed, it is appropriate to use a topical anesthetic (proparacaine or tetracaine) to facilitate the exam. Important findings include lagophthalmos (inability to close the eyelids completely); eyelash abnormalities, such as trichiasis (eyelashes that grow toward the eye and touch the cornea or conjunctiva); foreign bodies; surgical changes such as filtering blebs (subconjunctival aqueous humor collections secondary to a glaucoma procedure) or LASIK flaps; purulent discharge; hypopyon or anterior chamber inflammation; corneal epithelial defects; dendritiform lesions; and corneal opacities. An infiltrate appears as an opacity in the cornea, whereas an ulcer additionally includes stromal loss with an overlying epithelial defect that stains with fluorescein.

Infiltrates and ulcers can be distinguished from stromal edema or scars by the presence of opacity. Using an offset slit beam, an examiner cannot see through an infiltrate or an ulcer to the iris beneath, but the examiner can visualize the iris in the case of edema or scarring. In general, viral epithelial keratitis presents with branching corneal staining patterns known as "dendrites," whereas bacterial infiltrates tend to be well circumscribed. The borders of fungal infiltrates are "feathery" with satellite lesions, and *Acanthamoeba* infections typically present as a ring-shaped infiltrate. It should be noted that viral infections, particularly HSV and VZV, may predispose to superinfection with other pathogens.

Although the majority of community-acquired keratitis can be managed empirically, further diagnostic testing is indicated when the corneal infiltrate is large, central, or penetrates deeply into the corneal stroma. Further testing is also indicated in chronic or refractory cases of keratitis and in those cases with features suggestive of fungal, amoebic, or mycobacterial infection. This testing includes corneal smears and cultures, perhaps supported by conjunctival culture in cases of acute, purulent keratoconjunctivitis suspicious for gonococcal infection. Given the risk of corneal perforation, sample collection from the cornea should generally be attempted only by an ophthalmologist. Infectious material may be obtained using a sterile spatula, forceps, a sterile cotton, or calcium alginate swab. Standard culture plates should include blood agar, chocolate agar, Sabouraud dextrose agar, and thioglycolate broth. If the patient is a contact lens wearer, the lenses and case should be cultured as well.

Organisms

The most common infectious cause of keratitis is HSV-1. Other viral causes include VZV and, less commonly, Epstein-Barr virus and adenovirus. Bacterial keratitis is most often due to gram-positive cocci, specifically *Staphylococcus* spp., and gram-negative rods.

Other culprits include fungi (both yeast and molds, accounting for approximately 1,500 cases per year), typically *Fusarium, Aspergillus spp., or Candida spp.* Parasites (eg, *Acanthamoeba*) and nematodes (eg, *Onchocerca*) represent additional causes; *Acanthamoeba* trophozoites encyst within the cornea, often resulting in persistent or recurrent infection, whereas *Onchocerca volvulus* microfilariae live primarily in skin and migrate to the cornea from the conjunctiva.

Treatment

Topical antibiotic drops achieve high tissue concentrations and are the treatment of choice in most cases of keratitis. Empiric coverage should be prescribed regardless of suspected etiology and tailored later only under the care of an ophthalmologist. Adding ophthalmic ointment (eg, erythromycin or bacitracin) can improve patient comfort in the setting of an epithelial defect. The choice of therapy and dosing schedule may be considered according to this algorithm, which reflects the current practices of Johns Hopkins Ophthalmology:

- For small (≤ 1.0 mm) peripheral infiltrates with no ulceration, risk of visual loss is low, and frequent (q1 to 2 hours) broad-spectrum topical antibiotics (eg, fluoroquinolones or cefazolin PLUS tobramycin or gentamycin) are appropriate for initial therapy. Moxifloxacin has better gram-positive coverage, while gatifloxacin and ciprofloxacin have better *Pseudomonas* and *Serratia* coverage. In contact lens wearers, consider adding tobramycin or ciprofloxacin ophthalmic ointment four times a day.
- Medium (1.0–1.5 m) peripheral infiltrates or smaller ulcers should be treated with even more frequent dosing: q1 hour around the clock for at least the first 24 hours using the same regimen.
- Vision threatening ulcers (larger than 1–2 mm, in the visual axis, or unresponsive to initial therapy) require fortified antibiotics, which must be compounded in a pharmacy equipped for their preparation. We typically begin with fortified tobramycin (14 mg/mL; gentamycin 1 gtt of 14 mg/mL can also be used) 1 gtt q1 hour plus vancomycin (25 mg/mL; cefazolin 50 mg/mL can also be used) 1 gtt q1 hour around the clock for at least the first 24 hours. It is worth considering a loading dose by administering 1 drop every 5 to 15 minutes for 30 to 60 minutes before starting q1 hour dosing.
- Viral keratitis without superinfection can be managed with topical 1% trifluridine eight times per day, although we preferentially prescribe oral antiviral therapy with valacyclovir 1g TID (better ocular penetration) or acyclovir 800 mg five times daily instead, which avoids the epithelial toxicity associated with topical antivirals. One can also consider ganciclovir ointment five times daily, although this relatively new therapy has not been compared with trifluridine or oral therapy in any large, randomized, controlled study.
- Optimal topical therapy for fungal keratitis is a topic of debate in the ophthalmology community. Common first line agents have included topical natamycin and amphoteracin B, but triazoles, such as voriconazole and posaconazole, are gaining popularity. Antifungal therapy is only initiated by ophthalmology once filamentous organisms are identified in culture.

Other keys to effective treatment include discontinuing contact lens use and protecting the eye with a rigid shield *without* a patch, as patching provides a reservoir for infection. Cycloplegia with atropine 1 gtt daily to BID (twice daily), homatropine 1 gtt BID, or cyclopentolate 1 gtt TID improves photophobia and can decrease pain. Oral pain medication (anti-inflammatory drugs or narcotics in select cases) can also offer relief. Oral antibiotic therapy with fluoroquinolones (or third-generation cephalosporins) may benefit patients concerning for impending perforation.

Follow-up with ophthalmology should occur daily until the corneal epithelium heals and it is clear that the infiltrate is decreasing in size and density. Ophthalmology can then direct slow tapering of antibiotic therapy as indicated. Hospital admission may be indicated for imminently vision-threatening infections, concerns about patient adherence to therapy or follow-up, suspected topical anesthetic misuse or abuse, or need for systemic antibiotics.

Use of topical corticosteroids to minimize corneal inflammation and scarring once an acute infection is controlled remains controversial in the ophthalmology community and should never be initiated by non-ophthalmologists. In particular, topical steroids are recommended in stromal keratitis caused by HSV infection but must be used with great care.

Other Key Issues

HSV-associated stromal keratitis is the most common cause of infectious corneal blindness in the United States, yet its presentation can be fairly subtle. Stromal haze can be mistaken for a scar by an inexperienced observer, as there are no overlying epithelial defects. For this reason, symptoms out of proportion to exam findings or a history concerning for viral infection is an indication for prompt referral to ophthalmology.

Suggested Readings and References

1. American Academy of Ophthalmology Cornea/External Disease Panel. Preferred Practice Pattern®Guidelines. *Bacterial keratitis*. San Francisco, CA: American Academy of Ophthalmology; 2013. www.aao.org/ppp
2. Basic and clinical science course (BCSC) Section 8: *External disease and cornea*. San Francisco, CA: American Academy of Ophthalmology; 2011.
3. FlorCruz NV, Peczon IV. Medical interventions for fungal keratitis. *Cochrane Database of Systematic Reviews*. 2008:Issue 1.
4. Gerstenblith AT, Rabinowitz MP. *The Wills Eye Manual: Office and Emergency Room Diagnosis and Treatment of Eye Disease*. 6th ed. Philadelphia, PA: Wolters Kluwer/Lippincott Williams & Wilkins; 2012.
5. Suwan-apichon O, Reyes JMG, Herretes S, Vedula SS, Chuck RS. Topical corticosteroids as adjunctive therapy for bacterial keratitis. *Cochrane Database of Systematic Reviews*. 2007:Issue 4.

Endophthalmitis

M. DeAugustinas, A Kiely

Summary Box

Disease Description: Inflammation of the interior structures of the eye, by definition involving both anterior (aqueous) and posterior (vitreous) chambers, typically with severe injection, corneal edema (clouding), hypopyon (layered pus in the anterior chamber), and eyelid edema.

Organisms:

Traumatic: *Bacillus cereus*, gram-negative bacteria

Post-op acute: Coagulase-negative *Staphylococcus, S. aureus, Streptococcus* spp., and gram-negatives

Post-op chronic: *P. acnes*, coagulase-negative *Staphylococcus, Corynebacterium*, and fungi

Endogenous: *Candida* in fungal infection; *Streptococcus* spp. in endocarditis, *Bacillus* in IV drug users

Treatment: Prompt intravitreal injection of antibiotics by an ophthalmologist. Systemic therapy only in in endogenous infections, continuing until cultures clear. Third-generation PO fluoroquinolones and azoles give good ocular penetration; IV amphotericin or caspofungin should be used in severe fungal cases.

Other Key Issues: This is an ophthalmic emergency. Same day ophthalmology consult/referral is mandatory. Vision is threatened over the course of hours.

Disease Description

Epidemiology

Endophthalmitis refers to inflammation of both the anterior and posterior intraocular chambers and their structures. This vision-threatening condition occurs in three principal scenarios (listed in order of decreasing incidence): penetrating ocular trauma, after intraocular surgery, and in systemically infected (often immunocompromised) patients.

In penetrating trauma, the incidence of endophthalmitis is 2% to 7%, higher in cases where an intra-ocular foreign body (IOFB) is present.

Post-operative endophthalmitis occurs in only 0.07% to 0.1% of ophthalmic surgery patients and can be divided into three categories: acute-onset (within 6 weeks of intraocular surgery), chronic or delayed-onset (greater than 6 weeks from surgery, typically cataract extraction), and bleb-associated (months or even years after filtering surgery for glaucoma). Typically, when it occurs, endophthalmitis is an acute event occurring after surgery or injury, but it is important not to miss chronic endophthalmitis, particularly because bleb-associated infections can be even more virulent and vision-threatening than other types of post-operative endophthalmitis.

Endogenous infections occur when systemically infected patients seed the eye with circulating infectious material. Endogenous infections are rare, accounting for only 10% of all cases, but can be devastating, particularly in the setting of immune compromise.

Presenting Features

Endophthalmitis presents with marked intraocular inflammation (characterized by severe injection, corneal edema, and eyelid edema), often with hypopyon. Patients report pain and significant vision loss out of proportion to typical post-operative complaints.

Diagnostic Considerations

Critical historical elements include a comprehensive, detailed history of any ocular surgery (particularly glaucoma surgery), including the date and nature of the surgery. An accurate measurement of visual acuity can also be very important, as this can change management under certain circumstances (see "Treatment" following).

Diagnostic Tests

Ophthalmologic screening should include accurate visual acuity measurements. Physical exam will often reveal hypopyon, corneal clouding, and sometimes leukocoria. One should lift the upper eyelid to look for a purulent bleb, which will appear as an elevation of the conjunctiva with purulent material inside. Slit lamp findings can include a characteristic peripheral white plaque within the lens capsule in the case of *P. acnes* infection.

It is recommended that all patients with candidemia have a baseline fundoscopic examination, ideally within 72 hours of diagnosis, as ocular involvement can occur early and may be asymptomatic or cause only painless "floaters." Ocular involvement in candidemia increases to up to 37% of patients without appropriate systemic therapy. A repeat fundoscopic examination is recommended 2 weeks after the initial examination.

Diagnosis requires culturing intraocular contents (aqueous humor from the anterior chamber or a vitreous biopsy). A diagnosis of endophthalmitis without a clear cause (eg, a history of trauma or surgery) should prompt a systemic workup, as one can find an extraocular disease focus in 90% of endogenous cases.

Organisms

Microbiology

Cultured organisms in cases of endophthalmitis vary depending on the circumstances of the infection.

- Acute-onset, post-operative endophthalmitis is typically caused by coagulase-negative *Staphylococcus*, *S. aureus*, *Streptococcus* spp., or gram-negative organisms.
- Chronic/delayed-onset cases include infections with *Propionibacterium acnes*, coagulase-negative *Staphylococcus*, *Corynebacterium* spp., and fungi. Bleb-associated infections are more often caused by *Streptococcus* spp., *Haemophilus* spp., and gram-positive organisms.
- Twenty-five percent of traumatic endophthalmitis (particularly with a contaminated intraocular foreign body) is attributable to *Bacillus cereus*, which is rarely seen in other ocular infections and can

progress rapidly to vision loss and, often, loss of the eye. In animal models, *Bacillus* exotoxin can extinguish visual function within 12 hours. Other causes of traumatic endophthalmitis include gram-negative organisms.

- Endogenous bacterial endophthalmitis is most commonly seen with bacteremia caused by endocarditis, meningitis, and both gastrointestinal and urinary tract infections. It can be caused by a variety of species: *Staphylococcus* spp., *Streptococcus* spp. in endocarditis, *Bacillus* in IV drug users, Serratia, and gram-negatives (including *N. meningitides, H. influenzae, E. coli* and *Klebsiella*).
- Endogenous fungal endophthalmitis is typically caused by *Candida* (most common), *Aspergillus* spp., *Cryptococcus neoformans*, or rarely *Coccidiodes* spp. and is associated with indwelling catheters, chronic antibiotic use, hyperalimentation, gastrointestinal surgery (consider *Aspergillus* after orthotopic liver transplant), and immunosuppression (including diabetes).

Treatment

Treatment typically involves the administration of intravitreal antibiotics. However, a bleb infection that has not yet evolved to endophthalmitis ("blebitis") can initially be managed with aggressive topical antibiotics. In the case of trauma, prompt removal of any IOFB and wound closure reduce the risk of developing endophthalmitis. As rapid diagnosis and treatment are essential for preserving vision, suspected cases of endophthalmitis should be referred emergently to ophthalmology (same day).

The Endophthalmitis Vitrectomy Study (EVS) demonstrated that if visual acuity has dropped to only the perception of light, patients with acute-onset, post-operative endophthalmitis fair better with vitrectomy surgery than with vitreous biopsy and antibiotic injection alone. Patients with the perception of hand motions or better had equivalent outcomes with either intervention. This study also suggested that there is no role for intravenous antibiotics in post-operative cases.

Endogenous endophthalmitis, on the other hand, clearly warrants systemic therapy. Although prompt ophthalmologic consult is necessary in endogenous endophthalmitis, less severe bacterial and fungal cases may resolve with systemic therapy alone. Third-generation oral fluoroquinolones and azoles show particularly good ocular penetration and may be considered for empiric treatment while waiting for ophthalmology. Severe fungal cases may require IV amphotericin or caspofungin.

Suggested Readings and References

1. Basic and clinical science course (BCSC) Section 9: *Intraocular inflammation and uveitis*. San Francisco, CA: American Academy of Ophthalmology; 2011.
2. Basic and clinical science course (BCSC) Section 12: *Retina vitreous*. San Francisco, CA: American Academy of Ophthalmology; 2011.
3. Endophthalmitis Vitrectomy Study Group. Results of the Endophthalmitis Vitrectomy Study: a randomized trial of immediate vitrectomy and of intravenous antibiotics for the treatment of postoperative bacterial endophthalmitis. *Arch Ophthalmol*. 1995;113:1479–1496.

Section VI

Cardiovascular Infections

Infective Endocarditis

Ajar Kocher

Summary Box

Disease Description: Infective endocarditis (IE) is an infection of the heart's innermost layer, the endothelium, leading to an all-cause mortality of 20% to 30%. Fever and a new murmur are the most prominent clinical findings. The most common predisposing condition is mitral valve prolapse, implicated in 70% to 75% of cases of IE.

Organism: *Streptococci* and *Staphylococci* cause 80% of IE cases.

Diagnosis: Blood cultures and echocardiograms are critical for IE diagnosis. Transesophageal echocardiogram (TEE) is the preferred diagnostic tool for prosthetic valve endocarditis and Cardiovascular Implantable Electronic Devices (CIED) infections.

Treatment: Acute native valve endocarditis (NVE) should be treated with vancomycin (15 mg/kg IV q12 hours) and gentamicin (1 mg/kg IV or IM q8 hours). Subacute NVE should be treated with ceftriaxone (2 g IV or IM every 24 hours) and gentamicin. Prosthetic valve endocarditis (PVE) should be treated with vancomycin, cefepime (1-2 gm IV q 12 hours), and gentamicin. Antibiotic duration is most often 4 to 6 weeks from the first day of negative cultures.

Other Key Issues:

IE complicated by heart failure and cerebral emboli has a high rate of morbidity and mortality.

Large vegetations, mobile lesions, mitral valve vegetations, and infection by *S. aureus* and fungi are more likely to result in embolic phenomena.

Indications for surgery include severe heart failure, persistent infection, fungal infection, heart block, and abscess formation.

Disease Description

Epidemiology

IE is an infection of the heart's innermost layer, the endothelium. Most cases require a predisposing injury to the endocardium to serve as a nidus for thrombus development, which in turn acts as nidus for bloodstream microorganisms.[1] These intravascular microorganisms can result from dental and other invasive procedures, infected vascular catheters, and skin lesions. However, most episodes of IE result from transient bacteremia during menial tasks such as chewing and brushing one's teeth.[1] The most common predisposing condition for IE is mitral valve prolapse, which is implicated in 70% to 75% of cases of IE.[2] Other risk factors include rheumatic heart disease, bicuspid aortic valve, congenital heart disease, prosthetic heart valves, immunocompromise, intravenous drug use (IVDU), presence of a pacemaker or an implantable cardioverter defibrillator, and hemodialysis.[3]

Although the total number of annual cases of infective endocarditic have remained stable for the past 30 years, there has been a shift in the typical patient profile. In the current era, there are more elderly patients, intravenous drug users, and prosthetic valve patients with IE.[1] The mortality of all causes of IE is 20% to 30%.[4] Factors associated with poor prognosis include the following: heart failure, aortic valve involvement, prosthetic valve, advanced age, abscess formation, human immunodeficiency virus with CD4 count < 200, embolic complications, comorbidities, and *Staphylococcus* infection.[3]

Diagnosis

As the presentation of IE is so diverse, it is imperative that physicians adopt a high index of suspicion. To facilitate the diagnosis, the Duke criteria (see Tables 18.1 and 18.2) were developed in 1994 and later modified in 2000.[5] There are both major and minor criteria; definite clinical diagnosis occurs with two

Table 18.1 Duke Criteria[a]

Major Criteria	Minor Criteria
Positive blood cultures for microorganisms typical for IE in 2 separate cultures	Fever 38°C
Persistently positive blood cultures for microorganisms typical for IE at least 12 hours apart or at least three cultures positive with at least 1 hour in between cultures.	Predisposing condition (heart condition or history of intravenous drug use)
A single positive blood culture for Coxiella burnetii (or anti-phase 1 IgG antibody titer greater than 1:800)	**Vascular phenomena** • Major arterial embolus • Septic pulmonary infarct • Mycotic aneurysm • Intracranial hemorrhage • Conjunctival hemorrhages • Janeway lesions
Evidence of endocardial involvement (Positive echocardiogram) • Oscillating intracardiac mass on valve or supporting structures, in the path of regurgitant jets, or on implanted material, in the absence of an alternative explanation • Abscess • New partial dehiscence of prosthetic valve • New valvular regurgitation (increase or change in preexisting murmur not sufficient)	**Immunologic phenomenon** • Glomerulonephritis • Osler nodes • Roth spots • Rheumatoid factor
	• Positive blood culture, but does not meet major criterion or provide serologic evidence of active infection with organisms consistent with IE

Abbreviations: IE, infective endocarditis; IgG, immunoglobulin G.

[a]Typical microorganisms are considered to be *viridans streptococci, S. bovis, S. aureus, enterococci* (without a primary focus), and HACEK organisms (*Haemophilus* spp., *Actinobacillus actinomycetemcomitans, Cardiobacterium hominis, Eikenella corrodens*, and *Kingella* spp. (adapted from *Circulation*, June 2005).

Table 18.2 Definitive or Possible IE

Definitive IE	Possible IE
2 major criteria	1 major criterion and 1 minor criterion
1 major criteria + 3 minor criteria	3 minor criteria
5 minor criteria	
Pathological lesions present: vegetation or abscess (intracardiac or embolized) confirmed by histology or culture	

Abbreviation: IE, infective endocarditis.

major criteria, one major and three minor, or five minor criteria. Possible clinical diagnosis results from one major and one minor criterion or three minor criteria.[5]

Clinical Context of IE

Prosthetic Valve: PVE is divided into early PVE, which occurs within the first 60 days of surgery and late PVE beyond the first 60 days. Early PVE tends to be due to an intraoperative or nosocomial complication, so the most common pathogens include coagulase-negative *Staphylococcus* (CoNS) and *S. aureus*.[2] There is no significant difference in incidence and severity between mechanical and bioprosthetic valves, nor is there a difference between mitral and aortic valves.[2]

Intravenous drug use: The median age of IVDU patients is 30 to 40 years, and the most commonly infected valves are the tricuspid valve (> 50%) and the aortic valve (25%).[6] The culprit pathogens of IVDU-associated IE include *S. aureus, P. aeruginosa,* and fungi.[7]

CIED: Risk factors for CIED infections include pocket size, device type, number of leads, revision or replacement of device, and renal insufficiency. The most common pathogens are *S. aureus* and CoNS.[8]

Diagnosis

The manifestations of IE are highly variable based on the infecting microorganism, affected valve, predisposing condition, and time course (acute vs. subacute).

Physical Exam: Fever is the most common finding in IE.[3] New regurgitant murmurs, in the correct clinical context, are highly suggestive of IE. Murmurs may be absent with tricuspid involvement and with infected CIED. Signs of heart failure occur in approximately 50% of IE patients.[9] Furthermore, a comprehensive neurological exam must be completed on every patient with IE to evaluate for cerebral emboli. Formal fundoscopic examinations should be performed looking for Roth spots, chorioretinitis, and endophthalmitis. IE may also present with immune-complex phenomena such as Osler nodes (painful, raised red lesions on the hands and feet). Exam manifestations of embolic phenomena include petechiae on buccal and conjunctival mucosa, splinter hemorrhages, and splenomegaly.[2] The etiology of Janeway lesions (nontender macular lesion on palms and soles) is unclear. One theory is that they are also embolic phenomena; another is that they are necrotic microabscesses confined to the dermis.

Laboratory evaluation: Several abnormalities may be present, such as leukocytosis, anemia, elevated erythrocyte sedimentation rate or C-reactive protein, positive rheumatoid factor, and a false positive venereal disease research laboratory test or Lyme antibody.[1] Urinalysis should be evaluated for hematuria and casts secondary to glomerulonephritis. Blood cultures are imperative for diagnosis and treatment. Prior to the initiation of antibiotics, three sets of blood cultures should be obtained from three different venipuncture sites, 30 minutes apart.[2] For the main causative agents, the first two blood cultures will be in 90% of cases and must be repeated after the initiation of antibiotics to assess treatment efficacy.[1]

Electrocardiogram evaluation: Clinicians must pay attention to conduction abnormalities, such as new atrioventricular conduction slowing (ie, PR prolongation), which is a poor prognostic sign suggestive of a myocardial abscess undergoing transmural spread across the aortic root.[3] Similarly, new fascicular and bundle branch blocks in the setting of IE may indicate an infection that has spread to previously healthy fascicles or bundle branches.

Echocardiography: Ultrasonography can identify vegetations; characterize the lesions by size and mobility; and discover complications such as abscesses, fistulae, and the extent of valvular dysfunction.[2] Transthoracic echocardiogram has low sensitivity of 29% to 63% but high specificity (close to 100%). TEEs are better studies to assess prosthetic valve endocarditis, CIED infections, posterior structures, fistulae, leaflet perforation, paravalvular leaks, and abscesses.[10]

Left Heart Catheterization: Cardiac catheterization is required prior to operative management of IE to assess for concurrent coronary artery disease and the need for coronary artery bypass grafting.

Organisms

Streptococcal and Staphylococcal organisms cause 80% of IE cases.[1] *S. Auerus* is associated with higher complication rates, more embolic phenomena, and increased mortality. *S. Auerus* is also the most common cause of IE in injection drug users, diabetics, tricuspid IE, and nosocomial IE.[1] *S. lugdunensis* usually requires surgical intervention because it preferentially attaches to native valves and is associated with abscess formation and valve destruction.[11] *Streptococcus anginosus* tends to form abscesses and spread via the blood stream to other organ systems, thus requiring a longer antibiotic course. *Pseudomonas aeruginosa* carries a high fatality rate and usually mandates surgical management.[3] Fungi (*Candida, Aspergillus,* and *Histoplasma* spp.) are associated with prosthetic valves, indwelling intravascular hardware, immunosuppression, and IVDU. Fungal vegetations are often large and thus pose a higher risk of embolic complications.[3]

Culture Negative Infective Endocarditis (CNIE) is defined as endocarditis without positive blood cultures after three samples. It accounts for 10% of IE.[1] Common offenders of CNIE include fungi, anaerobes, *Legionella, Tropheryma whipplei, Chlamydia psittaci, Coxiella, Brucella, Bartnoella,* and the HACEK bacteria (*Haemophilus, Actinobacillus, Cardiobacterium, Eikenella, Kingella*). It is critical to isolate a pathogen via polymerase chain reaction, serology, and histology because many of the aforementioned organisms do not respond to empiric antibiotics.[1]

Treatment

Medical: Antibiotic therapy should be targeted to the isolated organism and customized to utilize bactericidal agents. Aminoglycosides are often used for their synergistic effect with beta-lactam agents. Due to the complexity of treatment regimens, IE cases should be managed by a multidisciplinary team with involvement of cardiology, infectious disease, and cardiothoracic surgery.[2]

Acute NVE should be treated with vancomycin and gentamicin. (Vancomycin 15 mg/kg IV q12 hours [adjust for 1-hour peak serum concentration of 30–45 mcg/mL and trough levels of 10–15 mcg/mL] and gentamicin 1 mg/kg IV or IM q8 hours [adjust for peak serum concentration of 3–4 mcg/mL and trough levels of < 1 mcg/mL].)[2] Subacute NVE should be treated with ceftriaxone (2 g IV or IM every 24 hours) and gentamicin. PVE should be treated with vancomycin, cefepime (1–2 gm IV q12 hours) and gentamicin.[2] Antibiotic duration is most often 4 to 6 weeks from the first day of negative cultures. Fungal IE should be treated with amphotericin B and flucytosine.[2] Even after a valve infected with fungal species is removed, there is data to support long-term antifungal suppressive therapy with fluconazole to prevent recurrence.[12] Treatment of CIED infections often involves removal of the entire device in addition to empiric vancomycin targeting the most common source pathogen, CoNS, which is often resistant to oxacillin.[8]

Surgical Treatment

Surgery plays a pivotal role in the management of IE and is indicated in about 25% to 33% of cases.[3] Class I indications for NVE include fungal infection; severe valvular disease causing heart failure, aortic regurgitation, or mitral regurgitation that results in elevated left ventricular end-diastolic pressure; persistent infection defined as fever and/or bacteremia extending beyond 7 to 10 days of antibiotic therapy; and certain complications, which include heart block, periannular abscess, aortic abscess, and fistula formation.[2] Operating on a lesion that is at a high risk of embolization is controversial. However, vegetations greater than 10 mm should be strongly considered for operative management.[13]

The optimal timing of surgery is an area that is currently under active investigation. New data suggests that patients with native mitral or aortic valve endocarditis with a vegetation greater than 10 mm benefit from surgery within the first 48 hours of diagnosis.

Prophylaxis

Only high-risk patients require prophylaxis to prevent IE. This includes patients with prosthetic heart valves, a history of prior infective endocarditis, certain unrepaired congenital heart diseases, and cardiac transplant patients with valvulopathy.[2] Procedures requiring antibiotic prophylaxis include dental procedures that manipulate the gingival tissue, periapical region of teeth, or perforate of oral mucosa. Prophylaxis is also needed for the following: tonsillectomy, adenoidectomy, invasive respiratory procedures involving incision, and procedures performed on infected skin.[2] The first line agent for prophylaxis is amoxicillin 2 g by mouth 1 hour prior to the procedure.

Complications

Heart failure is a common complication of IE (55% of cases) and the leading cause of death in IE.[2] Septic emboli (25%–50% of cases) cause a variety of clinical manifestations. From highest to lowest frequency, these complications include the following: cerebral, splenic, renal, pulmonary, peripheral vasculature, coronary, and ocular.[9] Neurological consequences of IE include cerebral emboli, encephalopathy, and, less commonly, meningitis and brain abscess. Cerebral emboli require special attention due to the risk of hemorrhagic conversion, particularly in the setting of exposure to high doses of heparin during intraoperative cardiac procedures. Mycotic aneurysms, found in the setting of IE and headache, merit a delay in surgical intervention until the aneurysm is addressed through resection or clipping.

The risk of embolization correlates with the size of vegetation (a vegetation greater than 10 mm has a threefold higher risk of embolization compared to lesions less than 10 mm), mobility of vegetation, localization to the mitral valve, and culprit microorganism (*S. auerus* and fungi have higher rates of embolization).[9] The risk of embolic events tapers after 1 to 2 weeks of antimicrobial therapy.[9] As discussed previously, peri-valvular abscesses can erode the heart's conduction system and cause atrioventricular block and other electrophysiological complications. Infections involving prosthetic valve sutures may unseat the valve causing dehiscence and subsequent profound heart failure.[3]

Suggested Readings and References

1. Moreillon, P. and Y.A. Que, *Infective endocarditis*. Lancet, 2004. **363**(9403): p. 139–49.
2. American College of Cardiology/American Heart Association Task Force on Practice, G., et al., *ACC/AHA 2006 guidelines for the management of patients with valvular heart disease: a report of the American College of Cardiology/American Heart Association Task Force on Practice Guidelines (writing committee to revise the 1998 Guidelines for the Management of Patients With Valvular Heart Disease): developed in collaboration with the Society of Cardiovascular Anesthesiologists: endorsed by the Society for Cardiovascular Angiography and Interventions and the Society of Thoracic Surgeons*. Circulation, 2006. **114**(5): p. e84–231.
3. Habib, G., et al., *Guidelines on the prevention, diagnosis, and treatment of infective endocarditis (new version 2009): the Task Force on the Prevention, Diagnosis, and Treatment of Infective Endocarditis of the European Society of Cardiology (ESC). Endorsed by the European Society of Clinical Microbiology and Infectious Diseases (ESCMID) and the International Society of Chemotherapy (ISC) for Infection and Cancer*. Eur Heart J, 2009. **30**(19): p. 2369–413.
4. Mylonakis, E. and S.B. Calderwood, *Infective endocarditis in adults*. N Engl J Med, 2001. **345**(18): p. 1318–30.
5. Li, J.S., et al., *Proposed modifications to the Duke criteria for the diagnosis of infective endocarditis*. Clin Infect Dis, 2000. **30**(4): p. 633–8.
6. Mathew, J., et al., *Clinical features, site of involvement, bacteriologic findings, and outcome of infective endocarditis in intravenous drug users*. Arch Intern Med, 1995. **155**(15): p. 1641–8.
7. Gordon, R.J. and F.D. Lowy, *Bacterial infections in drug users*. N Engl J Med, 2005. **353**(18): p. 1945–54.
8. Baddour, L.M., Y.M. Cha, and W.R. Wilson, *Clinical practice. Infections of cardiovascular implantable electronic devices*. N Engl J Med, 2012. **367**(9): p. 842–9.
9. Habib, G., *Management of infective endocarditis*. Heart, 2006. **92**(1): p. 124–30.
10. Shively, B.K., et al., *Diagnostic value of transesophageal compared with transthoracic echocardiography in infective endocarditis*. J Am Coll Cardiol, 1991. **18**(2): p. 391–7.
11. Liu, P.Y., et al., *Staphylococcus lugdunensis infective endocarditis: a literature review and analysis of risk factors*. J Microbiol Immunol Infect, 2010. **43**(6): p. 478–84.
12. Smego, R.A., Jr. and H. Ahmad, *The role of fluconazole in the treatment of Candida endocarditis: a meta-analysis*. Medicine (Baltimore), 2011. **90**(4): p. 237–49.
13. Kang, D.H., et al., *Early surgery versus conventional treatment for infective endocarditis*. N Engl J Med, 2012. **366**(26): p. 2466–73.

Chapter 19

Myocarditis and Pericarditis

Kevin Alexander

Summary Boxes

Infectious Myocarditis	Infectious Pericarditis
DISEASE DESCRIPTION	DISEASE DESCRIPTION
Signs/Symptoms	Sign/Symptoms
• Possible viral prodrome	• Acute, sharp, retrosternal, and pleuritic chest pain that may radiate to the shoulder
• Heart failure symptoms (progressive dyspnea, fatigue, and chest pain)	• Worse when lying flat, better when leaning forward
• Left ventricular dysfunction on echocardiogram	• May have fever and hemodynamic instability
Diagnosis	Diagnosis
• Gold standard: endomyocardial biopsy (EMB) and immunohistochemical analysis	• Pericardial friction rub
• Cardiac magnetic resonance imaging (MRI), cardiac markers, and electrocardiogram (ECG)	• ECG: diffuse ST elevations and PR depressions
Complications	• Cardiac markers, chest x-ray, and echocardiogram
• Heart failure (arrhythmias, cardiogenic shock, and sudden cardiac shock)	• Pericardiocentesis if cardiac tamponade or recurrent pericarditis with effusion
• Chronic myocarditis	Complications
ORGANISMS	• Most cases: self-limited
• Mainly viruses (ie, coxsackievirus and parvovirus B19)	• Recurrence, tamponade, and constrictive pericarditis
• Other pathogens: bacteria and fungi	ORGANISMS
TREATMENT	• Mainly viruses
• Supportive treatment	• Other pathogens: bacteria and fungi
• General heart failure therapy	TREATMENT
• Antibiotics and antivirals (when pathogen is identified)	• NSAIDs (nonsteroidal anti-inflammatory drugs)
• Heart transplant for severe cases may be indicated	• Colchicine
	• Pericardiocentesis (effusion)
	• Antibiotics if a bacterial pathogen is identified (*Mycobacterium tuberculosis* most common bacterial cause worldwide)

Infectious Myocarditis

Disease Description
Epidemiology
Infectious myocarditis is a primary, inflammatory cardiomyopathy that can lead to cardiomyocyte toxicity via direct myocyte invasion, toxin production, and/or stimulation of a chronic inflammatory response through antigenic mimicry. Its incidence is difficult to determine due to significant disease heterogeneity and the lack of a noninvasive gold standard for diagnosis.

Diagnosis
The gold standard for diagnosing myocarditis is still EMB with immunohistochemical analysis. According to an American Heart Association/American College of Cardiology/European Society of Cardiology joint statement, EMB has a Class IB indication for patients with the following: (1) less than 2 weeks of new heart failure with a normal or dilated left ventricle and hemodynamic decompensation; or (2) 2 weeks to 3 months of new heart failure symptoms with a dilated left ventricle and failure to respond to standard therapy within 2 weeks, new ventricular arrhythmias, or new second- or third-degree heart block.[1] A histological diagnosis can be made using the Dallas Criteria, which requires the presence of a lymphocytic infiltrate with associated myocardial necrosis.[2] Immunohistochemical stains may occasionally identify a specific viral etiology for myocarditis.

Other serological markers and imaging can aid in the diagnosis and rule out other causes of heart failure. Cardiac MRI has been used to identify differences in gadolinium enhancement between healthy and inflamed myocardium and may help to identify targets for EMB.[3] Patients may acutely present with elevated markers of myocardial injury (troponin I is usually greater than creatine kinase myocardial band [CK-MB]) and elevated nonspecific markers of inflammation, such as C-reactive protein (CRP) and erythrocyte sedimentation rate (ESR).[4] ECG findings include nonspecific T-wave changes, ST-segment depression or elevation, bundle branch blocks, and tachyarrhythmias.[5] Echocardiographic analysis of myocarditis usually reveals nonspecific findings, but it can be helpful to identify other causes of heart failure (ie, myocardial infarction, valvular disease, and right ventricular dysfunction) and pericardial effusions.

Typical Disease Course
Patients typically present with several days to weeks of heart failure symptoms, including progressive dyspnea, fatigue, and chest pain (especially if pericarditis is also present) as well as signs of left ventricular dysfunction on echocardiography. Sometimes, these signs and symptoms are preceded by a clear viral prodrome. A subset of patients with acute myocarditis will develop fulminant myocarditis, which is characterized by cardiogenic shock, often requiring inotrope therapy and mechanical circulatory support. Interestingly, survivors of fulminant myocarditis are more likely to completely recover than those with a more indolent presentation.[6]

Complications
Most complications arise from heart failure and include arrhythmias, cardiogenic shock, and sudden cardiac death. Patients with acute myocarditis may also progress to chronic myocarditis and develop a dilated cardiomyopathy.

Organisms

Myocarditis is most commonly caused by viruses. Coxsackievirus B was the first pathogen to be linked to myocarditis. More recently, parvovirus B19, adenoviruses, enteroviruses, and human immunodeficiency virus (HIV) have been found to be common causes. Less frequently, hepatitis B and C, Epstein-Barr virus, cytomegalovirus, influenza, and herpes viruses have been implicated.

Depending on the patient's history, there are several important non-viral causes to consider, including Chagas disease (South America), Lyme disease (tick exposure), and toxoplasmosis (immunocompromised). Bacterial and fungal causes of myocarditis are rare and often secondary to direct invasion from a systemic infection. *Corynebacterium diphtheriae* infections commonly involve the heart. *Neisseria meningitidis*, *Legionella* spp., *Mycoplasma* spp., *Staphylococcus aureus*, and *Streptococcus* spp. are other bacterial pathogens implicated in bacterial myocarditis. Fungal etiologies include *Candida*, *Aspergillus*, *Histoplasma*, *Blastomyces*, *Coccidioides*, and *Cryptococcus* species.

Treatment

Often, the causative pathogen is not identified; in cases where one is identified, appropriate anti-infective agents may be used. Treatment is primarily supportive. General heart failure therapy, including beta blockers, angiotensin converting enzyme inhibitors, diuretics, and aldosterone antagonists, should be used. Heart transplantation may ultimately be indicated for patients with a chronic dilated cardiomyopathy that is refractory to medical therapy.

Infectious Pericarditis

Disease Description

Epidemiology
Acute infectious pericarditis involves inflammation of the parietal and visceral layers of the pericardial sac that surround the heart. Although the exact incidence of acute pericarditis is unknown, an epidemiological study found acute pericarditis in 5% of emergency department patients with non-myocardial infarction chest pain.[7]

Diagnosis
The diagnosis is primarily clinical. Many patients (85%) have a pericardial friction rub.[8] Pulsus paradoxus may be present in cases of cardiac tamponade. Pulsus paradoxus is a drop in systemic arterial pressure of *greater* than 10 mmHg with inspiration and can be found in moderate to severe cardiac tamponade as well as occasionally with constrictive pericarditis or chronic obstructive pulmonary disease exacerbations/asthma attacks. ECG often reveals characteristic diffuse ST-segment elevations and PR-segment depressions. Patients often have markers of myocardial injury and inflammation (elevated troponin, CK-MB, white blood cell count, ESR, and CRP). In the case of purulent pericarditis, blood cultures may be positive for the offending organism, indicating a systemic infection. Chest radiography may reveal signs of a pericardial effusion. Echocardiography can also identify an effusion and signs of serious sequelae, including cardiac tamponade and constrictive pericarditis. Pericardiocentesis is indicated for cardiac tamponade or recurrent pericarditis with an effusion. The fluid should be submitted for cell counts, cytology, triglycerides, and adenosine deaminase as well as bacterial, fungal, and mycobacterial cultures.

Typical Disease Course
Patients most commonly present with acute-onset, sharp, retrosternal, and pleuritic chest pain that is worse when lying supine and improved by leaning forward. The pain can radiate to the arms, shoulders, or neck. Radiation to the trapezius muscles is the most specific, likely because the phrenic nerve travels through the pericardium. Patients may also have a fever and show signs of systemic illness. Hemodynamic compromise may be seen in those with cardiac tamponade.

Complications
Most cases of pericarditis are self-limited. However, recurrent pericarditis can be seen in 24% of patients and usually occurs within 2 weeks.[9] Cardiac tamponade develops in up to 60% of patients with purulent or tuberculosis pericarditis.[10] In a subset of patients, constrictive pericarditis is a long-term complication of acute pericarditis. Purulent and tuberculous pericarditis have higher incidences of leading to constrictive pericarditis compared to viral pericarditis.[11]

Organisms

Similar to infectious myocarditis, viruses are the major cause of infectious pericarditis. The most common pathogens are coxsackieviruses, adenoviruses, *human herpesvirus 6*, HIV, cytomegalovirus, Epstein-Barr virus, and *parvovirus B19*. *Mycobacterium tuberculosis* remains the most common bacterial cause of pericarditis worldwide, but it is becoming far less common in developed countries. Other bacteria, such as *Staphylococcus, Streptococcus, Neisseria*, and *Haemophilus* species, are common causes of purulent pericarditis. Purulent pericarditis often arises from a post-cardiac surgery infection, sepsis, or direct extension of a lung infection, or infectious endocarditis. Causes of fungal pericarditis include *Histoplasma* (most common among immunocompetent patients), *Candida, Aspergillus*, and *Coccidioides* species.

Treatment

Indications for hospitalization include fever greater than 38.0°C, signs of cardiac tamponade or a large pericardial effusion, immunosuppressed state, current anticoagulation therapy, and troponinemia suggestive of myocarditis.[12] First line symptomatic treatment includes NSAIDs and colchicine. When added to NSAID therapy, colchicines has been shown to reduce the risk of recurrent pericarditis and to reduce treatment failure in recurrent pericarditis.[13,14] Common regimens include colchicine 0.6 mg every 12 hours and aspirin 650 to 1000 mg every 6 hours or ibuprofen 800 mg every 8 hours with a gradual taper. Corticosteroids may be used for those who do not respond. Because infectious pericarditis usually has a viral etiology, antibiotics are only started if blood or pericardial effusion cultures demonstrate a bacterial or fungal cause. Purulent pericarditis and cardiac tamponade should be treated with drainage via either pericardiocentesis or a pericardiotomy. Pericardial resection is the only treatment for constrictive pericarditis.

Suggested Readings and References

1. Cooper LT, et al. The role of endomyocardial biopsy in the management of cardiovascular disease: a scientific statement by from the American Heart Association, the American College of Cardiology, and the European Society of Cardiology. *J Am Coll Cardiol*. 2007;50:1914–1931.

2. Aretz HT, Billingham ME, Edwards WD, et al. Myocarditis: a histopathologic definition and classification. *Am J Cardiovasc Pathol*. 1987;1:3–14.

3. Laissy JP, Messin B, Varenne O, et al. MRI of acute myocarditis: a comprehensive approach based on various imaging sequences. *Chest*. 2002;122:1638–1648.

4. Smith SC, Ladenson JH, Mason JW, Jaffe AS. Elevations of cardiac troponin I associated with myocarditis. Experimental and clinical correlates. *Circulation*. 1997;95:163–168.

5. Schultheiss HP, Kühl U, Cooper LT. The management of myocarditis. *Eur Heart J*. 2011;32:2616–2625.

6. McCarthy RE 3rd, Boehmer JP, Hruban RH, et al. Long-term outcome of fulminant myocarditis as compared with acute (nonfulminant) myocarditis. *N Engl J Med*. 2000;342:690–695.

7. Troughton RW, Asher CR, Klein AL. Pericarditis. *Lancet*. 2004;363:717–727.

8. Zayas R, Anguita M, Torres F, et al. Incidence of specific etiology and role of methods for specific etiologic diagnosis of primary acute pericarditis. *Am J Cardiol*. 1995;75:378–382.

9. Tingle LE, Molina D, Calvert CW. Acute pericarditis. *Am Fam Physician*. 2007;76:1509–1514.

10. Permanyer-Miralda G. Acute pericardial disease: approach to the aetiologic diagnosis. *Heart*. 2004;90:252–254.

11. Imazio M, Brucato A, Maestroni S, et al. Risk of constrictive pericarditis after acute pericarditis. *Circulation*. 2011;124:1270–1275.

12. Imazio M, Demichelis B, Parrini I, et al. Day-hospital treatment of acute pericarditis: a management program for outpatient therapy. *J Am Coll Cardiol*. 2004;43:1042–1046.

13. Imazio M, Bobbio M, Cecchi E, et al. Colchicine as first-choice therapy for recurrent pericarditis: results of the CORE (COlchicine for REcurrent pericarditis) trial. *Arch Intern Med*. 2005;165:1987–1991.

14. Imazio M, Bobbio M, Cecchi E, et al. Colchicine in addition to conventional therapy for acute pericarditis: results of the COlchicine for acute PEricarditis (COPE) trial. *Circulation*. 2005;112:2012–2016.

Catheter-Associated Infections

Swathi Eluri

Summary Box

Disease Description: Infection whose source is an indwelling catheter

Organisms: Coagulase-negative *Staphylococcus*, *Staphylococcus aureus*, Enterococci, gram-negative bacilli, and *Candida* spp.

Treatment:
Oral first line: n/a
Second line: n/a
Parenteral: Vancomycin 15 mg/kg q12 hours for methicillin-resistant Staphylococcus aureus (MRSA); Nafcillin or Oxacillin 2 g q4 hours for methicillin-susceptible Staphylococcus aureus (MSSA); Ceftriaxone1 to 2 g IV q24 hours for *E. coli* and *Klebsiella*; cefepime 2 g IV q12 hours or meropenem 1g IV q8 hours for *Pseudomonas*; ambisome 0.3 to 1 mg/kg per day or fluconazole 400 to 600 mg IV q24 hours for *Candida* spp.

Other Key Issues: Chlorhexidine/silver sulfadiazine coated catheters, hand hygiene, 0.5% chlorhexidine for skin preparation, full barrier precautions during line insertion, and line insertion site are all effective in reducing infection.

107

Disease Description

Infections associated with the use of catheters include catheter-associated and catheter-related infections. Catheter-associated infections, which often present as sepsis, include primary bloodstream infections that occur in the presence of intravascular catheters. They are not related to an infection at another site. A catheter-related infection is a more specific definition that is defined as a primary bloodstream infection with documented colonization of the device, skin exit site, and microbiologically proven device-related bloodstream infection. Catheters are defined by the vessel in which they are cannulated (central or peripheral), the site of insertion, and the catheter's pathway from skin to vessel. The risk of infection depends on catheter type and the number of days the catheter has been in place.[1]

Risk factors after insertion for catheter-related infection include prolonged hospitalization, prolonged duration of catheterization, heavy microbial colonization at the insertion site or catheter hub, internal jugular and femoral catheterization, neutropenia, premature birth, total parenteral nutrition (TPN) through the catheter, and poor catheter care.[2] Patients hospitalized for greater than 7 days have been shown to have a twofold to threefold higher risk of infection by a resistant pathogen. Patients of female gender are at lower risk. Cuffed devices have been shown to have lower infection risk than non-cuffed central venous catheters.

Epidemiology

Nosocomial infections are the leading cause of morbidity and mortality in hospitalized patients. Of these nosocomial infections, 10% to 20% are associated with the use of intravascular devices. It is estimated that 200,000 to 400,000 blood stream infections associated with intravascular catheters occur annually in hospitalized patients in the United States.[3] Approximately 51% occur in the intensive care unit (ICU).[4] According to the Centers for Disease Control and Prevention (CDC), there has been a 58% decrease in catheter-related blood stream infections in the United States during the 9-year period between 2001 and 2009.[5] More recently, the CDC reported that infection rates were 32% lower than expected in 2010. This trend shows that the new preventative measures taken to reduce catheter-associated infections have made a significant impact in decreasing infection rates. Despite the decrease in the infection rate, the total cost of catheter-related blood stream infections in the United States has been estimated to be as high as 2.3 billion dollars annually.[6]

Presenting Features

Catheter-related bloodstream infections can have presenting features both locally and systemically. The most common manifestation is fever. Patients can also present with symptoms of bacteremia, such as chills, rigors, hypotension, or confusion without an obvious source. Local infections occur in about 30% of cases and present at the catheter exit site with erythema, induration, purulence, or tenderness within 2 cm of the line exit site. Tunnel infections present greater than 2 cm from the exit site and along the subcutaneous tract of the catheter. Pocket infections can also be seen with implanted intravascular devices. Although local signs are highly suggestive of a catheter-related infection, the absence of these features does not rule out the presence of a systemic infection.

Diagnostic Considerations

The first step in the diagnosis of a suspected catheter-related infection is to draw simultaneous aerobic and anaerobic blood cultures from both the vascular catheter and a peripheral vein prior to the initiation of antibiotics. Ideally, the distal port of the catheter should be used to obtain cultures.[7] There is no indication to obtain blood from all ports unless a peripheral culture cannot be drawn. In that case, two sets of cultures from each port should be drawn. Because the yield of the culture depends on the amount of blood drawn, it is generally recommended that 20 to 30 mL be drawn from a single site at any one time. Both the skin surface and catheter hub should be cleaned with alcohol, tincture of iodine, or alcoholic chlorhexidine (> 0.5%). In the presence of localized purulence or exudates from the catheter exit site, the fluid should be sent for gram stain and culture.[6]

Complications

In rare cases, patients with systemic catheter-related infections can develop endocarditis, osteomyelitis, or suppurative thrombophlebitis.

Diagnostic Tests

Drawing paired blood cultures from the venous catheter and a peripheral vein simultaneously has been shown to be both sensitive and specific (75% and 97% for short-term catheters, 93% and 100% for long-term catheters, respectively) for the diagnosis of catheter-related infection.[8] To diagnose a catheter-related blood stream infection, there needs to be greater than threefold more colony forming units

(CFU) from the catheter in comparison to the peripheral culture. Differential time to positivity is also widely used. According to this method, a catheter-related infection can be diagnosed with a sensitivity of 94% and specificity of 91% if a positive blood culture drawn from the catheter is detected at least 120 minutes earlier than the peripheral blood culture.[9]

Other techniques that can be used are a catheter tip culture, which involves culturing a 5-cm segment of catheter by rolling it on an agar plate. A colony count of at least 15 CFU is considered evidence of colonization. However, this method is not as accurate for intraluminal bacterial colonization, as these bacteria likely will not contact the agar while rolling the catheter over it. Endoluminal brushing can detect intraluminal bacteria by placing a brush through the catheter hub and culturing it.[10] However, it is not as widely used due to complications, such as inciting arrhythmias, bacteremia, and embolization. Sound waves can also be applied to the catheter segment (ie, sonication) to detach the bacteria on the catheter tip. The resultant broth can then be cultured, using a colony count greater than 100 CFU/mL as the threshold for diagnosing a catheter-related infection.

Microbiology

Catheter-related infection can occur via the extraluminal or intraluminal route. The intraluminal route involves migration of pathogens through the catheter lumen after colonization of the catheter hub. This type of infection is more prevalent in long-term catheters (greater than 10 days).[11] The extraluminal route is more commonly seen and involves microbes from the patient's skin migrating over the external surface of the line. The source of these organisms can be the patient's endogenous skin flora or extrinsic catheter contamination during catheter placement or manipulation. In some instances, there can be hematogenous seeding of organisms from other body sites or from contaminated infusates.[12] In these cases, microorganisms adhere to the catheter and form a biofilm, which tend to be more resistant to host defenses and antimicrobials. The organisms may subsequently colonize the extraluminal or intraluminal surface of the catheter, resulting in bloodstream infections.

Organisms

The most commonly reported causative pathogens are coagulase-negative *Staphylococcus* spp. (34%), *Staphylococcus aureus* (10%), *Enterococci* spp. (16%), and *Candida* spp. (8%).[11,13] Gram-negative bacilli, such as *Klebsiella pneumoniae* account for 19% of reported infections and *E. coli* for 21% of infections reported to the CDC with increasing resistance to third-generation cephalosporins for both organisms. *Pseudomonas aeruginosa* species are becoming resistant to imipenem and ceftazidime.[14] MRSA accounts for more than 50% of ICU infections, but the incidence of MRSA central-line associated blood stream infections have has decreased by 49.6% between 1997 and 2007.[15]

Treatment

The initial management of catheter-related infection includes starting empiric antibiotic therapy with vancomycin 15 mg/kg q12 hours dosing because gram-positive cocci are the most common causative pathogens, especially in health care settings with an increased prevalence of MRSA. For MSSA, nafcillin or oxacillin 2 g q4 hours can be used. Additional coverage for gram-negative bacilli and *Candida* species should be provided in the following groups: ICU patients with femoral lines, TPN, transplant patients, hematologic malignancy, and those who are already on prolonged broad-spectrum antibiotics. Empiric gram-negative coverage should be tailored to local resistance patterns and organisms. Typical treatment regimens for *E. coli* and *Klebsiella* spp. include a third-generation cephalosporin, such as ceftriaxone 1 to 2 g IV q24 hours.[11] Pseudomonal coverage should be provided for neutropenic patients, severely ill patients with sepsis, and those with known prior colonization with cefepime 2 g IV q12 hours or meropenem 1g IV q8 hours. For Candidal infections, ambisome 0.3 to 1 mg/kg per day or fluconazole 400 to 600 mg IV q24 hours can be used for treatment.

For uncomplicated infections, a 7 to 14 day antibiotic course after the first negative blood culture is recommended.[7] Complicated infections, characterized by suppurative thrombophlebitis, endocarditis, or osteomyelitis, require a 4- to 8-week course of treatment. Successful treatment is indicated by clearance of blood cultures after a course of antibiotics. Failure is defined as persistently positive cultures despite antibiotics or recurrent infections with the same organism.

The primary treatment of catheter-related bloodstream infection also includes the removal of the infected catheter for source control. Catheter removal is generally recommended for all short-term catheters. If the organism is coagulase-negative *Staphylococcus*, removing the line is optional, and patients are treated with a 10- to 14-day course of antibiotics. If treatment with antibiotics fails or the clinical condition deteriorates, however, the line should immediately be removed. Long-term catheters should be removed if the infection-causing pathogen is *S. aureus*, a gram-negative bacillus, a *Candida* spp., or a *Mycobacterium* spp. Additionally, catheter removal is advised in all complicated infections and if cultures remain positive for greater than 72 hours.[7]

Other Key Issues

Multiple hospitals across the nation have started to implement standardized quality control interventions to minimize catheter-related bloodstream infections. These interventions focus on good hand hygiene, use of 0.5% chlorhexidine for skin preparation, full barrier precautions during line insertion, minimizing unnecessary lines, and carefully choosing the line insertion site. New tools, such as the use of ultrasound in both ICUs and hospital floors for line insertion, have made an impact in reducing associated infections. Multiple studies have shown that ultrasound-guided line placement by an experienced operator results in a decrease in mechanical complication and the number of attempts.[16] This, in turn, reduces the risk of infection.

Additionally, studies have shown that preparing the skin with 0.5% chlorhexidine or alcohol containing chlorhexidine solutions has been shown to reduce line-related infections.[17] There is no strong clinical evidence to show that chlorhexidine-impregnated sponge dressings make an impact on infection rates. On the other hand, catheters coated with chlorhexidine/silver sulfadiazine or minocycline/rifampin are effective in reducing catheter colonization and catheter-related blood stream infections.[18] The use of these antibiotic-coated catheters is generally recommended for high-risk patients, those in the ICU, or those on total parenteral nutrition.[19]

The latest guidelines also strongly recommend the use of antimicrobial lock solutions in patients with recurrent catheter-associated infections and high-risk groups, such as those on TPN, dialysis, or onco-logic patients.[20] Finally, the use of sutureless devices to secure the catheter is a category II recommendation because the preservation of skin integrity surrounding the device decreases the risk of infection.[21]

Suggested Readings and References

1. Maki DG, Kluger DM, Crnich CJ. *The risk of bloodstream infection in adults with different intravascular devices: a systematic review of 200 published prospective studies. Mayo Clin Proc.* 2006;81:1159–1171.
2. Lorente L, et al. Central venous catheter-related infection in a prospective and observational study of 2,595 catheters. *Crit Care.* 2005;9:R631–R635.
3. Mermel LA. Prevention of intravascular catheter-related infections. *Ann Intern Med.* 2000;132:391–402.
4. Wisplinghoff H, et al. Nosocomial bloodstream infections in US hospitals: analysis of 24,179 cases from a prospective nationwide surveillance study. *Clin Infect Dis.* 2004;39:309–317.
5. Vital signs: central line-associated blood stream infections—United States, 2001, 2008, and 2009. *MMWR Morb Mortal Wkly Rep.* 2011;60:243–248.
6. Pronovost P, et al. An intervention to decrease catheter-related bloodstream infections in the ICU. *N Engl J Med.* 2006;355:2725–2732.
7. Mermel LA, et al. Clinical practice guidelines for the diagnosis and management of intravascular catheter-related infection: 2009 Update by the Infectious Diseases Society of America. *Clin Infect Dis.* 2009;49:1–45.
8. Safdar N, Fine JP, Maki, DG. Meta-analysis: methods for diagnosing intravascular device-related bloodstream infection. *Ann Intern Med.* 2005;142:451–466.
9. Blot F, et al. Diagnosis of catheter-related bacteraemia: a prospective comparison of the time to positivity of hub-blood versus peripheral-blood cultures. *Lancet.* 1999;354:1071–1077.
10. Raad I, Hanna H, Maki D. Intravascular catheter-related infections: advances in diagnosis, prevention, and management. *Lancet Infect Dis.* 2007;7:645–657.
11. Mermel LA, et al. Guidelines for the management of intravascular catheter-related infections. *Clin Infect Dis.* 2001;32:1249–1272.
12. Maki DG, Mermel LA. Infections due to infusion therapy. *CINA-AGINCOURT.* 1999;15:71–95.
13. O'Grady NP, et al. Guidelines for the prevention of intravascular catheter-related infections. *Am J Infect Control.* 2011;39(suppl 1):S1–S34.
14. Gaynes R, Edwards JR, Overview of nosocomial infections caused by gram-negative bacilli. *Clin Infect Dis.* 2005;41:848–854.
15. Burton DC, et al. Methicillin-resistant Staphylococcus aureus central line-associated bloodstream infections in US intensive care units, 1997-2007. *JAMA.* 2009;301:727–736.

16. Hind D, et al. Ultrasonic locating devices for central venous cannulation: meta-analysis. *BMJ*. 2003;327:361.

17. Reduction in central line-associated bloodstream infections among patients in intensive care units—Pennsylvania, April 2001-March 2005. *MMWR Morb Mortal Wkly Rep*. 2005;54:1013–1016.

18. Darouiche RO, et al. A comparison of two antimicrobial-impregnated central venous catheters. Catheter Study Group. *N Engl J Med*. 1999;340:1–8.

19. Heard SO, et al. Influence of triple-lumen central venous catheters coated with chlorhexidine and silver sulfadiazine on the incidence of catheter-related bacteremia. *Arch Intern Med*. 1998;158:81–87.

20. Cober MP, Kovacevich DS, Teitelbaum DH. Ethanol-lock therapy for the prevention of central venous access device infections in pediatric patients with intestinal failure. *JPEN J Parenter Enteral Nutr*. 2011;35:67–73.

21. Yamamoto AJ, et al. Sutureless securement device reduces complications of peripherally inserted central venous catheters. *J Vasc Interv Radiol*. 2002;13:77–81.

Septic Thrombophlebitis

Sudip Saha

Summary Box

Disease Description: Venous thrombosis resulting from the inflammation induced by bacteremia

Organisms:
  Staphylococcus aureus
  Streptococci
  Enterobacteriaceae
  Fusobacterium necrophorum

Treatment:
  Parenteral: vancomycin + ceftriaxone (cefepime if concern for *Pseudomonas*)
  Oral First line: clindamycin[2]

Disease Description

Septic (suppurative) thrombophlebitis is venous thrombosis that occurs in the setting of bacteremia. There is usually a degree of perivascular inflammation seen on histology.[1]

Epidemiology

Septic thrombophlebitis is typically catheter-associated. The bacteremia is usually of greater than 72 hours duration in the setting of appropriate antimicrobial therapy.[2] Septic thrombophlebitis occurs most commonly in the setting intravenous catheters.[3] However, most cases of infection related to intravenous catheters are not complicated by septic thrombophlebitis. In a case series of 102 intravenous catheter-related infections, only 7% were complicated by septic thrombophlebitis. The incidence is higher in specific patient populations. Those with severe burns, frequent exposure to broad-spectrum antibiotics, high skin inoculum of organisms that typically cause this condition, and loss of skin integrity are at increased risk.[4]

Jugular vein septic thrombophlebitis, also known as Lemierre's syndrome, is a subset of septic thrombophlebitis that deserves special consideration.[5] This condition can affect otherwise young, healthy adults and is often preceded by dental infections, infectious mononucleosis, and pharyngitis with tonsillar and peritonsillar involvement.[6] The infection involves the carotid sheath vessels and can affect many structures, including the parapharyngeal space, anterior neck muscles, internal jugular vein, internal carotid artery, vagus nerve, and lymph nodes in this area. Commonly, those at particular risk have had pharyngitis or septic pulmonary emboli.[7]

Presenting Features

Catheter-related septic thrombophlebitis: This condition typically presents with persistent bacteremia (about 72 hours) despite appropriate antimicrobial therapy. There is evidence of erythema, tenderness, and/or drainage at the site of an intravenous catheter. Complications of catheter-related thrombophlebitis include secondary infections, such as septic emboli, pneumonia, empyema, osteomyelitis, and joint infection. In larger vessels like the inferior or superior vena cava, systemic symptoms (ie, fevers, chills, rigors, and hypotension) can be present as can tissue edema in sites distal to the thrombus due to both inflammation and inadequate venous drainage.[2]

Jugular vein septic thrombophlebitis: Clinical presentation includes high fevers (typically greater than 39°C), rigors, respiratory distress, ulceration or erythema of the oropharynx, and tenderness and swelling of the neck. Special consideration should be given to septic emboli from the jugular vein to the pulmonary system, which can cause empyema and/or secondarily spread to distal sites, such as bones and joints.[8]

Diagnostic Tests

Catheter-related septic thrombophlebitis: Microbiological diagnosis is made on the basis of blood cultures, direct culture of the vein itself (if a surgical approach is taken), or, sometimes less reliably, when an aspirate from the vein is expressed. Aspiration from the vein has the potential for skin flora contamination. Duplex ultrasonography should be used to evaluate for the presence of thrombus within the venous system.[2]

Jugular vein septic thrombophlebitis: Microbiological diagnosis is similarly made on the basis of blood cultures and direct culture from the vein itself if a procedural approach is taken. The best tool to evaluate jugular vein septic thrombophlebitis is high resolution CT (computed tomography) with IV (intravenous) contrast. In addition to indirectly detecting thrombus via filling defects, CT with IV contrast can reveal local soft tissue swelling worrisome for pharyngitis and/or tonsillar infection, which precedes frank bacteremia. Duplex ultrasonography can also be used but may be less accurate in regions underlying the clavicle or mandible.[5]

Organisms

Catheter-related septic thrombophlebitis: The most common pathogen is *S. aureus*. Other less common pathogens include *Streptococcus* spp., Enterobacteriaceae spp., nosocomial pathogens, and polymicrobial infections in the setting of burns. Although fungi are less common pathogens, are seen, especially in larger vessels (ie, inferior or superior vena cava) and in association with catheters used for total parenteral nutrition.[9]

Jugular vein septic thrombophlebitis: The typical organisms in jugular vein septic thrombophlebitis are typically normal oropharyngeal flora. *Fusobacterium necrophorum*, an anaerobic organism, is the most common pathogen in this disorder. Other less common pathogens include other *Fusobacterium* spp., *Porphyromonas asaccharolytica*, *Eikenella corrodens*, *Streptococcus* spp., or *Bacteroides* spp.[5]

Treatment

Catheter-related septic thrombophlebitis: Primary treatment of this condition includes removal of infected materials (ie, IV catheter and/or the infected thrombus), intravenous antibiotics, and possible anticoagulation.[10] In the setting of sepsis or severe infection that is not responding to antimicrobials, surgical excision of the affected vein should be considered.[11] In the case of larger venous systems, such as the inferior or superior vena cava, thrombectomy can also be considered. Peripheral vein septic thrombophlebitis should be treated with antimicrobials that have activity against *Staphylococcus* spp. and Enterobacteriaceae spp., such as vancomycin and ceftriaxone, respectively. Pharmaceutical management is not well studied, but commonly accepted practices include a 2- to 4-week course of antibiotics with narrowing of antibiotic coverage based upon culture data. Finally, anticoagulation can be considered because a thrombus is present. However, in the setting of removing the inciting agent (ie, venous catheter), the benefit and duration of anticoagulation is not well understood. Currently accepted practices include considering anticoagulation in appropriate candidates who demonstrate extension of thrombus over time.[1]

Jugular vein septic thrombophlebitis: Primary treatment similarly includes removing infected materials, intravenous antibiotics, consideration of surgical management, and possible anticoagulation. Given the predominance of anaerobes and oropharyngeal flora, antibiotic therapy should include beta-lactamase resistant beta lactams, such as ampicillin-sulbactam, piperacillin-tazobactam, ticarcillin-clavulanate, or a cabapenem. Surgical drainage of pulmonary abscesses or peritonsillar/neck abscesses should be considered.

Suggested Readings and References

1. Mermel LA, Allon M, Bouza E, et al. Clinical practice guidelines for the diagnosis and management of intravascular catheter-related infection: 2009 update by the Infectious Diseases Society of America. *Clin Infect Dis.* 2009;49:1–45.

2. Arnow PM, Quimosing EM, Beach M. Consequences of intravascular catheter sepsis. *Clin Infect Dis.* 1993;16:778–784.

3. Andes DR, Urban AW, Acher CW, Maki DG. Septic thrombosis of the basilic, axillary, and subclavian veins caused by a peripherally inserted central venous catheter. *Am J Med.* 1998;105:446–450.

4. Pruitt BA Jr, McManus WF, Kim SH, Treat RC. Diagnosis and treatment of cannula-related intravenous sepsis in burn patients. *Ann Surg.* 1980;191:546–554.

5. Sinave CP, Hardy GJ, Fardy PW. The Lemierre syndrome: suppurative thrombophlebitis of the internal jugular vein secondary to oropharyngeal infection. *Medicine (Baltimore).* 1989;68:85–94.

6. Golpe R, Marín B, Alonso M. Lemierre's syndrome (necrobacillosis). *Postgrad Med J.* 1999;75:141–144.

7. Anton E. Lemierre syndrome caused by Streptococcus pyogenes in an elderly man. *Lancet Infect Dis.* 2007;7:233.

8. Khan EA, Correa AG, Baker CJ. Suppurative thrombophlebitis in children: a ten-year experience. *Pediatr Infect Dis J.* 1997;16:63–67.

9. Strinden WD, Helgerson RB, Maki DG. Candida septic thrombosis of the great central veins associated with central catheters: clinical features and management. *Ann Surg.* 1985;202:653–658.

10. Gillespie P, Siddiqui H, Clarke J. Cannula related suppurative thrombophlebitis in the burned patient. *Burns.* 2000;26:200–204.

11. Kniemeyer HW, Grabitz K, Buhl R, et al. Surgical treatment of septic deep venous thrombosis. *Surgery.* 1995;118:49–53.

Pulmonary Infections

Community-Acquired Pneumonia

Ryan Circh

Summary Box

Disease Description: Community-acquired pneumonia (CAP) is defined as an acute infection of the pulmonary parenchyma in someone who has not recently had close contact with the health care system.

Organisms: Most common pathogens: *Streptococcus pneumonia, Mycoplasma pneumonia, Haemophilus influenza, Chlamydophila pneumonia, Legionella pneumophila,* and *Influenzavirus* genera
  Less common pathogens: Gram-negative bacilli, oral anaerobes, *Klebsiella pneumoniae,* methicillin-resistant *Staphylococcus aureus* (MRSA), and fungi

Treatment: Treat for a minimum of 5 days or until the patient has been afebrile for 48 to 72 hours, whichever is longer.

Outpatient:
  Healthy: Macrolides, such as Azithromycin 500 mg PO (oral administration) on day 1 followed by 250 mg PO daily on days 2 to 5
  Comorbidities: Beta lactam such as Amoxicillin 1 g PO tid or Augmentin 2 g PO bid PLUS azithromycin as previously

Inpatient:
    Beta lactam, such as Ceftriaxone 1 g IV (intravenous) q24 hours PLUS azithromycin 500 mg IV or PO daily
    Inpatient intensive care unit (ICU): Ceftriaxone 1 g IV q24 hours PLUS azithromycin 500 mg IV q24 hours
    MRSA: Vancomycin with goal trough of 12–20 mcg/dL or linezolid 600 mg IV q12 hours
    Influenza A: Oseltamivir 75 mg PO bid (twice a day)

Other Key Issues: Prompt antibiotics and admission to the correct level of care are essential in emergency management. No single clinical finding, lab test, or diagnostic image is reliable for ruling pneumonia in or out, but radiologic evidence can be extremely useful in confirming the diagnosis of CAP in immunocompetent patients. Clinical decision tools like CURB-65 and PORT score can help identify low-risk patients when making decisions about whether or not to admit.

Disease Description

Epidemiology

CAP is the most common infectious cause of death in the United States and the sixth most common cause of death overall. Mortality rates at 30 days are nearly 23% for patients who are hospitalized for CAP, and one-year all-cause mortality in those diagnosed with CAP is 28%. Disease prevalence typically peaks in the winter months.[2]

Presenting Features

Common presentations include abrupt fever, chills, productive cough, purulent sputum, dyspnea, pleuritic chest pain, and the absence of rhinorrhea and sore throat. On exam, patients are often tachypneic and tachycardic. Common findings include coarse rales, bronchial breath sounds, focal areas of decreased breath sounds, dullness to percussion, and increased tactile fremitus. Elderly or immunocompromised patients may lack many of these characteristic symptoms and may additionally have altered mental status.[5]

Diagnostic Considerations

There is no single clinical, radiographic, or laboratory test that is sensitive or specific enough to rule CAP in or out.[1,3,4] Clinical findings that are associated with a positive chest x-ray include fever, tachycardia, tachypnea, rales, decreased breath sounds, sputum production, and absence of rhinorrhea and sore throat.[4]

The PORT score and CURB-65 are two well-validated clinical scoring systems to aid physicians in identifying low-risk patients.[6,7] Box 22.1 shows their recommendations. CURB-65 (confusion, uremia, respiratory rate, low blood pressure, age 65 years or greater) may be an efficient system to use in the emergency department.

PORT score and CURB-65 are strong predictors of low-risk patients. They are less useful for correctly identifying those who will require ICU management. To date, the best scoring systems for determining the need for early ICU admission are the 2007 Infectious Diseases Society of America/American Thoracic Society's (IDSA/ATS) minor severity criteria and the Risk of Early Admission to the Intensive Care Unit index (REA-ICU index).[8] Severity criteria are listed in Box 22.2. According to the REA-ICU index, patients should be admitted to the ICU if they have one major or three minor criteria.[1]

Historically, CAP was diagnosed as typical versus atypical. Recommendations from the 2007 IDSA/ATS guidelines state that CAP should no longer be categorized as typical versus atypical but rather as outpatient versus inpatient when evaluating patients for CAP.[1]

Typical Disease Course

Patients can present at any stage of infection, making it difficult to determine the trajectory of their clinical course during the initial assessment. Approximately 10% of admissions are directly to an ICU setting, and another 30% of non-ICU admissions will end up in the ICU during the course of hospitalization.[9]

Box 22.1 Clinical Scoring Systems: PORT Score and CURB-65

PORT Score*

Class I/II score (< 70): outpatient treatment

Class III score (71–90): observe, short admission, or outpatient management with close follow-up

Class IV score (91–130): inpatient treatment

Class V score (> 130): ICU

CURB-65 (confusion, uremia, respiratory rate, low blood pressure, age 65 years or greater)

Low risk score (0–1): outpatient treatment

Moderate risk score (2): inpatient versus outpatient management with good follow-up

Severe risk score (> 3): inpatient, consider ICU

*A full discussion of the PORT score goes beyond the scope of this chapter. Its elements and a discussion of its uses and limitations is readily available on several online calculators, including mdcalc.com.

> **Box 22.2 REA-ICU Index**
>
> Admit to the ICU if three minor or one major criteria is met.
>
> **Minor Criteria (3 required)**
>
> 1. Respiratory rate > 30 breaths/minute
> 2. PaO2/FiO2 ratio < 250
> 3. Multilobar infiltrates
> 4. Confusion/disorientation
> 5. Uremia (blood urea nitrogen > 20 mg/dL)
> 6. Leukopenia (white blood cell < 4000)
> 7. Thrombocytopenia (platelets < 100, 000)
> 8. Hypothermia (core temp < 36°C)
> 9. Hypotension requiring aggressive fluid resuscitation
>
> **Major Criteria (1 required)**
>
> Invasive mechanical ventilation
>
> Septic shock with need for vasopressors

Complications

CAP can present with significant complications, which often depend upon the infecting pathogen. Hypoxia can result from ventilation-perfusion mismatch, requiring supplemental oxygen and assisted ventilation. MRSA, anaerobes, and gram-negative bacilli can cause necrotizing pneumonia and abscess formation, which requires drainage. Bacteremia can occur and lead to sepsis and septic shock.

Diagnostic Tests

An opacity seen on imaging that represents a consolidation or segmental infiltrate is central to the diagnosis of CAP. Such findings will typically be found on posterior-anterior and lateral chest radiographs. If the chest radiograph is inconclusive, dry computed tomography (CT) scan of the chest is a more sensitive modality. CT may also be recommended when there is concern for cavitations or masses causing bronchial obstruction.

In a patient with a high clinical suspicion for CAP, but a consolidation cannot be found on imaging, empiric antibiotics should be considered. In these patients, it may be too early in the disease course to see evidence of pneumonia on initial imaging; consolidation will typically develop 1 to 2 days after admission. Other causes of false negative radiographs include neutropenia, dehydration, and *Pneumocystis jiroveci* infection.[10]

Bedside ultrasound can be utilized when chest x-ray cannot determine consolidation versus effusion. In an experienced operator's hands, lung ultrasound can achieve a sensitivity and specificity of 98% and 95%, respectively, which is better than chest x-ray when diagnosing pneumonia.[11]

There is no definitive lab test to confirm CAP, but certain laboratory tests can be helpful.[1] These include a white blood cell count, serum lactate, procalcitonin, blood cultures, sputum cultures, urine antigen tests, and rapid viral antigens.

Organisms

Microbiology

For CAP to develop, a breakdown in a patient's host defenses is typically required. Most commonly, this is due to an immunocompromised state or a recent viral illness. Other causes include exposure to a particularly virulent organism, an overwhelming inoculum, aspiration, and hematogenous spread.

Primary and secondary organisms

Several organisms are linked to CAP. The most frequent pathogens are *S. pneumoniae*, *H. influenzae*, *M. pneumoniae*, *L. pneumophila*, *C. pneumoniae*, and respiratory viruses. Less common pathogens include gram-negative bacilli, oral anaerobes, fungi, and MRSA. Very unusual and situation-specific etiologies include *Hantavirus*, *Yersinia pestis*, *Bacillus anthracis*, *Francisella tularensis*, *Chlamydia psittaci*, and *Coxiella burnetti*.

Table 22.1 Outpatient Treatment Dosage[a]

Outpatient	Medication		Dose	Route	Frequency
Healthy	Macrolides	Azithromycin	500 mg day 1, 250 mg after	PO	Daily
		Doxycycline	100 mg	PO	BID
Comorbidities	Amoxicillin/clavulanic acid PLUS azithromycin (dosed as previous)		2 g	PO	BID
	Moxifloxacin		400 mg	PO	Daily
	Levofloxacin		750 mg	PO	Daily

Abbreviations: PO, oral administration; BID, twice a day.
[a]Doses are based on normal renal and hepatic function.

Treatment[1,5,12]

Assessment of the airway, breathing, and circulation is essential. Adequate fluid resuscitation, early appropriate antibiotics, and careful attention to monitoring are still mainstays of treatment.

Patients in respiratory distress should be placed on bilevel positive airway pressure to assist gas exchange and should be intubated if they fail to improve. Markers of failure include unimproved respiratory rate, pulse oximetry, or CO_2 levels after an hour of noninvasive ventilation. Risk factors for patients who will need intubation are PaO_2/FiO_2 less than 150 and bilateral pulmonary infiltrates. When the patient is intubated, tidal volumes of 6 mL/kg of ideal body weight (acute respiratory distress syndrome protocol) is recommended. The number needed to treat with low tidal volume mechanical ventilation in CAP is nine.[1]

Outpatient: Outpatient treatment should be reserved for healthy patients and those with good follow-up. Avoiding first-line use of fluoroquinolones is recommended due to increasing resistance. Suggested regimens include using a macrolide as first line, with a minimum duration of treatment of 5 days. The patient should be afebrile for 48 to 72 hours before stopping antibiotics.[5] For more severe infections, consider adding a beta-lactam/beta-lactamase inhibitor (see Table 22.1).

Inpatient: Dual therapy and IV administration are preferred over monotherapy and oral treatment. Monotherapy and oral antibiotics should be reserved for only short, mild-moderate severity admissions. Dual therapy should also be used when there is concern for multi-drug resistant pathogens and for more severe disease[1] (see Table 22.2).

Specific Patients

Influenza A: Start treatment within 48 hours of symptom onset to decrease the duration of symptoms and the likelihood of lower respiratory complications. Treatment may be used in those presenting beyond 48 hours who are going to be hospitalized in order to decrease viral shedding in (see Table 22.3).

Aspiration: Coverage should only be added for large volume aspiration, severe gingival disease, and diminished levels of consciousness (eg, intoxication, seizure, and altered mental status). Ceftriaxone, cefepime, and moxifloxacin have adequate coverage for most oral anaerobes (see Table 22.3).

Key Considerations

Pneumonia can be a devastating disease. Prompt antibiotics and admission to the correct level of care are essential to emergency management. No single clinical finding, lab test, or diagnostic image is reliable

Table 22.2 Inpatient Treatment Dosage

Inpatient	Medication	Dose	Route	Frequency
Non-ICU	Ceftriaxone PLUS	1 g	IV	q24 h
	Azithromycin	500 mg	IV/PO	daily
PCN allergy	Moxifloxacin	400 mg	IV/PO	q24 h
	Levofloxacin	750 mg	IV/PO	q24 h
ICU	Ceftriaxone PLUS Azithromycin	1 g	IV	q24 h
	OR Moxifloxacin			

Abbreviations: ICU, intensive care unit; IV, intravenous; h, hours; PO, oral administration; PCN, penicillin.

Table 22.3 Treatment for Specific Patients				
MRSA	Linezolid	600 mg	IV/PO	q12 h
	Vancomycin	Goal trough 15–20 mcg/dL		
Influenza	Oseltamivir	75 mg	PO	BID
	Zanamivir	10 mg	inhalation	BID
Aspiration	Clindamycin	600 mg	IV	q8 h

Abbreviations: MRSA, methicillin-resistant *Staphylococcus aureus*; IV, intravenous; PO, oral administration; h, hours.

for ruling pneumonia in or out, but radiologic evidence can be extremely useful in confirming the diagnosis of CAP in immunocompetent patients. Repeat radiological studies are indicated if a patient fails to do well on appropriate therapy. Clinical decision tools like CURB-65 and PORT scores can help identify low-risk patients when making decisions about whether or not to admit.

Suggested Readings and References

1. Mandell LA, Wunderink RG, Anzueto A, et al. Infectious Diseases Society of America/American Thoracic Society consensus guidelines on the management of community-acquired pneumonia in adults. *Clin Infect Dis.* 2007;44(suppl 2):S27–S72.
2. File TM, Marrie TJ. The burden of community-acquired pneumonia in North American adults. *Postgrad Med.* 2010;122:130–141.
3. Bartlett JG. Diagnostic approach to community-acquired pneumonia in adults. Uptodateonline.com.
4. Metlay JP, Fine MJ. Testing strategies in initial management of patients with community-acquired pneumonia. *Ann Intern Med.* 2003;138:109–118.
5. Harwood-Nuss' Clinical Practice of Emergency Medicine. Chapter 73 Pneumonia.
6. Fine JF, Auble TE, et al. A prediction rule to identify low-risk patients with community-acquired pneumonia. *N Engl J Med.* 1997;336:243–250.
7. Lim WS, Baudouin SV, George RC, et al. BTS guidelines for the management of community acquired pneumonia in adults: update 2009. *Thorax.* 2009;64(suppl 3):iii1–iii55.
8. Renaud B, Labarere J, Coma E, et al. Risk stratification of early admission to the intensive care unit of patients with no major criteria of severe community-acquired pneumonia: development of an international prediction rule. *Crit Care.* 2009;13:R54.
9. Renaud B, Santin A, Coma E, et al. Association between timing of intensive care unit admission and outcomes for emergency department patients with community-acquired pneumonia. *Crit Care Med.* 2009;37:2867–2874.
10. Bartlett JG. Diagnostic tests for agents of community-acquired pneumonia. *Clin Infect Dis.* 2011;52(suppl 4):S296–S304.
11. Cortellaro F, Colombo S, Coen D, Duca PG. Lung ultrasound is an accurate diagnostic tool for the diagnosis of pneumonia in the emergency department. *Emerg Med J.* 2012;29:19–23.
12. 2012–2013 Johns Hopkins Antibiotic Guidelines Handbook.

Hospital Acquired Pneumonia

Joshua Lupton

Summary Box

Disease Description: Pneumonia consists of inflammation of the pulmonary parenchyma and is typically caused by bacteria or viruses. It is can be subdivided clinically into community-acquired pneumonia (CAP) and hospital-acquired pneumonia (HAP), which also includes health care-associated community-acquired pneumonia (HCAP) as well as ventilator-associated pneumonia (VAP).

Organisms: The most common causative organisms of CAP is *Streptococcus pneumonia*. For HAP and HCAP, the most common organism is methicillin-resistant *Staphylococcus aureus* (MRSA), but consideration should be given to other multidrug resistant bacterial organisms, including *Pseudomonas aeruginosa* and *Acinetobacter* species.

Treatment: Treatment varies between CAP, HCAP, and HAP.
  Outpatient oral first line: Azithromycin 500 mg once, 250 mg PO QD for 5 to 14 days OR
    doxycycline 100 mg PO BID for 5 to 14 days
  Inpatient oral first line: levofloxacin 750 mg PO QD for 5 to 14 days
  Inpatient parenteral first line, low drug resistance risk*: levofloxacin 750 mg IV q24 hours for
    7 to 21 days
  Inpatient parenteral first line, high drug-resistance risk: levofloxacin 750 mg IV q24 hours +
    impenem 500 mg IV q6 hours + vancomycin 15 mg/kg q12 hours for 7 to 21 days

Other Key Issues: The majority of organisms causing HCAP and HAP are multiple drug-resistant (MDR) pathogens, and treatment should be adjusted accordingly. Patients with chronic lung diseases such as Chronic Obstructive Pulmonary Disease and cystic fibrosis, or those that are immunocompromised, are at an increased risk for drug-resistant pathogens and more severe disease. Aggressive treatment and broader empirically covered treatment may be necessary in these special populations.

*Low drug resistance risk depends on geographical and patient-specific factors. Assume patients with suspected HCAP or HAP are high drug-resistance risk until culture testing confirms sensitivity.

Disease Description

Pneumonia consists of inflammation of the pulmonary parenchyma, which typically results from a microbial infection. Pneumonia is broadly classified by both the causative agent—typically bacterial, viral, or fungal—as well as by the location of acquisition: either CAP, HCAP, or HAP.

HAP is defined as a new pneumonia (not present on admission) that occurs 48 hours or more after admission to a hospital. It is associated with high mortality.

HCAP is defined as a pneumonia that is acquired from a health care facility that is not a traditional hospital setting and typically affects patients who have comorbidities. This population includes nursing home and long term care residents, patients undergoing same-day procedures, patients receiving home- or hospital-based intravenous therapy within 30 days, and patients undergoing dialysis within the prior 30 days or hospitalization for 2 or more days within the last 90 days.

The addition of HCAP category in the Infectious Diseases Society of America/American Thoracic Society (IDSA/ATS) guidelines reflects an attempt to highlight a population that may be at risk for multidrug-resistant organisms, and, as such, inclusion criteria may likely be revised in future recommendations.

Epidemiology

In the United States, pneumonia caused approximately 16.9 deaths per 100,000 people in 2013.[1]

CAP is the most common cause of infection-related death worldwide.[2] A recent systematic review concluded that the majority of CAP hospital admissions occurred in the winter (26%) and spring (34%) months compared to summer or fall.[3]

Current literature suggests that HAP is now tied with surgical site infections as the most common hospital-acquired infection in the United States, affecting an estimated 157,500 patients in the United States in 2011.[4] HAP affects nearly 1 in 15 intensive care unit (ICU) patients, making it the second most common nosocomial infection, with the vast majority thought to originate from VAP.[5] VAP is defined as a HAP that occurs 48 hours or more after endotracheal intubation; it is thought to occur in up to 20% of patients requiring greater than 48 hours of mechanical ventilation. In these patients, there is a twofold increase in mortality compared to similar patients that do not develop VAP.[6] In addition to health consequences, HAP represents significant financial costs, with VAP alone estimated to have cost the US health care system an additional $3 billion in 2012.[7]

HCAP occurs in patients that have had at least one contact with the health care system in the past 90 days typically among those residing in a long-term care facility, with regular IV therapy, with immunosuppression, or with a history of recent treatment at a hospital.[8] Aspiration is thought to be the cause of up to 30% of HCAP in patients presenting from continuing care facilities.[9]

Presenting Features

Pneumonia can present along a spectrum of disease severity, but the majority of patients with CAP or HCAP present with some constellation of cough, fever, sputum production, and pleuritic chest pain (Box 23.1).[2,10,11] Often there are rales on lung examination and infiltrate, frequently lobar, on chest x-ray.[2,10,11] These features are also apparent in HAP, but they must occur more than 48 hours after admission to a hospital (Figure 23.1).[8] More specifically, HAP is classified by the IDSA as having lung infiltrate on chest x-ray with at least two of the following: fever, leukocytosis, leukopenia, or purulent secretions. As VAP is strongly associated with mechanical ventilation, the development of a fever in a patient on mechanical ventilation for more than 48 hours should raise strong suspicion for HAP[6,8] (see Figure 23.1).

Diagnostic Tests

Laboratory tests can be of some assistance in the diagnosis of CAP; however, for approximately half of CAP cases, a definitive diagnosis cannot be made.[2] Some studies suggest that a definitive diagnosis is obtained from blood cultures for less than 10% of patients. Blood cultures, when indicated for patients

Box 23.1 Symptoms Concerning for Pneumonia
Cough
Fever
Sputum production
Pleuritic Chest pain

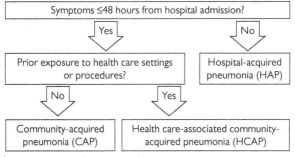

Figure 23.1 Flow-chart for determining clinical pneumonia subset.

with more severe CAP warranting hospitalization, can be useful in establishing a causative organism to target treatments. One can use clinical decision models to help determine when to obtain blood cultures, but generally these should only be done when the results are likely to alter clinical management decisions.[10]

Although blood cultures are optional for outpatient treatment of CAP, these should be conducted for anyone with suspected HCAP or HAP. For HCAP and HAP, approximately one-quarter of blood cultures are negative. For severely ill inpatients with suspected CAP, HCAP, or HAP, additional tests can include sputum culture and urinary testing for *Legionella pneumophila* and *Streptococcus pneumoniae* antigens.

Combined with traditional culturing of blood, urine, and sputum samples, polymerase-chain-reaction (PCR) techniques afford better opportunities to determine the causative organism in pneumonia. A recent study found that combining PCR detection with conventional methods improved diagnostic yield to 80% from 49.6%.[12] Although PCR is more effective in detecting pathogens (particularly viruses), a causative organism will still not be found in a significant proportion of patients. Nevertheless, given the broad causes of CAP, HCAP, and HAP, it is important for a clinician to attempt to find the causative organism in hospitalized patients, and PCR affords additional opportunities to do so. When using PCR, special care must be taken to not overlook potential concurrent infection with bacteria when the initial PCR test is positive for a virus.[11]

The IDSA requires infiltrates on chest x-ray or other imaging for the diagnosis of pneumonia.[13] The standard imaging study for diagnosing pneumonia is the chest x-ray. Computed tomography imaging is only recommended in patients with high clinical suspicion of pneumonia but with normal or nonspecific chest x-ray findings. Ultrasound by trained clinicians can have a high sensitivity (94%) and specificity (96%) at diagnosing pneumonia and may represent an alternative in the future to the chest x-ray.[14] Still, chest x-ray is the imaging of choice for confirming and monitoring pneumonia.

Organisms

The most common cause of CAP worldwide is *Streptococcus pneumoniae*.[15] Other bacterial causes of CAP include *Haemophilus influenzae*, *Staphylococcus aureus*, other *Streptococci* spp., *Mycoplasma pneumoniae*, *Legionella* species (most notably *Legionella pneumophila*), *Chlamydophila pneumoniae*, *Mycobacterium tuberculosis*, *Coxiella burnetii*, *Francisella tularensis*, *Chlamydophila psittaci*, and other gram-negative bacilli. The most common causative agent for pneumonia varies greatly by geographical region. In the United States, there is no one cause responsible for a majority of CAP.

The majority of viral CAP is caused by the influenza virus, but other viral causes of CAP include respiratory syncytial virus, parainfluenza viruses, adenovirus, *human metapneumovirus*, varicella, severe acute respiratory syndrome, and Middle East respiratory syndrome.[15] Fungal causes of CAP include histoplasmosis, coccidioidomycosis, and blastomycosis.[16]

The most common causes of HAP internationally and in the United States are MRSA (approximately one-third of HAP), methicillin-sensitive *Staphylococcus aureus* (MSSA), *Pseudomonas aeruginosa*, *Klebsiella* species, and *Enterobacter* species.[8,17] However, in half of patients with HAP, the infection is polymicrobial; in one-quarter of patients, cultures are negative.[8] MRSA is also the most common cause (up to 40%) of HCAP, with *Pseudomonas aeruginosa* and MSSA the next two most common etiologies, respectively.[8] Approximately one-third of HCAP and HAP are caused by MRSA and 10% to 20% by *Pseudomonas aeruginosa*,[8,17] necessitating broader empirical coverage to include drug-resistant organisms.

Treatment

For hospitalized patients, empiric antimicrobial therapy for HAP should be given as soon as pneumonia is suspected. Empiric treatment for HAP should be fluoroquinolone or cephalosporin if there is low risk for drug resistance (Table 23.1).[18,19] In a high-risk, drug–resistant microbial setting, which increasingly describes most US hospitals, empiric HAP therapy should include coverage for MRSA, gram-negative rods, and atypical bacteria (Table 23.1).[18] Treatment typically ranges from 7 to 21 days, although if that HAP organism is known, treatment length can be reduced as appropriate. It is important to consistently assess the clinical response to treatment for HAP. Temperature, oxygenation, and organ function should improve after 48 to 72 hours of treatment.[18] White blood cell counts and chest x-rays should also show improvement in this time frame.

The first step in the treatment of patients with acute CAP is to decide appropriate disposition.[10] Several published guidelines help score pneumonia severity, including the Pneumonia Severity Index, the CURB-65 score, SMART-COP, and guidelines from the IDSA.[13] In short, if a patient has septic shock or respiratory failure requiring mechanical ventilation, they should be directly admitted to the ICU. According to a 2009 cohort study of 453 adults, delayed transfer to the ICU resulted in twice the mortality (23.4% vs 11.7%) compared to direct ICU transfer.[20]

The second step is to determine the likely causative organism of the CAP. If the presenting symptoms suggest an uncomplicated bacterial cause, then first-line treatment is empirical antimicrobial therapy.[13] If severity is mild and the patient can be treated in the outpatient setting, empiric therapy is usually all that is needed, and the specific causative organism need not be determined. The IDSA's guidelines recommend a macrolide or doxycycline as the first-line therapy for outpatient CAP treatment (Table 23.2). For hospitalized patients, including those in the ICU, initial empiric therapy with a quinolone or a combination of a beta-lactam and a macrolide are the first-line therapeutic recommendations from the IDSA (Table 23.2).[13] Although duration of antibiotic therapy is under debate, it is generally accepted to treat empirically for a minimum of 5 days and no more than 14 days.[11] Evidence suggests that treatment durations longer than 7 days are no more effective at curing the infection than treatment for 7 days or less.[21,22]

If the presenting symptoms suggest an uncomplicated viral cause, then first-line treatment is either symptom management or oseltamivir. This distinction depends on the prevalence of influenza in the community and the results of any PCR tests. If influenza is common, then empiric oseltamivir is most appropriate. Additionally, oseltamivir should be considered in patients with non-viral CAP, HCAP, or HAP if there are symptoms of influenza or concern for influenza infection.[11]

First-line empiric treatment for inpatient CAP is either a respiratory fluoroquinolone or the combination of a macrolide and a beta-lactam like azithromycin. If *Pseudomonas aeruginosa* is suspected or confirmed, an antipseudomonal beta-lactam should be given with a fluoroquinolone. The duration of inpatient antimicrobial treatment should be at least 5 days. For patients presenting with suspected HCAP, there should be a higher clinical suspicion for MRSA. In this instance, vancomycin or linezolid should be added to the preceding empirical treatment regimens for hospitalized CAP patients (see Table 23.2).[10]

Other Key Issues

Patients that have diseases or conditions that weaken the immune system or pulmonary function are at increased risk for pneumonia. Of note, patients with Chronic Obstructive Pulmonary Disease, cystic fibrosis, or those who are immunocompromised are at an increased risk for developing CAP, HCAP, or HAP caused by *Pseudomonas aeruginosa, Haemophilus influenzae, Klebsiella pneumoniae,* and *Moraxella*

Table 23.1 Treatment of HCAP and HAP	
Low Risk for Drug Resistance	High Risk for Drug Resistance
Levofloxacin	Low-risk regimen
750 mg IV q24 h	—PLUS—
7–10 days	Impenem
—OR—	500 mg IV q6 h
Ceftriaxone	PLUS
1–2 g IV qd	Vancomycin
7–10 days	15 mg/kg q12 h
	7–21 days

Abbreviations: IV, intravenous; h, hours; qd, every day.

Table 23.2 Treatment of CAP	
Outpatient Treatment	Inpatient Treatment
Azithromycin	Levofloxacin
500 mg PO day 1	750 mg PO qd
250 mg PO qd	5–14 days
5–14 days	—OR—
—OR—	Amoxicillin
Doxycycline	1g PO TID
100 mg PO BID	5–14 days
5–14 days	—PLUS—
	Outpatient regimen

Abbreviations: PO, oral administration; qd, every day; TID, three times a day; BID, two times a day.

catarrhalis. For empirical treatment of pneumonia in this patient population, antimicrobials with activity against beta-lactamase producing organisms should be given.[10] If *Pseudomonas aeruginosa* is suspected, switching to two drugs in the antipseudomonal beta-lactam class or carbapenem is recommended by the IDSA.[13]

There is currently a vaccine available against *Streptococcus pneumonia,* and all patients should be offered this vaccine before discharge from the hospital.[10] However, despite the use of this vaccine, *Streptococcus pneumonia* is still the number one causative organism of CAP and should remain high on the differential diagnosis of patients presenting with suspected CAP.

Pneumonia may also present differently in the elderly, who are already more susceptible to CAP, HCAP, and HAP due to decreased mobility and increased comorbidities. Additionally, the CAP admission guideline scores for severity are not as appropriate in the elderly.[23] In elderly patients with comorbidities presenting from the community, clinicians must have a high suspicion for HCAP given the patients' likely increased exposure to health care.

Suggested Readings and References

1. Centers for Disease Control. *Deaths: Final data for 2013.* 2014;64(2).

2. Remington LT, Sligl WI. Community-acquired pneumonia. *Curr Opin Pulm Med.* 2014;20:215–224.

3. Murdoch KM, Mitra B, Lambert S, Erbas B. What is the seasonal distribution of community acquired pneumonia over time? A systematic review. *Australas Emerg Nurs J.* 2014;17:30–42.

4. Magill SS, Edwards JR, Bamberg W, et al. Multistate point-prevalence survey of health care-associated infections. *N Engl J Med.* 2014;370:1198–1208.

5. Alp E, Guven M, Yildiz O, Aygen B, Voss A, Doganay M. Incidence, risk factors and mortality of nosocomial pneumonia in intensive care units: A prospective study. *Ann Clin Microbiol Antimicrob.* 2004;3:17.

6. Safdar N, Dezfulian C, Collard HR, Saint S. Clinical and economic consequences of ventilator-associated pneumonia: a systematic review. *Crit Care Med.* 2005;33:2184–2193.

7. Zimlichman E, Henderson D, Tamir O, et al. Health care-associated infections: A meta-analysis of costs and financial impact on the US health care system. *JAMA Intern Med.* 2013;173:2039–2046.

8. Quartin AA, Scerpella EG, Puttagunta S, Kett DH. A comparison of microbiology and demographics among patients with healthcare-associated, hospital-acquired, and ventilator-associated pneumonia: A retrospective analysis of 1184 patients from a large, international study. *BMC Infect Dis.* 2013;13:561.

9. Reza Shariatzadeh M, Huang JQ, Marrie TJ. Differences in the features of aspiration pneumonia according to site of acquisition: community or continuing care facility. *J Am Geriatr Soc.* 2006;54:296–302.

10. Watkins RR, Lemonovich TL. Diagnosis and management of community-acquired pneumonia in adults. *Am Fam Physician.* 2011;83:1299–1306.

11. Musher DM, Thorner AR. Community-acquired pneumonia. *N Engl J Med.* 2014;371:1619–1628.

12. Huijskens EG, Rossen JW, Kluytmans JA, van der Zanden AG, Koopmans M. Evaluation of yield of currently available diagnostics by sample type to optimize detection of respiratory pathogens in patients with a community-acquired pneumonia. *Influenza Other Respir Viruses.* 2014;8:243–249.

13. Mandell LA, Wunderink RG, Anzueto A, et al. Infectious diseases society of America/American Thoracic Society consensus guidelines on the management of community-acquired pneumonia in adults. *Clin Infect Dis.* 2007;44(suppl 2):S27–72.

14. Hu QJ, Shen YC, Jia LQ, et al. Diagnostic performance of lung ultrasound in the diagnosis of pneumonia: a bivariate meta-analysis. *Int J Clin Exp Med.* 2014;7:115–121.

15. Johansson N, Kalin M, Tiveljung-Lindell A, Giske CG, Hedlund J. Etiology of community-acquired pneumonia: increased microbiological yield with new diagnostic methods. *Clin Infect Dis.* 2010;50:202–209.

16. Valdivia L, Nix D, Wright M, et al. Coccidioidomycosis as a common cause of community-acquired pneumonia. *Emerg Infect Dis.* 2006;12:958–962.

17. Jones RN. Microbial etiologies of hospital-acquired bacterial pneumonia and ventilator-associated bacterial pneumonia. *Clin Infect Dis.* 2010;51(suppl 1):S81–87.

18. American Thoracic Society, Infectious Diseases Society of America. Guidelines for the management of adults with hospital-acquired, ventilator-associated, and healthcare-associated pneumonia. *Am J Respir Crit Care Med.* 2005;171:388–416.

19. Wilke M, Grube R. Update on management options in the treatment of nosocomial and ventilator assisted pneumonia: review of actual guidelines and economic aspects of therapy. *Infect Drug Resist.* 2013;7:1–7.

20. Renaud B, Santin A, Coma E, et al. Association between timing of intensive care unit admission and outcomes for emergency department patients with community-acquired pneumonia. *Crit Care Med.* 2009;37:2867–2874.

21. Li JZ, Winston LG, Moore DH, Bent S. Efficacy of short-course antibiotic regimens for community-acquired pneumonia: a meta-analysis. *Am J Med.* 2007;120:783–790.

22. Havey TC, Fowler RA, Daneman N. Duration of antibiotic therapy for bacteremia: a systematic review and meta-analysis. *Crit Care.* 2011;15:R267.

23. Simonetti AF, Viasus D, Garcia-Vidal C, Carratala J. Management of community-acquired pneumonia in older adults. *Ther Adv Infect Dis.* 2014;2:3–16.

Chapter 24

Pleural Effusions (Parapneumonic Process and Empyema)

Timothy Niessen

Summary Box

Disease Description: Pleural effusions occur when an influx of fluid into the pleural space exceeds its removal. An exudative effusion results from leaky barriers and is often associated with infections. Parapneumonic effusions are exudative pleural effusions adjacent to pulmonary infections.

Organisms: Streptococci, Staphylococci, gram-negative bacilli, and anaerobes are common organisms.

Treatment:
- Empiric therapy is typically directed at both *Streptococcus pneumoniae* and anaerobes:
  - ampicillin-sulbactam 1.5 to 3 g IV every 6 hours OR
  - ceftriaxone 2 g/day IV plus metronidazole 500 mg IV or PO every 8 hours
- Severe disease (broaden coverage to also include methicillin-resistant *Staphylococcus aureus* [MRSA] and *Pseudomonas aeruginosa*):
  - vancomycin 15 mg/kg IV every 12 hours OR
  - linezolid 600 mg IV or orally twice daily
    - PLUS either
  - cefepime 1–2 g every 8–12 hours plus metronidazole 500 mg IV or orally every 8 hours OR
  - meropenem 1 g IV every 8 hours

Diagnostic tests: Chest imaging, thoracentesis (pleural fluid examination)

Treatment: For parapneumonic process, antibiotic selection is similar but distinct for pneumonia due to the acidic and hypoxic environment of the pleural environment. In some cases, after antibiotic therapy and thoracentesis has been initiated, surgical intervention may be necessary: tube thoracostomy, video-assisted thoracoscopic surgery (VATS), open decortications, and open thoracostomy.

Other Key Issues: Approximately 15% of patients with pleural effusions are without a diagnosis even after an exhaustive workup.

Box 24.1 Light's Criteria for Exudative Effusions
Pleural fluid protein / serum protein > 0.5
or
Pleural fluid lactate dehydrogenase (LDH) / serum LDH > 0.6
or
Pleural fluid LDH > two-thirds upper limit of normal serum LDH

In health, a very small volume of fluid occupies the space between the visceral and parietal pleura of the lung. Pleural effusion occurs when an influx of fluid into this pleural space exceeds its removal. Fluid may accumulate due to impaired clearance by the pleural lymphatic system or due transudative or exudative processes. Transudative effusions typically result from a change in oncotic forces (eg, such as occurs in congestive heart failure, cirrhosis, or nephrotic syndrome). Exudative effusions occur as a consequence of leaky barriers, such as those associated with pulmonary infections, malignancy, pulmonary embolism, or inflammation. Light's criteria can help distinguish transudative from exudative effusions (Box 24.1).[1]

A parapneumonic effusion is an accumulation of exudative fluid in the setting of pneumonia, lung abscess, or bronchiectasis. Parapneumonic effusions are common, occurring in 20% to 57% of bacterial pneumonias.[2,3,4] Risk factors for parapneumonic effusion include chronic lung disease, immune compromise, gastroesophageal reflux disease, intravenous drug use, alcoholism, malnutrition, aspiration, and thoracic or esophageal procedures.[5,6] Most parapneumonic effusions are sterile and resolve with treatment of the underlying pneumonia. However, when inadequately treated, they may evolve through the exudative, fibrinopurulent, and organizing phases of empyema formation. With treatment, empyema has a mortality of 22% and substantial associated morbidity reflected by prolonged hospitalization, persistent sepsis, and respiratory embarrassment.[7] With the increasing incidence of empyema from 1996–2008 from 3.04 to 5.98 per 100,000 people, early identification and drainage of infected pleural effusions remains important.[8]

The symptoms of a parapneumonic effusion are variable and nonspecific. They may include persistent cough, dyspnea, pleuritic chest pain, fever, weight loss, anorexia, and malaise. Distinguishing these symptoms from the primary focus of infection may be difficult. More indolent presentations may suggest anaerobic infection, particularly in those with risk factors for aspiration. Findings of dullness to percussion, decreased breath sounds, decreased fremitus, and asymmetric chest expansion suggest effusion but are inadequate to diagnose or exclude concurrent pleural effusion.[9] The standard posterior-anterior and lateral chest x-ray may demonstrate effusions larger than 200 cc. The lateral decubitus view is more sensitive for small effusions; it is also useful to determine size and to confirm that the fluid is free flowing. Chest ultrasound may detect effusions as small as 5 cc and can further characterize effusions based on echogenicity to help delineate septations thereby facilitating thoracentesis.[10] Chest CT with contrast may be required to fully evaluate loculated effusions. Chest CT helps also allows for better evaluation of the lung pleura (for thickening or nodularity), lung parenchyma, and mediastinum. The "split pleurae sign," pleural thickening and enhancement, and attenuation of the extrapleural subcostal fat are radiographic features that distinguish pleural infection from a peripheral pulmonary abscess. The role of magnetic resonance imaging and positron emission tomography imaging of parapneumonic effusions is not clearly defined.[11]

Most parapneumonic effusions should be sampled by thoracentesis, although a free-flowing effusion that is less than 10 mm on a lateral decubitus film may be clinically monitored.[12] Ultrasound guidance increases successful fluid aspiration while decreasing complications and is recommended. Diagnostic studies should include pleural fluid and serum total protein, lactate dehydrogenase (LDH) glucose, pH, cell counts, gram stain and culture (aerobic and anaerobic) as well as additional cultures (mycobacterial, fungal) and cytology as indicated. Bedside inoculation of infected pleural fluid into blood culture bottles increases diagnostic yield.[13] Peripheral blood cultures should also be obtained and are positive in as many as 15% of cases and may be the only culture data available to guide therapy.

Parapneumonic pleural effusions can be stratified by risk for poor outcome according to imaging and laboratory criteria ranging from very low-risk, simple effusion to high-risk, complex empyema (Table 24.1).[14,15] A typical parapneumonic effusion is sterile, has a normal glucose and pH, and is likely to resolve with treatment of the underlying infection. Complicated parapneumonic effusions reflect bacterial invasion into the pleural space and are identified when the effusion is large, loculated, and associated with thickened pleura; the pleural fluid pH is low (< 7.2), glucose is low (<60), or LDH is

Table 24.1 Categorizing Risk for Poor Outcome in Patients with Parapneumonic Pleural Effusion[a]

Pleural Space Anatomy			Pleural Fluid Bacteriology			Pleural Fluid Chemistry[b]		Category	Risk of Poor Outcome	Drainage
A_0	Minimal, free-flowing effusion (< 1cm on lateral decubitus)[c]	AND	B_x	unknown	AND	C_x	pH unknown	1	Very low	No
A_1	Small to moderate free-flowing effusions (> 1 cm and < ½ hemithorax)	AND	B_0	negative	AND	C_0	pH ≥ 7.20	2	Low	No
A_2	Large, free-flowing effusion (≥ ½ hemithorax), or loculated effusion, or effusion with thickened parietal pleura	OR	B_1	positive	OR	C_1	pH < 7.20	3	Moderate	Yes
			B_2	frank pus				4	High	Yes

Abbreviations: P, pleural fluid glucose; B, bacteriology, C, chemistry.

[a]Chest, 2000 rubric.

[b]pH determined using a blood gas analyzer is the preferred pleural fluid chemistry test. If unavailable, pleural fluid glucose should be used (P_0 ≥ 60 mg/dL; P_1 glucose < 60 mg/dL).

[c]Effusions of this size do not require thoracentesis for evaluation and are likely to resolve.

elevated (> 1000 units/L). In some cases, the effusion may be culture or gram-stain positive, but frank pus will not be aspirated. Complicated parapneumonic effusions generally require drainage. Several noninfectious causes of effusions such as malignancy, lupus, and rheumatoid pleurisy can masquerade as a complicated parapneumonic effusion.

Empyema occurs when frank pus occupies the pleural space and requires drainage. Causative pathogens are identified in only 60% of clinically infected pleural fluid samples due to sampling error, exposure to antibiotics prior to sampling, and difficulty in culturing causative organisms.[5,7] A positive gram stain or culture is not required to diagnose empyema.

The microbiologic causes of empyema are similar to but distinct from underlying bacterial pneumonia due to the acidic and hypoxic of the empyema. Anaerobic infection is important and has been identified in as many as 76% of cases.[16] The bacteriology of community-acquired infection differs from hospital-acquired infection. In one experimental cohort MIST1 (First Multicenter Intrapleural Sepsis Trial) (REF 7 below). cohort, culture and ribosomal RNA sequencing revealed that community acquired pleural infections were most frequently due to streptococcal infection (*S. pneumonia*, 21%; *S. intermedius* group, 24%; *S. pyogenes*, 3%; other streptococci species, 5%). Anaerobic infections—including Fusobacterium, *Bacteroides, Peptostreptococcus, Prevotella* spp., *Clostridium* spp., or mixed anaerobes—were identified in 20% of samples. Gram-negative bacilli (9%) and *Staphylococcus aureus* (8%) were also common. Although important respiratory pathogens, there was no evidence of *Mycoplasma* spp. or *Legionella* spp. in this study of pleural effusions. The bacteriology of hospital-acquired infections revealed more frequent *Staphylococci* (35%) and gram-negative organisms (23%) as well as increased antibiotic resistance (40%).[6] Mycobacterial infection was found in 9% at one center and is an easily overlooked but important cause of empyema. Tuberculous pleural disease should be considered if risk factors are present.[5] Mycobacterial stains and cultures from pleural fluid are notoriously insensitive; a high index of suspicion and pleural biopsy is often required to confirm tuberculous pleural disease. Fungal empyema remains rare but may be an emerging cause with especially poor outcomes.

Antibiotic selection should target the underlying infectious organism according to culture and susceptibility results. Initial empiric therapy should take into account local antibiotic policies, resistance patterns, and, importantly, should include anaerobic coverage.[12] Empiric therapy often includes beta-lactams with beta lactamase inhibitors (ampicillin-sulbactam 1.5 to 3 g IV every 6 hours); cephalosporins (cefotaxime, 1 to 2 g every 8 hours IV or IM); or ceftriaxone, 1 to 2 g IV q24 hours in combination with metronidazole 500 mg IV or PO, carbapenems (meropenem 1 g IV every 8 hours), or clindamycin. Aminoglycosides should be avoided because they poorly penetrate the pleural space and are not active in acidic environments. In patients with penicillin allergy, clindamycin in combination with ciprofloxacin or a cephalosporin can be considered. Macrolide antibiotics are not routinely required. Hospital-acquired infections or cases with high suspicion for MRSA infection should include vancomycin or similar coverage for antibiotic-resistant *Staphylococci* until culture and sensitivity results are known. Parenteral therapy may be transitioned to oral therapy when drainage is achieved and hemodynamics have normalized. Goals of therapy are to sterilize the pleural space, to evacuate loculations, and to achieve adequate lung expansion. The optimal duration is not well defined and is tailored to the clinical scenario with organism sensitivity, clinical response, extent of disease, adequacy of drainage, and immune status. Courses range from 2 to 6 weeks from the time of drainage.

Timely drainage of complicated parapneumonic effusions or empyema is critical. Options for drainage include serial thoracentesis, tube thoracostomy, VATS, open decortications, and open thoracostomy.[12,17] Although large bore chest tubes have traditionally been favored due to concerns that smaller tubes are more easily occluded, small bore chest tubes (< 14F) cause less discomfort without significantly affecting outcomes.[18] Regular flushing of the smaller bore tubes may prevent occlusion. Intrapleural instillation of fibrinolytic and mucolytic agents may improve pleural drainage and reduce surgical intervention, although the use of fibrinolytics in adults has been controversial.[7,19] Early consultation with thoracic surgery for patients failing antibiotic therapy and chest tube drainage is warranted, especially for those patients with persistent sepsis and residual pleural collections.

Suggested Readings and References

1. Light RW, Macgregor MI, Luchsinger PC, Ball WC. Pleural effusions: the diagnostic separation of transudates and exudates. *Ann Intern Med.* 1972;77:507–513.

2. Light RW, Girard WM, Jenkinson SG, George RB. Parapneumonic effusions. *Am J Med.* 1980;69:507–512.

3. Taryle DA, Potts DE, Sahn SA. The incidence and clinical correlates of parapneumonic effusions in pneumococcal pneumonia. *Chest.* 1978;74:170–173.

4. Fine NL, Smith LR, Sheedy PF. Frequency of pleural effusions in mycoplasma and viral pneumonias. *N Engl J Med.* 1970;283:790–793. doi:10.1056/NEJM197010082831505.

5. Marks DJB, Fisk MD, Koo CY, et al. Thoracic empyema: a 12-year study from a UK tertiary cardiothoracic referral centre. *PLoS ONE.* 2012;7:e30074. doi:10.1371/journal.pone.0030074.

6. Maskell NA, Batt S, Hedley EL, Davies CWH, Gillespie SH, Davies RJO. The bacteriology of pleural infection by genetic and standard methods and its mortality significance. *Am J Respir Crit Care Med.* 2006;174:817–823. doi:10.1164/rccm.200601-074OC.

7. Maskell NA, Davies CWH, Nunn AJ, et al. U.K. Controlled trial of intrapleural streptokinase for pleural infection. *N Engl J Med.* 2005;352:865–874. doi:10.1056/NEJMoa042473.

8. Grijalva CG, Zhu Y, Nuorti JP, Griffin MR. Emergence of parapneumonic empyema in the USA. *Thorax.* 2011;66:663–668. doi:10.1136/thx.2010.156406.

9. Wong CL, Holroyd-Leduc J, Straus SE. Does this patient have a pleural effusion? *JAMA.* 2009;301:309–317. doi:10.1001/jama.2008.937.

10. Tsai T-H, Yang P-C. Ultrasound in the diagnosis and management of pleural disease. *Curr Opin Pulm Med.* 2003;9:282–290.

11. Heffner JE, Klein JS, Hampson C. Diagnostic utility and clinical application of imaging for pleural space infections. *Chest.* 2010;137:467–479. doi:10.1378/chest.08-3002.

12. Davies HE, Davies RJO, Davies CWH, BTS Pleural Disease Guideline Group. Management of pleural infection in adults: British Thoracic Society Pleural Disease Guideline 2010. *Thorax.* 2010;65(suppl 2):ii41–53. doi:10.1136/thx.2010.137000.

13. Menzies SM, Rahman NM, Wrightson JM, et al. Blood culture bottle culture of pleural fluid in pleural infection. *Thorax.* 2011;66:658–662. doi:10.1136/thx.2010.157842.

14. Light RW. A new classification of parapneumonic effusions and empyema. *Chest.* 1995;108:299–301.

15. Colice GL, Curtis A, Deslauriers J, et al. Medical and surgical treatment of parapneumonic effusions: an evidence-based guideline. *Chest.* 2000;118:1158–1171.

16. Bartlett JG, Gorbach SL, Thadepalli H, Finegold SM. Bacteriology of empyema. *Lancet.* 1974;1(7853):338–340.

17. Corcoran JP, Hallifax R, Rahman NM. New therapeutic approaches to pleural infection. *Curr Opin Infect Dis.* 2013;26:196–202. doi:10.1097/QCO.0b013e32835d0b71.

18. Rahman NM, Maskell NA, Davies CWH, et al. The relationship between chest tube size and clinical outcome in pleural infection. *Chest.* 2010;137:536–543. doi:10.1378/chest.09-1044.

19. Rahman NM, Maskell NA, West A, et al. Intrapleural use of tissue plasminogen activator and DNase in pleural infection. *N Engl J Med.* 2011;365:518–526. doi:10.1056/NEJMoa1012740.

Lung Abscess

Kevin Gibbs

Summary Box

Disease Description: A lung abscess is a circumscribed collection of necrotic lung paren-chyma that typically presents with subacute pulmonary symptoms.

Organisms:
  Oral anaerobes
  Microaerophilic *Streptococcus* spp.
  Staphylococcus aureus
  Klebsiella pneumoniae
  Pseudomonas aeruginosa

Treatment:
  Oral first line: Clindamycin
  Second line: Amoxicillin-clavulanate, moxifloxacin
  Parenteral: Clindamycin, beta-lactam/beta-lactamase inhibitor, carbapenems

Other Key Issues: Indications for percutaneous drainage or surgery include large cavity size (greater than 6 cm), highly resistant organisms, failure to respond to antibiotics, or life-threatening hemoptysis.

Disease Description

Epidemiology

Lung abscesses are intraparenchymal collections of purulent and necrotic tissue caused by infectious organisms. These typically polymicrobial abscesses have decreased in frequency in the modern antibiotic era. However, despite the widespread use of antimicrobial therapies, mortality from lung abscess remains high (10%–20%). Lung abscesses are classified as either primary or secondary based on etiology. Primary abscesses, which represent approximately 80% of all cases, occur in the setting of normal lung parenchyma and intact host immune defenses. In contrast, secondary abscesses arise in the setting of predisposing conditions, such as immunosuppression or bronchial obstruction. Lung abscesses can further be subdivided by chronicity. Abscesses present for less than one month are classified as acute, whereas those lasting more than one month are chronic.

Primary lung abscess is classically a disease of middle-aged men with a 5:1 male to female ratio. It occurs most commonly in the fifth and sixth decades of life. Infection and subsequent abscess formation result from large volume aspiration of oral secretions. Therefore, conditions that predispose to aspiration also predispose to lung abscess. Such conditions include all causes of depressed sensorium (with alcohol intoxication being the most common cause) as well as both mechanical and neurologic causes of dysphagia. The burden of oral anaerobes also plays an important role in disease pathogenesis. Individuals with poor dentition have higher oral anaerobe concentrations within the gingival margin, increasing both the size of the inoculum when aspiration occurs and the subsequent risk of lung abscess formation. The importance of dentition in lung abscess is underscored by the observation that edentulous patients have a lower incidence of aspiration pneumonia and lung abscess.

Diagnosis

On clinical grounds alone, it can be difficult to differentiate a lung abscess from pneumonia. Patients with lung abscess typically have a longer duration of symptoms (on average, 14 days with abscess versus 3 days with pneumonia). Patients with lung abscess generally appear less acutely ill and have fewer rigors or shaking chills. However, both groups can present with high fevers and cough. Chest radiography is critical in distinguishing lung abscess from pneumonia. In the former, chest radiographs will show a cavitary lung lesion with an air-fluid level, usually in a dependent distribution (superior segment of the lower lobes or posterior segments of the upper lobes). Chest computed tomography (CT) provides additional meaningful data and should be obtained if the chest radiograph is suggestive of abscess. CT can help distinguish an abscess from a cavitary mass or pleural-based process and can identify coexisting infectious complications, such as empyema. Additionally, CT scan can provide prognostic information because larger abscess volumes and right lower lobe location may portend worse outcomes.

Typical Disease Course

Patients with lung abscesses typically have a subacute course of symptoms. An aspiration event leads to inoculation, infection, and subsequent polymicrobial pneumonia. Symptomatic individuals who present for medical care early in their course respond well to community-acquired pneumonia therapies. If the infection remains untreated, however, the individual can go on to develop a necrotizing infection and abscess (typically one week after the aspiration event). Once formed, abscesses cause both systemic and pulmonary symptoms. Pulmonary complaints predominately involve cough and purulent sputum production. The classic finding of particularly foul-smelling sputum occurs in 50% of cases. Constitutive symptoms include fever, leukocytosis, night sweats, weight loss, and malaise.

Complications

Hemoptysis (due to bronchial artery neoangiogenesis and breakdown in the abscess wall) and pleuritis may also be present. Empyema (which occurs in 30% of cases) represents the major complication of lung abscess. Constitutive symptoms include fever, leukocytosis, night sweats, weight loss, and malaise.

Organisms

Oral anaerobes cause the majority of primary lung abscesses, accounting for 80% to 100% of cases in observational series (with the notable exception of cases reported in Taiwan, where *Klebsiella* is the dominant organism). Abscesses are typically polymicrobial, with *Peptostreptococcus*, microaerophilic *Streptococcus*, *Bacteroides*, and *Prevotella* species all being frequent isolates. Monomicrobial abscesses can develop due to virulent strains of traditional pathogens, such as S. *aureus*, *Klebsiella*, and *Pseudomonas*, but these are comparatively rare. The preponderance of anaerobic pathogens poses a significant diagnostic challenge for microbiological diagnosis. Moreover, traditional sputum cultures are ineffective for isolating anaerobes. Percutaneous and transtracheal aspirations have historically been performed, but these techniques are neither routinely available nor clinically feasible.

Treatment

Because culture data is lacking from most lung abscesses, antibiotic therapy must be empiric, and changes in treatment regimens must be dictated by clinical symptoms. Clindamycin has been effective in multiple small-scale studies for the treatment of lung abscess and is the first-line therapy for abscess treatment. For outpatients, clindamycin 150 to 300 mg orally every 6 hours is the preferred regimen. Amoxicillin/clavulanate and moxifloxacin are reasonable alternatives in patients intolerant of clindamycin because both agents have adequate in vitro anaerobe coverage and in vivo clinical experience to support their use. In contrast to the aforementioned agents, metronidazole has proven particularly ineffective in treating lung abscesses, likely due to inadequate streptococcal coverage, so it should not be used as monotherapy. In hospitalized patients, a regimen of clindamycin 600 mg intravenous every 8 hours is appropriate. Patients at high risk for nosocomial pathogens (particularly *Pseudomonas*) may warrant empiric coverage with antipseudomonal agents that also have broad anaerobe coverage, such as certain carbapenems or piperacillin/tazobactam, until aerobic cultures have returned. Once the patient has clinically improved, the individual may be transitioned to an oral regimen. On appropriate regimens, patients typically demonstrate clinical improvement within days of initiating therapy. Prolonged symptoms or signs of ongoing infection are concerning for antibiotic treatment failure.

The duration of antibiotic therapy for lung abscess remains somewhat controversial. Recommendations vary from 3 weeks to longer courses based on clinical improvement and radiographic resolution of the abscess cavity. Although no clear consensus exists, lung abscess treatment is extended beyond the courses typical of other bacterial lung infections.

Other Key Issues

The role for invasive drainage also remains poorly elucidated. Options for drainage include CT-guided percutaneous procedures, endoscopically placed drains, and surgical resection (the latter of which was the historical treatment for lung abscess before antibiotics). Drainage and/or surgery should be considered in cases of antibiotic failure, life-threatening hemoptysis, large cavity diameter (greater than 6 cm), or highly resistant organisms. Surgical candidacy depends on the patient's functional status, comorbidities, and ability to tolerate lung resection.

Summary
Lung abscesses are a relatively rare pulmonary infection predominately caused by aspiration of oral anaerobes. These infections are typically polymicrobial and difficult to accurately culture, requiring empiric therapy with antibiotics with broad anaerobic coverage. Most patients respond well to antimicrobials, but mortality remains high in the subset who fails medical therapy.

Suggested Readings and References

Bartlett JG. Anaerobic bacterial infections of the lung. *Anaerobe* 18;2012:235–239.

Bartlett JG, Gorbach SL. Treatment of aspiration pneumonia and lung abscess. *JAMA* 1975 Dec 1;1234(9):935–937.

Desai H, Agrawal A. Pulmonary emergencies: pneumonia, acute respiratory distress syndrome, lung abscess, and empyema. *Med Clin N Am* 2012;96:1127–1148.

Hirshberg B, Sklair-Levi M, Nir-Paz R, Ben-Sira L, Krivoruk V, Kramer MR. Factors predicting mortality of patients with lung abscess. *Chest* 1999;115:746–750.

Yazbeck MF, Dahdel M, Kalra A, BZrowne AS, Pratter MR. Lung abscess: Update on microbiology and management. *Am J Ther* 2014 May–Jun;21(3):217–221.

Chapter 26

Influenza

Gabrielle Jacquet and Andrea Dugas

Summary Box

Disease Description: Influenza is a highly contagious acute viral infection. It is transmitted via respiratory droplets and hand to eye/nose/mouth contact.

Organisms: Type A, B, and C RNA *Orthomyxoviridae*

Treatment: Illness is self-limiting in a vast majority of cases. Supportive treatment is indicated. Antivirals are warranted in patient populations who have or at high risk of severe disease or influenza-related complications.

Other Key Issues: Infection control and preventing transmission to other patients and health care workers in the emergency department

Disease Description

Influenza is a viral syndrome caused by a highly contagious viral infection. Whereas most cases result in acute febrile respiratory symptoms and are self-limited, substantial morbidity and mortality can result in susceptible populations, including patients who are at the extremes of age (less than 2 or greater than 64 years of age), have chronic medical conditions, or are immunocompromised, pregnant, residing in a nursing home, obese, or of Native American dissent.

Epidemiology

Influenza is believed to be responsible for over 200,000 hospitalizations and up to 50,000 associated all-cause deaths within the United States each year. Outbreaks emerge in a seasonal distribution with a marked increase in the winter months. There is substantial year to year variability with increased morbidity and mortality during severe epidemics or pandemics.

The early recognition of influenza by providers in is paramount for reducing morbidity and mortality and for preventing transmission to other patients and health care personnel.

Presenting Features and Complications

General Features: Influenza typically presents as a sudden onset illness with respiratory symptoms as well as fever, rigors, malaise, myalgia, and/or fatigue.

Cardiovascular Manifestations: The most common cardiovascular manifestation of influenza is tachycardia; however, influenza has also been associated with additional cardiovascular complications, such as myocardial infarction and heart failure.

Pulmonary Manifestations: Influenza most commonly presents with respiratory symptoms from either the upper or lower respiratory system. Cough, rhinorrhea, sore throat, and shortness of breath are common. Influenza can lead to lower airway disease, such as a viral pneumonia or lead to superimposed bacterial lung infections (classically, MRSA pneumonia). Additionally, influenza infection can exacerbate symptoms of preexisting respiratory illness, including chronic obstructive pulmonary disease (COPD) and asthma.

Renal Manifestations: Rhabdomyolysis and acute renal failure have been documented in cases of influenza, but this is not common.

Hematologic Manifestations: Leukopenia and relative lymphopenia are common but nonspecific laboratory findings.

Neurologic Manifestations: Influenza commonly presents with a headache and generalized fatigue. The main neurologic complication of influenza is a viral encephalopathy.

Gastrointestinal Manifestations: Anorexia, nausea, and vomiting are common with influenza infection and are more likely in the pediatric population and those infected with influenza B.

Diagnostic Considerations and Tests

Definitions: The United States Centers for Disease Control (CDC) has created a case definition for influenza-like illness (ILI) that is used in conjunction with the agency's extensive surveillance programs (see Box 26.1). Although useful as a case definition and critical to surveillance efforts, this set of symptoms is not sufficient for diagnosis and has a poor diagnostic sensitivity. Despite numerous attempts, there are not a clear set of symptoms that may be used to reliably diagnose influenza.

Diagnostic Tests: There are several diagnostic tests available for influenza. Viral culture or reverse transcription polymerase chain reaction (RT-PCR) have the highest sensitivity and specificity; however, they take several hours to days to complete, reducing their usefulness in the ED setting. There are several options for rapid influenza tests. There are more than 10 rapid antigen-based tests approved by the US Food and Drug Administration (FDA). They differ in their ability to distinguish between influenza A and B viruses and in their ability to work with different specimen types (eg, throat swab vs nasal swab) as well as in their sensitivity and specificity. Based on the influenza type, these antigen-based rapid tests have poor sensitivity, ranging from 10% to 70%, with good specificity (90%–95%) when compared to RT-PCR. Similar to the rapid antigen-based tests, there are several options for direct immunofluorescence assays (DFA), which have slightly improved sensitivity (50%–80%) but a longer turnaround time. Given the poor

---

Box 26.1 Definition of Influenza-Like Illness (ILI)

- Temperature ≥ 37.8°C (100°F) AND
- Cough and/or sore throat in the absence of a known cause other than influenza

sensitivity of both the rapid antigen tests and the DFA tests, the CDC has stated that these tests are not sufficient for excluding the diagnosis of influenza. There are several rapid PCR-based assays emerging that have a high sensitivity (90%–100%), high specificity (95%–100%), and turnaround time of 1 to 2 hours.

Further studies, such as complete blood count, serum electrolytes, throat culture, and chest radiograph, should be considered and ordered as per clinical suspicion.

Differential Diagnosis: A number of viruses beside influenza can be responsible for ILI. These include *respiratory syncytial virus*, picornaviruses (small RNA viruses that include enteroviruses and rhinoviruses), parainfluenza, and adenovirus.

Organisms

Influenza viruses A, B, and C are associated with influenza in humans. Type A and B infections tend to be more severe, so testing and treatment guidelines tend to focus on these infections. Type C influenza usually causes illness that tends to be substantially milder than what is seen with infection with the former two categories.

Treatment

A majority of cases of influenza are self-limited and require no treatment other than supportive care. However, there is a subset of the population at risk of severe disease who will benefit from timely antiviral treatment. Antiviral treatment is recommended for those with severe or progressive illness, especially those requiring hospital admission, or those with lower respiratory tract disease. Additionally, antiviral treatment is warranted for inpatient populations at high risk for complications following infection with influenza (see Box 26.2). Antiviral treatment is the most effective when initiated within 48 hours of symptom onset. This window is increased for those with severe disease requiring hospital admission, as some studies have suggested benefit up to 5 days from symptom onset. Finally, fastidious infection control procedures should be implemented in all suspected cases of influenza to minimize spread of the illness to other patients and health care workers.

Antivirals: There are currently two classes of influenza antivirals approved by the FDA. The adamantanes (amantadine and rimantadine), are active against Influenza A only and are no long recommended for clinical use due to substantial resistance in circulating influenza strains. The neuraminidase inhibitors are active against both Influenza A and Influenza B and include three approved medications: oral oseltamivir (Tamiflu), inhaled zanamivir (Relenza), and intravenous peramivir (Rapivab; see Box 26.3).

Box 26.2 Persons at High Risk for Influenza Complications

On the basis of epidemiologic studies of seasonal influenza or 2009 H1N1, persons at higher risk for influenza complications include

- Children aged <5 years (especially those aged < 2 years);
- Adults aged ≥ 65 years;
- Persons with chronic pulmonary (including asthma), cardiovascular (except hypertension alone), renal, hepatic, hematologic (including sickle cell disease), and metabolic disorders (including diabetes mellitus) or neurologic and neurodevelopment conditions (including disorders of the brain, spinal cord, peripheral nerve, and muscle such as cerebral palsy, epilepsy [seizure disorders], stroke, intellectual disability [mental retardation], moderate to severe developmental delay, muscular dystrophy, or spinal cord injury;
- Persons with immunosuppression, including that caused by medications or by human immunodeficiency virus infection;
- Women who are pregnant or postpartum (within 2 weeks after delivery);
- Persons aged ≤ 18 years who are receiving long-term aspirin therapy;
- American Indians/Alaska Natives;
- Persons who are morbidly obese (ie, body mass index ≥ 40); and
- Residents of nursing homes and other chronic-care facilities.

Box 26.3 Antivirals for Treatment and Chemoprophylaxis of Influenza

Current CDC recommended antiviral regimens for treatment of influenza in adults 18 and older:
- Zanamivir
  - 10 mg (two 5-mg inhalations) twice daily for 5 days
- Oseltamivir
  - 75 mg twice daily for 5 days
  - This medication is not recommended for use in patients with underlying respiratory disease (eg,. asthma, COPD)
- Peramivir
  - One 600 mg dose via intravenous infusion over 15 to 30 minutes

Current CDC recommended antiviral regimens for treatment of influenza in children:
- Zanamivir (children ≥ 7 years of age)
  - 10 mg (two 5-mg inhalations twice daily)
  - Treatment is for 5 days
- Oseltamivir
  - If younger than 1 year old
  - 3 mg/kg per dose twice daily
  - If 1 year or older, dose varies by child's weight:
    - 15 kg or less: the dose is 30 mg twice a day
    - > 15 to 23 kg: the dose is 45 mg twice a day
    - > 23 to 40 kg: the dose is 60 mg twice a day
    - > 40 kg: the dose is 75 mg twice a day
  - Treatment is for 5 days
  - This medication is not recommended for use in patients with underlying respiratory disease (eg, asthma, COPD)

Current CDC recommended antiviral regimens for influenza chemoprophylaxis in adults 18 and older:
- Zanamivir
  - 10 mg (two 5-mg inhalations) once daily for 7 days
- Oseltamivir
  - 75 mg once daily for 7 days

Current CDC recommended antiviral regimens for influenza chemoprophylaxis in children:
- Zanamivir (5 years or older)
  - 10 mg (two 5-mg inhalations) once daily for 7 days
- Oseltamivir
  - If child is younger than 3 months old, use of oseltamivir for chemoprophylaxis is not recommended unless situation is judged critical due to limited data in this age group.
  - If child is 3 months or older and younger than 1 year old
  - 3 mg/kg per dose once daily
  - If 1 year or older, dose varies by child's weight:
    - 15 kg or less: the dose is 30 mg once a day
    - > 15 to 23 kg: the dose is 45 mg once a day
    - > 23 to 40 kg: the dose is 60 mg once a day
    - > 40 kg: the dose is 75 mg once a day
  - All chemoprophylaxis regimens are for 7 days

Antivirals: Antiviral treatment is recommended for those at high risk of complications from influenza. It is also recommended for all persons within a household as chemoprophylaxis when one family member develops suspected or confirmed influenza and another cohabitant is at high risk of complications secondary to infection (see Box 26.2).

Other Key Issues

Pregnant Women: Although appropriate antiviral medications are classified by the FDA as class C, the current standard of care holds that the potential benefits of treatment outweigh any possible risks to the fetus. Pregnant women with ILI with suspected influenza should be considered for prompt treatment with antiviral medications on an empiric basis, regardless of rapid influenza diagnostic test results or vaccination status.

Bacterial Coinfection: Although influenza is known to cause viral pneumonia, it also damages the respiratory epithelium, increasing the risk of bacterial coinfection. Potential bacterial coinfection should be considered in those with severe illness, pneumonia, and otitis media.

Vaccination and Prophylaxis

The CDC now recommends that everyone over the age of 6 months get vaccinated based on the recommendation from CDC's Advisory Committee on Immunization Practices (ACIP) for "universal" flu vaccination in the United States.

Chemoprophylaxis for close contacts is not always necessary for those who have been vaccinated.

Other Key Points

The CDC periodically publishes recommendations for infection control. The most published recent recommendation elements include but are not limited to minimizing potential exposures, careful attention to respiratory hygiene (including cough etiquette), hand hygiene, adherence to standard precautions, and minimizing visitors for patients who are in isolation for influenza.

Suggested Readings and References

1. Thompson WW, Comanor L, DK Shay. Epidemiology of seasonal influenza: use of surveillance data and statistical models to estimate the burden of disease. *J Infect Dis.* 2006;194(suppl2):S82–S91. doi:10.1086/507558.

2. Harper S, Bradley J, et al. Seasonal influenza in adults and children—diagnosis, treatment, chemoprophylaxis, and institutional outbreak management: Clinical Practice Guidelines of the Infectious Diseases Society of America. *Clin Infect Dis.* 2009;48:1003–1032.

3. Lofgren E, Fefferman NH, et al. Influenza seasonality: underlying causes and modeling theories. *J Virol.* 2007;81:5429–5436

4. Fowlkes A, Giorgi A, et al. Viruses associated with acute respiratory infections and influenza-like illness among outpatients from the Influenza Incidence Surveillance Project, 2010–2011. *J Infect Dis.* 2014;209:1715–1725.

5. Kelly H, Birch C. The causes and diagnosis of influenza-like illness. *Aust Fam Physician.* 2004;33:305–309.

6. Fiore A, Fry A, et al. Antiviral agents for the treatment and chemoprophylaxis of influenza: recommendations of the Advisory Committee on Immunization Practices (ACIP). *MMWR Morb Mortal Wkly Rep.* 2011;60:1–25.

7. Afilalo M, Stern E, Oughton M. Evaluation and management of seasonal influenza in the emergency department. *Emerg Med Clin North Am.* 2012;30:271–305.

8. Shey-Ying C, Yee-Chun C, et al. Field performance of clinical case definitions for influenza screening during the 2009 pandemic. *Am J Emerg Med.* 2012;30:1796–1803.

9. Louie JK, Salibay CJ, et al. Pregnancy and severe influenza infection in the 2013-2014 influenza season. *Obstet Gynecol.* 2015;125:184–192.

10. Thompson WW, Shay DK, Weintraub E, et al. Mortality associated with influenza and respiratory syncytial virus in the United States. *JAMA.* 2003;289:179–186.

11. Thompson WW, Shay DK, Weintraub E, et al. Influenza-associated hospitalizations in the United States. *JAMA.* 2004;292:1333–1340.

12. McGeer A, Green KA, Plevneshi A, et al. Antiviral therapy and outcomes of influenza requiring hospitalization in Ontario, Canada. *Clin Infect Dis.* 2007;45:1568–1575.

13. Muthuri SG, Myles PR, Venkatesan S, Leonardi-Bee J, Nguyen-Van-Tam JS. Impact of neuraminidase inhibitor treatment on outcomes of public health importance during the 2009-10 influenza A(H1N1) pandemic: a systematic review and meta-analysis in hospitalized patients. *J Infect Dis.* 2013;207:553–563.

14. Hsu J, Santesso N, Mustafa R, et al. Antivirals for treatment of influenza: a systematic review and meta-analysis of observational studies. *Ann Intern Med.* 2012;156:512–524.

15. Centers for Disease Control and Prevention (CDC). Evaluation of rapid influenza diagnostic tests for detection of novel influenza A (H1N1) Virus—United States, 2009. *MMWR Morb Mortal Wkly Rep.* 2009;58:826–829.

16. Call SA, Vollenweider MA, Hornung CA, Simel DL, McKinney WP. Does this patient have influenza? *JAMA*. 2005;293:987–997.

17. Ebell MH, White LL, Casault T. A systematic review of the history and physical examination to diagnose influenza. *J Am Board Fam Pract*. 2004;17:1–5.

18. Sambol AR, Iwena PC, Pieretti M, et al. Validation of the Cepheid Xpert Flu A real time RT-PCR detection panel for emergency use authorization. *J Clin Virol*. 2010;48:234–238.

19. Uyeki T. Diagnostic testing for 2009 pandemic influenza A (H1N1) virus infection in hospitalized patients. *N Engl J Med*. 2009;361:e114.

Atypical Pulmonary Infections

Rod Rahimi

Summary Box

Disease Description: Legionellosis or Legionnaires' disease (LD) is a common cause of community-acquired pneumonia and can cause rapidly progressive respiratory failure and septic shock.

Organisms: *Legionella pneumophila* (and other *Legionella* species)

Treatment:
  Oral first line: Respiratory fluoroquinolone
  Second line: Newer macrolides
  Parenteral: Respiratory fluoroquinolone

Other Key Issues: Given the potential for outbreaks of LD, documented cases should be reported to the local or state health department.

Disease Description

In the late 1930s and early 1940s, Hobart Reimann first began using the term "atypical pneumonia" to describe mild forms of pneumonia in which the "mortality rate is practically nil," contrasting these cases with the high mortality associated with "typical" pneumonia in the pre-antibiotic era.[1,2] Whereas the original use of the term represented a clinical definition, a microbiological definition was subsequently developed describing lower respiratory tract infections caused by "atypical" bacterial pathogens, namely, those that cannot be readily identified via Gram stain or routine bacterial culture.

Although there is no current consensus on which bacterial pathogens are included under the heading of atypical pneumonias, *Legionella* species, *Mycoplasma pneumonia*, and *Chlamydia pneumoniae* traditionally fall into this category. Due to the perpetuation of the original clinical definition and the fact that pneumonia secondary to *Mycoplasma* or *Chlamydia* is usually not severe, some have developed a conceptual marriage between the terms "atypical pneumonia" and "walking pneumonia," meaning that the patient is not bedbound due to the illness. However, patients with severe community-acquired Legionnaires' disease (LD) can develop rapid respiratory failure. Without appropriate antibiotic therapy and subsequent intensive care unit (ICU) admissions for patients with severe LD, a mortality rate of 33% can be expected.[3] As a result, we encourage divorcing the term atypical pneumonia from the notion of low-acuity illness. Given its ability to produce outbreaks and critical illness, *Legionella* can create infectious disease emergencies and thus will be the focus of this discussion of atypical pneumonia.

Epidemiology

LD was first described after an infectious outbreak involving delegates to the American Legion convention in Philadelphia in 1976. *Legionella* was initially viewed as an unusual cause of pneumonia. However, subsequent epidemiological studies have demonstrated that it is fairly common, causing 2% to 9% of all community-acquired pneumonias that require hospitalization.[4-7] *Legionella* species flourish in man-made water systems, and outbreaks are often associated with direct contact with various aerosol-producing devices, such as cooling towers, showers, mist spraying devices in grocery stores, whirlpool spas, industrial plants, fountains, and evaporative condensers.[8] In Norway, an outbreak of LD from an industrial air scrubber suggested that *Legionella* can be transmitted across impressive distances, possibly greater than 10 km.[9]

Presenting Features

The incubation period for LD is approximately 2 to 14 days. Respiratory symptoms, such as cough and dyspnea, generally predominate. Nnonspecific symptoms can include fever, malaise, myalgia, anorexia, and headache. Unfortunately, there are no characteristic presenting clinical or radiological features, and the severity of illness can range from mild to severe. However, Fernández-Sabé and colleagues have identified certain features via multivariate analysis that are more common in LD than other bacterial pneumonias. These include male sex, heavy alcohol use, previous beta-lactam therapy, axillary temperature greater than 39°C, myalgia, and gastrointestinal symptoms.[10] There is also evidence that severe hyponatremia and hypophosphatemia is associated with LD.[11,12] Finally, LD should be considered as a cause of rapidly progressive, community-acquired pneumonia in an otherwise healthy adult.

Risk Factors

Cigarette smoking and chronic lung disease are the most common risk factors for LD.[13-15] Given the intracellular lifecycle of *Legionella*, it is not surprising that patients with suppressed adaptive immune responses are at increased risk for LD, particularly those patients who have undergone organ transplantation.[16-18] Patients who have received an organ transplant and are undergoing treatment for allograft rejection with more than one immunosuppressive agent are at risk for LD.[17] Interestingly, for reasons that are unclear, human immunodeficiency virus/AIDS does not seem to increase the risk for LD.[19]

Diagnostic Tests

There are numerous diagnostic tests of variable utility for LD.[20] The most commonly used diagnostic method for LD is the *Legionella* antigen urine assay.[21] In a meta-analysis, the pooled sensitivity of this assay was 0.74 (95% confidence interval [CI], 0.68–0.81) and specificity was 0.99 (95% CI, 0.984–0.997).[22] This assay is run on an easily obtainable urine specimen and usually can result in less than an hour. However, commercially available *Legionella* urine antigen assays generally only detect *Legionella pneumophila* serotype 1 (see the following for further discussion). As a result, formal culture remains important.

In a suspected case of LD, a urine sample should be submitted for the urinary antigen assay along with a respiratory specimen for culture. The microbiology laboratory should be aware of the suspected diagnosis of LD so that the respiratory sample can be grown on supplemented buffered charcoal yeast extract. Culture often takes 3 to 5 days. A direct fluorescence assay may also be used, but the sensitivity of this method remains poor.[23] Serological studies have not been found to be clinically useful given the long time frame needed for seroconversion.[24] Polymerase chain reaction amplification of *Legionella* nucleic acids is a reliable assay but often not available at many centers.[25]

Organism

Legionella species are small aerobic, non-spore-forming bacteria. *Legionella* usually does not appear on Gram stain, although it can stain as gram negative. There are approximately 50 species in the *Legionellaceae* family with more than 70 serogroups.[26] In an international collaborative survey of community-acquired LD, *Legionella pneumophila* was found to be the most common cause of human infections, causing greater than 90% of cases.[27] *L. pneumophila* serogroup 1 alone was responsible for greater than 80% of cases.[27]

Treatment

Whereas erythromycin was initially used to treat LD, trials have demonstrated that the newer macrolides (eg, clarithromycin and azithromycin) and the respiratory fluoroquinolones (eg, levofloxacin, gatifloxacin, and moxifloxacin) are the antimicrobial agents of choice.[28,29] Unfortunately, there are no randomized controlled trials comparing macrolides and fluoroquinolones in LD. However, there is evidence that patients who received fluoroquinolones experienced fewer complications and shorter hospital stays.[29] As a result, fluoroquinolones should be considered first-line agents.

It has recently been suggested that combination therapy with a newer macrolide and fluoroquinolone improves outcomes in severe community-acquired LD.[30] In cases of severe LD, administration of a fluoroquinolone within 8 hours of ICU admission was associated with improved outcomes.[3] Yu and colleagues collected evidence from six clinical trials and demonstrated that levofloxacin at 500 mg once daily for 10 to 14 days or 750 mg once daily for 5 days was effective in treating mild-to-moderate as well as severe LD.[13] For immunosuppressed patients with severe disease, longer treatment courses with levofloxacin should be considered. When azithromycin is used, it is reasonable to treat with an initial dose of 1 g followed by 500 mg daily for 7 to 10 days.

Other Key Issues to Consider

Given the potential for outbreaks of LD, documented cases should be reported to the local or state health department. Along with LD, *Legionella* may cause Pontiac Fever, an influenza-like illness without pneumonia, which is self-limiting and does not require treatment.[31]

Suggested Readings and References

1. Reimann HA. Landmark article Dec 24,1938: An acute infection of the respiratory tract with atypical pneumonia. A disease entity probably caused by a filtrable virus. By Hobart A. Reimann. *JAMA.* 1984;251:936–944.
2. Reimann HA, Havens PW, Price AH, Etiology of atypical ("virus") pneumonias: with a brief résumé of recent discoveries. *Arch Intern Med.* 1942;70:513–522.
3. A Gacouin, Le Tulzo Y, Lavoue S, et al. Severe pneumonia due to *Legionella pneumophila*: prognostic factors, impact of delayed appropriate antimicrobial therapy. *Intensive Care Med.* 2002;28:686–691.
4. Baum von H, Ewig S, Marre R, et al. Community-acquired Legionella pneumonia: new insights from the German competence network for community acquired pneumonia. *Clin Infect Dis.* 2008;46:1356–1364.
5. Fang GD, Fine M, Orloff J, et al. New and emerging etiologies for community-acquired pneumonia with implications for therapy: a prospective multicenter study of 359 cases. *Medicine (Baltimore).* 1990;69:307–316.
6. Marston BJ, Plouffe JF, File TM, et al. Incidence of community-acquired pneumonia requiring hospitalization: results of a population-based active surveillance study in Ohio. The Community-Based Pneumonia Incidence Study Group. *Arch Intern Med.* 1997;157:1709–1718.
7. Yu VL, Stout JE. Editorial commentary: community-acquired legionnaires disease: implications for underdiagnosis and laboratory testing. *Clin Infect Dis.* 2008;46:1365–1367.
8. Marrie TJ, Garay JR, Weir E. Legionellosis: why should I test and report? *CMAJ.* 2010;182:1538–1542.
9. Nygard K, Werner-Johansen O, Ronsen S, et al. An outbreak of legionnaires disease caused by long-distance spread from an industrial air scrubber in Sarpsborg, Norway. *Clin Infect Dis.* 2008;46:61–69.
10. Fernández-Sabé N, Rosón B, Carratalà J, et al. Clinical diagnosis of Legionella pneumonia revisited: evaluation of the Community-Based Pneumonia Incidence Study Group scoring system. *Clin Infect Dis.* 2003;37:483–489.

11. Woodhead MA, Macfarlane JT. Legionnaires' disease: a review of 79 community acquired cases in Nottingham. *Thorax*. 1986;41:635–640.

12. Yu VL, Kroboth FJ, Shonnard J, et al. Legionnaires' disease: new clinical perspective from a prospective pneumonia study. *Am J Med*. 1982;73:357–361.

13. Yu VL, Greenberg RN, Zadeikis N, et al. Levofloxacin efficacy in the treatment of community-acquired legionellosis. *Chest*. 2004;125:2135–2139.

14. Greig JE, Carnie JA, Tallis GF, et al. An outbreak of Legionnaires' disease at the Melbourne Aquarium, April 2000: investigation and case-control studies. *Med J Aust*. 2004;180:566–572.

15. Boer Den JW, Nijhof J, Friesema I. Risk factors for sporadic community-acquired Legionnaires' disease: a 3-year national case-control study. *Public Health*. 2006;120:566–571.

16. Singh N, Stout JE, Yu VL. Prevention of Legionnaires' disease in transplant recipients: recommendations for a standardized approach. *Transpl Infect Dis*. 2004;6(2):58–62.

17. Gudiol C, Garcia-Vidal C, Fernández-Sabé N, et al. Clinical features and outcomes of Legionnaires' disease in solid organ transplant recipients. *Transpl Infect Dis*. 2009;11(1):78–82.

18. Jacobson KL, Miceli MH, Tarrand JJ, Kontoyiannis DP. Legionella pneumonia in cancer patients. *Medicine (Baltimore)*. 2008;87:152–159.

19. Sandkovsky U, Sandkovsky G, Suh J, et al. Legionella pneumonia and HIV: case reports and review of the literature. *AIDS Patient Care STDs*. 2008;22:473–481.

20. Waterer GW, Baselski VS, Wunderink RG. Legionella and community-acquired pneumonia: a review of current diagnostic tests from a clinician's viewpoint. *Am J Med*. 2001;110:41–48.

21. Yu VL. Rapid diagnostic testing for community-acquired pneumonia: can innovative technology for clinical microbiology be exploited? *Chest*. 2009;136:1618.

22. Shimada T. Systematic review and meta-analysis: urinary antigen tests for legionellosis. *Chest*. 2009;136:1576.

23. She RC, Billetdeaux E, Phansalkar AR, Petti CA. Limited applicability of direct fluorescent-antibody testing for bordetella sp. and legionella sp. specimens for the clinical microbiology laboratory. *J Clin Microbiol*. 2007;45:2212–2214.

24. Marrie T, Costain N, La Scola B, et al. The role of atypical pathogens in community-acquired pneumonia. *Semin Respir Crit Care Med*. 2012;33:244–256.

25. Zarogoulidis P, Alexandropoulou I, Romanidou G, et al. Community-acquired pneumonia due to Legionella pneumophila, the utility of PCR, and a review of the antibiotics used. *Int J Gen Med*. 2011;4:15–19.

26. Fields BS, Benson RF, Besser RE. Legionella and Legionnaires' disease: 25 years of investigation. *Clin Microbiol Rev*. 2002;15:506–526.

27. Yu VL, Plouffe JF, Pastoris MC, et al. Distribution of Legionella species and serogroups isolated by culture in patients with sporadic community-acquired legionellosis: an international collaborative survey. *J Infect Dis*. 2002;186:127–128.

28. Plouffe JF, Breiman RF, Fields BS, et al. Azithromycin in the treatment of Legionella pneumonia requiring hospitalization. *Clin Infect Dis*. 2003;37:1475–1480.

29. Blázquez Garrido RM, Espinosa Parra FJ, Alemany Francés L, et al. Antimicrobial chemotherapy for Legionnaires disease: levofloxacin versus macrolides. *Clin Infect Dis*. 2005;40:800–806.

30. Rello J, Gattarello S, Souto J, et al. Community-acquired legionella pneumonia in the intensive care unit: impact on survival of combined antibiotic therapy. *Med Intesiva*. 2013 Jun-Jul;37(5):320–326.

31. Guyard C, Low DE. Legionella infections and travel associated legionellosis. *Travel Med Infect Dis*. 2011;9:176–186.

Pulmonary Tuberculosis

Bhakti Hansoti

Summary Box

Disease Description: 90% of those with tuberculosis (TB) have asymptomatic infection. 10% have progressive disease (most commonly primary lung presentation).

Organisms: *Mycobacterium tuberculosis* (MTB)

Treatment:
Oral first line: Daily combination therapy with Ethambutol (15–20 mg/kg), Rifampin (10 mg/kg), Isoniazide (5 mg/kg), and Pyrazinamide (15–30 mg/kg).
Second line: oral fluoroquinolones in combination with first line agents
Parenteral: intravenous aminoglycosidesin combination with first line agents

Other Key Issues: There is an overall global decline in prevalence. A higher rate of active TB is seen in patients that are immunocompromised.

Disease Description

Epidemiology

TB is most commonly known for its lung manifestations. More than 2 billion people (about one-third of the world population) are infected with MTB; the global incidence peaked in 2003 and now appears to be declining slowly. Poverty, human immunodeficiency virus (HIV), and drug resistance are major contributors to the global epidemic. Approximately 96% of cases occur in developing countries. In the United States, there has been a marked decline in TB infection rates to a reported 3.2 per 100 000 in 2012; the majority of cases occur in foreign-born individuals emigrating from countries with high rates of endemic TB or those with a concurrent immunocompromised state.

Presenting Features

Clinical manifestations of TB vary depending on the stage of the disease:

Primary TB: Clinical manifestations occur only in one-third of cases. Symptoms include fever and chest pain. If associated with enlarged bronchial lymph nodes, it may present with retrosternal pain and dull intracapsular pain.

Reactivation TB: Typical symptoms are insidious and may include cough, weight loss, fatigue, fever, night sweats, chest pain, dyspnea, and/or hemoptysis. These findings are less frequently observed in extremes of age. Symptoms tend to occur late in the course of the disease and may remain undiagnosed for several years.

Diagnostic Considerations

There are two kinds of tests that are used to determine if a person has been infected with MTB: the tuberculin skin test or a TB blood test. However, both of these tests only tell you if a person has been infected with the bacteria and not whether the person has latent TB infection (LTBI) or has progressed to active TB. Diagnosis of active TB disease is made by obtaining a clinical specimen that is growing M. Tuberculosis and correlating this with clinical disease using investigations such as chest x-ray.

Typical Disease Course

Most people (90%) infected with M. Tuberculosis have asymptomatic LTBI with only a 10% lifetime chance of progression to active TB disease (when the life cycle progresses to stage 4; see following).

Complications

Pulmonary complications of TB include hemoptysis (most frequent), pneumothorax, and bronchiectasis. Massive hemoptysis can occur due to involvement of the pulmonary arteries, bronchial arteries, or interosseus arteries. Pneumothorax appears to result from the rupture of a peripheral cavity or a subpleural caseous focus with liquefaction into the pleural space. TB can also cause extensive pulmonary destruction and is associated with an increased incidence of lung cancer and with secondary chronic pulmonary aspergillosis.

Diagnostic Tests

Chest Radiograph: In primary pulmonary TB, the chest radiograph is often normal. The most common radiographic abnormalities include hilar adenopathy, pleural effusions, and pulmonary infiltrates (typically in upper lobes).

Routine laboratory findings: Routine hematology and biochemistry studies are frequently normal. The C-reactive protein can be elevated in 85% of patients, but this test is nonspecific.

Computer Tomography: CT is more sensitive than plain chest radiographs for diagnosis. The most common findings consist of centrilobular 2- to 4-mm nodules or branching linear lesions representing intrabronchial and peribronchiolar caseation necrosis.

Clinical Specimens: The gold standard for diagnosis is a positive smear for acid-fast bacilli (AFB) and culture. Attempts should be made to collect a series of three sputum samples obtained at 8- to 24-hour intervals. Sputum may be obtained spontaneously or induced. Sputum is preferred over bronchoalveolar lavage (BAL) specimens due to safety and costs. However, if BAL is necessary due to lack of sputum, the yields with both types of specimens are comparable. The detection of AFB on microscopic examination of stained smears is the most rapid and least expensive; however, a positive result may represent nontuberculous mycobacteria rather than TC. Thus, a positive culture remains the required standard for definitive diagnosis.

Tuberculin skin test (TST): TST is used to identify individuals with previous sensitization to myco-bacterial antigens and is recommended only as a screening test for high-risk populations. It consists of intradermal injection of tuberculin material, which stimulates a delayed type hypersensitivity response mediated by T-cells and causes induration within 48 to 72 hours. The test is interpreted as positive depending on the area of induration in millimeters and the person's risk of being infected:

- Induration > 5 mm if the patient has HIV, has had recent contact with MTB-positive person, or is immunocompromised due to organ transplant/steroids.
- Induration > 10 mm if the patient is a recent immigrant, injection drug user, health care worker/ employee in high risk settings (eg, hospitals/prisons), child < 4 years of age, or has a concurrent high-risk clinical condition.
- Induration > 15 mm is considered positive in all persons.

If a person is identified as having a positive TST, then they must undergo further clinical and microbiology evaluation to rule out active tuberculosis.

Organism

Microbiology

MTB is a small aerobic, nonmotile bacillus. It is a facultative intracellular parasite that is transferred through the air. It is weakly gram positive and non-spore forming. MTB retains certain stains (Ziehl–Neelsen stain) even after being treated with an acidic solution; thus, it is classified as an AFB.

Primary and Secondary Organisms

The TB complex includes four other TB causing organisms: *M. bovis, M. Africanum, M. Canetti,* and *M. microti.*

Life Cycle

Stage 1 (1–7 days): Onset, the bacteria is inhaled by the host.

Stage 2 (7–21 days): Symbiosis, if the initial macrophage does not succeed in killing the bacteria, the bacteria will replicate until the macrophage bursts, further disseminating the bacteria.

Stage 3 (14–21 days): Initial caseous necrosis in TB develops when the bacteria kill the non-activated surrounding macrophages, run out of cells to divide in, and, thus, halt reproduction. Though the bacteria can no longer reproduce in the tubercle, they can remain alive for a long period of time. The tubercle appear to have caseous centers, as the host kills its own tissues to prevent the spread of the bacteria.

Stage 4 (after 21 days): There is an interplay of tissue damage and macrophage-activated immune response. Macrophages surround the tubercle; the tubercle then grows and can break off or spread to the bronchus or other parts of the lungs. If the tubercle reaches the blood stream and seeds it with MTB, this is called miliary TB. Resulting secondary lesions can occur anywhere in the body.

Stage 5: Liquefaction and cavity formation. Not all people progress to this stage. In this stage, the tuber-cles liquefy, which allows the disease spread faster.

Treatment

First-line recommendations (and alternatives based on allergy)

The initial phase for previously untreated tuberculosis includes four drugs:

Rifampin (RIF 10 mg/kg per day; max 600 mg)

Isoniazid (INH, 5 mg/kg per day; max 300 mg)

Pyrazinamide (PZA 15–30 mg/kg per day, max 2 g)

Ethambutol (EMB 15–20 mg/kg per day, max 1600 mg)

The above quadruple therapy (RIPE therapy) is recommended daily for 2 months. This is fol-lowed by a continuation phase of therapy, typically consisting of 4 to 7 months of INH and RIF either daily or biweekly. Alternative regimes do exist, and institutional guidelines should be considered.

Second-line recommendations and third-line recommendations

Treatment of TB caused by drug-resistant organisms should be done in close consultation with an expert. The major categories of second-line agents for treatment of resistant TB include fluoroquinolones (Levofloxacin, Moxifloxacin, or Ofloxacin) and/or injectable aminoglycosides (Amikacin or Streptomycin).

Evolving or emerging treatment developments and considerations

There has been an increasing emphasis on patient-centered case management, a core focus of which is directly observed therapy. There is also new evidence suggesting a role for using 2-month sputum cultures to identify patients at risk of relapse or multidrug-resistant TB. There is increasing evidence to support the use of fluoroquinolones when first-line drugs are not tolerated or when strains shows resistance to RIF, INH, or EMB.

Suggested Readings and References

1. World Health Organization website. http://www.who.int/topics/tuberculosis/en/. Accessed August 8, 2013.
2. Centers for Disease Control and Prevention website. http://www.cdc.gov/tb/. Accessed August 8, 2013.
3. Zumla A, Raviglione M, Hafner R, von Reyn CF. *N Engl J Med.* 2013;368:745–755.
4. Lawn S, Zumla A. Tuberculosis. *Lancet.* 2011;378:57–72.
5. Holtz T, Sternberg M, Kammerer S, et al. Time to sputum culture conversion in multidrug-resistant tuberculosis: predictors and relationship to treatment outcome. *Ann Intern Med.* 2006;144:650–659

Chapter 29

Acute Uncomplicated Bronchitis

Sarina Sahetya

Summary Box

Disease Description: Acute bronchitis is a respiratory illness characterized by a normal chest radiograph and predominantly by cough with or without sputum production that lasts for up to 3 weeks.

Organisms: Viral pathogens—*Influenzavirus A* and *B, human parainfluenza virus, human coronavirus, rhinovirus, human respiratory syncytial virus* (RSV), and *human metapneumovirus*
    Bacterial pathogens—*Bordetella pertussis, Mycoplasma pneumoniae, Chlamydia pneumoniae*

Treatment: Symptomatic relief with antitussives, mucolytics, and beta-2 agonists as clinically indicated. Antibiotics are not routinely indicated.
- Suspected *B. pertussis*: oral first line: Azithromycin 500 mg on first day, then 250 mg for 4 more days. Second-line: trimethoprim-sulfamethoxazole 1600 mg for 14 days.
- Suspected Influenza: oral first-line therapy: oseltamivir or zanamivir if presentation with 48 hours of symptom onset

Other Key Issues: Elderly patients and patients with comorbid health conditions, especially chronic lung or heart disease, may require empiric antibiotic therapy.

Disease Description

Epidemiology

Throughout the United States, acute cough is the most common complaint for which patients are seen in the ambulatory setting. According to a survey of outpatient physicians, the most common diagnosis given to these patients is acute uncomplicated bronchitis. This diagnosis accounts for over 10 million office visits and affects up to 5% of the general population each year. The majority of cases have a viral origin and resolve spontaneously within 3 weeks. However, 90% of patients present before this, within the first 2 weeks of their illness, seeking symptomatic relief.

Presenting Features

The American College of Chest Physicians defines acute bronchitis as an acute respiratory illness characterized predominantly by cough with or without sputum production that lasts up to 3 weeks. Over 80% of patients will report cough with or without phlegm within the first 2 days of their illness. Over 50% of patients will have cough productive of purulent sputum. Importantly, multiple studies have shown that the purulence of sputum is a poor predictor of bacterial infection. Instead, purulence indicates sloughing of tracheobronchial epithelium and inflammatory cells, rather than the presence of alveolar disease. Other presenting symptoms include rhinorrhea, congestion, sneeze, sore throat, and wheezing. Acute bronchitis is also frequently associated with systemic symptoms such as low-grade fever, myalgia, and fatigue within the first few days of onset. Constitutional symptoms rarely persist beyond the first stage of illness, and other diagnoses should be considered if this occurs.

Diagnostic Considerations

Distinguishing between acute bronchitis and pneumonia is imperative because pneumonia is associated with significant morbidity and mortality without therapy. The presence of systemic inflammatory symptoms—including tachycardia, tachypnea, fever—and physical exam findings of chest consolidation (ie, rales, egophony, fremitus, dullness to percussion) should increase clinical suspicion for pneumonia over acute bronchitis. Other potential diagnoses include postnasal drip syndrome, cough-variant asthma, chronic bronchitis, and gastroesophageal reflux.

Typical Disease Course

Bronchitis is characterized by self-limited inflammation of the airways. Within the first few days of illness, bronchitis cannot be distinguished from mild upper respiratory infections, such as the common cold. Acute bronchitis should be considered when cough persists for greater than 5 days. Cough and airway hyperresponsiveness characterize the extended period between 5 and 21 days. During this period, pulmonary function tests will often demonstrate a reduction in FEV1 (forced expiratory volume in 1 second) and an increase in bronchial hyperreactivity in affected patients. Cough will resolve in approximately 75% of patients within 3 weeks with a median duration of between 10 and 20 days. Cough lasting longer than 3 weeks should prompt providers to begin considering the other diagnoses mentioned previously. Airway hyperreactivity typically improves after 5 to 6 weeks.

Complications

Bacterial superinfection following an acute episode of bronchitis is the most common complication, but superinfection is relatively uncommon in healthy adults. Complications occur most frequently in patients with other comorbid conditions or in patients older than 65 years. Nonetheless, superinfection following an episode of acute bronchitis should be considered in any patient who begins exhibiting clinical signs of pneumonia (ie, tachycardia, tachypnea, and fever).

Diagnostic Tests

Chest radiographs should be utilized primarily to distinguish acute bronchitis from pneumonia or interstitial disease and should be used when there is sufficient concern for pneumonia. Additionally, because older patients may develop pneumonia without mounting a systemic inflammatory response, chest radiograph should be ordered in patients older than 75 years of age who present with tachypnea, decreased oxygen saturation, or decreased mental status. Chest radiography findings in acute bronchitis are generally nonspecific and may include signs of bronchial thickening. The presence of parenchymal infiltrate, interstitial thickening, or pleural effusion should raise clinical suspicion for an alternative diagnosis.

Practitioners continue to struggle to separate the majority of acute bronchitis cases, which have a viral origin, from the small number of episodes that have a bacterial origin and could benefit from antibiotics. In recent years, the measurement of procalcitonin has gained favor as a method for providing targeted antibiotic therapy to patients. Procalcitonin is released from tissues in response to the direct stimulation of cytokines by bacterial infections. Alternatively, procalcitonin release is inhibited by interferon-gamma, which is released in response to viral infections. Two clinical trials discovered that the use of procalcitonin dramatically decreased the number of patients receiving antibiotic therapy with no difference in adverse outcomes or symptom relief. Antibiotics were strongly discouraged in patients with procalcitonin levels less than 0.10 mcg/L, and antibiotic use was advocated in patients with levels greater than 0.50 mcg/L. More research will need to be conducted to validate usefulness of procalcitonin. However, procalcitonin may be a beneficial test to limit the overprescription of antibiotics in the outpatient setting.

Expectorated sputum cultures are not recommended because bacterial pathogens cause only a minority of acute bronchitis cases. The one exception is when the diagnosis of B. pertussis is suspected. In patients with suspected B. pertussis, definitive diagnosis should be attempted by obtaining a culture of the posterior nasopharynx in addition to PCR (polymerase chain reaction) testing. Consider testing for B. pertussis in patients with paroxysms of coughing lasting greater than 2 weeks, patients with weak or no immunity, or in communities with recent epidemics of B. pertussis. Diagnostic testing for other bacterial causes of acute bronchitis, such as M. pneumoniae and C. pneumoniae, is not indicated unless recent community outbreaks have been reported. Rapid tests for influenza have a sensitivity ranging from 40% to 60% and a specificity of 99%. The presence of fever, systemic symptoms, and appropriate seasonal timing should guide rapid influenza testing.

Organisms

In most studies, approximately 90% of acute bronchitis is caused by viral infections. The most common viral pathogens include Influenzavirus A and B, human parainfluenza virus, human coronavirus, rhinovirus, RSV, and human metapneumovirus. Common bacterial pathogens include atypical bacteria such as B. pertussis, M. pneumoniae, and C. pneumoniae.

Treatment

Most patients with acute bronchitis simply require symptomatic treatment and reassurance. Nevertheless, studies reveal that between 60% and 80% of patients receive unwarranted antibiotic therapy, which has led to a national campaign geared toward reducing antibiotic use in cases of acute bronchitis. A Cochrane review of nine randomized, controlled trials examining antibiotic use in acute bronchitis revealed a statistically significant but likely clinically insignificant reduction in duration of cough by half a day. There were no significant differences in the subjective assessment of "feeling ill" or in the incidence of adverse events associated with antibiotics. Accordingly, the American College of Chest Physician guidelines state that routine treatment with antibiotics for a presumed diagnosis of acute bronchitis is not justified and should not be offered to patients.

The exception to this recommendation is in cases of suspected B. pertussis infection. In the previously vaccinated host, B. pertussis may be characterized by a relatively benign course and can be indistinguishable from other pathogens. Accordingly, if treatment is going to be initiated for suspected B. pertussis, then confirmatory PCR and culture should first be obtained. First-line therapy consists of a 5-day course of a macrolide antibiotic, preferably azithromycin 500 mg on day 1 and then 250 mg on days 2 through 5. If macrolides cannot be given, then TMP-SMX 1600 mg daily or 800 mg twice daily should be given for a 14-day total course.

Antibiotic therapy for pertussis should be initiated within the first few weeks of symptoms because patients are unlikely to derive much benefit in the convalescent phase of infection. Patients with confirmed or highly probable B. pertussis infection should be isolated for 5 days from the start of treatment to reduce spread of infection in the community. In patients with suspected influenzavirus infection, treatment with the neuraminidase inhibitors oseltamivir or zanamivir within the first 48 hours of symptom onset can be considered. These second generation, anti-influenza agents have been shown to decrease symptom duration by approximately one day. The efficacy of mucolytics, antitussives, and bronchodilators is not supported by clinical evidence; but guidelines note that benefit may be obtained in certain subgroups. Moreover, these agents are unlikely to cause much harm.

Other Key Issues

The preceding recommendations for the treatment of acute bronchitis pertain to the management of otherwise healthy individuals. Patients with preexisting comorbidities, especially those with underlying lung pathology, often require routine antibiotic therapy directed toward both typical and atypical bacterial pathogens. Patients over 65 years of age with a history of admission to a hospital within the past year, diabetes mellitus, congestive heart failure, or current use of oral glucocorticoids should be considered at high risk for serious complications and can be treated empirically with antibiotic therapy. Persistent cough lasting greater than 3 weeks should prompt physicians to consider alternative diagnoses.

Suggested Readings and References

1. Gonzales R, Sande MA. Uncomplicated acute bronchitis. *Ann Intern Med.* 2000;133:981–991.

2. Braman SS. Chronic cough due to acute bronchitis: ACCP evidence-based clinical practice guidelines. *Chest.* 2006;129:95S.

3. Wenzel RP, Fowler AA III. Clinical practice: acute bronchitis. *N Engl J Med.* 2006;355:2125–2130.

4. Snow V, Mottur-Pilson C, Gonzales R, et al. Principles of appropriate antibiotic use for treatment of acute bronchitis in adults. *Ann Intern Med.* 2001;134:518–520.

5. Gonzales R, Bartlett JG, Besser RE, et al. Principles of appropriate antibiotic use for treatment of uncomplicated acute bronchitis: background. *Ann Intern Med.* 2001;134:521–529.

6. Smith SM, Fahey T, Smucny J, Becker LA. Antibiotics for acute bronchitis. *Cochrane Database Syst Rev.* 2014;CD000245.

7. Metlay J, Kapoor W, Fine M. Does this patient have community acquired pneumonia? diagnosing pneumonia by history and physical examination. *JAMA.* 1997;278:1440–1445.

8. Schuetz P, Chiappa V, Briel M, Greenwald JL. Procalcitonin algorithms for antibiotic therapy decisions: a systemic review of randomized controlled trials and recommendations for clinical algorithms. *Arch Intern Med.* 2011;171:1322–1331.

9. Schuetz P, Amin DN, Greenwald JL. Role of procalcitonin in managing adult patients with respiratory tract infections. *Chest.* 2012;141:1063–1073.

10. Becker LA, Hom J, Villasis-Keever M, van der Wouden JC. Beta2-agonists for acute bronchitis. *Cochrane Database Syst Rev.* 2011:CD001726.

Gastrointestinal Infections

Chapter 30

Viral Gastroenteritis

Ximena Tobar and Shannon B. Putman

Summary Box

Disease Description: Gastroenteritis is a diarrheal disease often associated with nausea, vomiting, headache, abdominal cramping, myalgia, and low-grade fever. Stools are often described as watery, with bouts of diarrhea and emesis.

Organisms: *Rotavirus, Norovirus*, Enteric *Adenovirus*, and *Astrovirus* are the most common causes of viral gastroenteritis. *Rotavirus* is one of the most common causes worldwide, and *Norovirus* is a leading cause of epidemic viral gastroenteritis.

Treatment: Therapy is mainly supportive. Appropriate oral or intravenous hydration is essential. Specific antiviral agents are not available.

Other Issues: Prevention and control of spread are key issues for viral gastroenteritis. A meta-analysis suggests handwashing alone may reduce the spread of infection by 47%. The use of alcohol-based hand sanitizers and daily disinfection of surfaces with quaternary ammonium wipes has reduced the spread of *Norovirus* and was found superior to handwashing alone.

Disease Description

Epidemiology

Viral gastroenteritis ranks as one of the most common infectious illnesses globally, and its incidence ranks behind only respiratory infections in the United States. Viral gastroenteritis causes significant mortality in developing countries; more than 500,000 deaths per year are attributed to rotavirus alone. Although viral gastroenteritis only causes several hundred deaths per year in the United States, it is associated with significant morbidity as well as financial burden due to hospitalizations, lost work days, and school absenteeism.

Viral gastroenteritis is incredibly prevalent, particularly in children. It accounts for 3% to 5% of all hospital days and 7% to 10% of all hospitalizations in children younger than 18 years old. In the United States, the average incidence of viral gastroenteritis in children less than 5 years old ranges from one to five episodes per child-year, resulting in 15 to 25 million episodes of acute gastroenteritis per year. This leads to 3 to 5 million doctors' visits and 200,000 hospitalizations. Prior to the widespread use of the *Rotavirus* vaccine in the United States, half of all hospitalizations for viral gastroenteritis were caused by *Rotavirus*. *Norovirus, Human Astrovirus,* and enteric *Adenovirus* account for 5% to 15% of hospitalizations for gastroenteritis symptoms. Although a specific virus is not identified in as many as 25% of cases, it is likely that these cases are caused by one of the common viral pathogens, which are not detected due to insufficient testing sensitivity. The majority of cases of viral gastroenteritis are transmitted via the fecal–oral route. Viral gastroenteritis is most common in the winter, with 70% to 90% of hospitalizations occurring during the colder months.

Viral gastroenteritis is quoted as the source of most infectious diarrheal illness as evidenced by stool cultures that are positive for bacterial pathogens in only 1.5% to 5.6% of cases. The risk of acute bacterial colitis increases with the presence of blood or mucus in the stool, high fever, and prolonged duration of symptoms.

Viral gastroenteritis occurs with two classic epidemiological patterns: endemic and epidemic infection. Endemic infection, exemplified by *Rotavirus A*, tends to affect infants and children younger than 4 years old who have not developed active immunity. As *Rotavirus A* is a ubiquitous infection, older children and adults typically have measurable antibody titers and rarely develop symptoms with later exposure. *Norovirus* classically causes epidemic outbreaks in communities and families. Transmission often occurs as a result of fecal contamination of food, and 50% of all food-related outbreaks have been associated with *Norovirus*. On cruise ships, over 90% of diarrheal illness outbreaks are thought to be due to *Norovirus*. The Kaplan criteria have been used to identify if an outbreak of acute gastroenteritis is likely to be caused by *Norovirus*. These criteria include the following: more than 50% of patients have vomiting, mean incubation is 24 to 48 hours, mean duration of illness is 12 to 60 hours, and no bacterial pathogen is isolated from stool cultures. These criteria are 99% sensitive and 68% specific for *Norovirus* epidemic outbreaks.

Presenting Features

Viral gastroenteritis typically presents with nausea, vomiting, diarrhea, headache, abdominal cramping, myalgia, and low-grade fever. Stools are often described as watery, and patients may report bouts of diarrhea and emesis occurring on an hourly basis. Symptoms begin 12 hours to 4 days after exposure and last from 3 to 7 days. Risk factors associated with a more severe presentation include first infection with a specific pathogen, large infecting inoculum, strain virulence factors, and an immunocompromised host.

Differential Diagnosis

The infectious differential for a patient presenting with nausea, vomiting, and diarrhea includes viral, bacterial, and parasitic infections. Blood or mucus in the stool is suggestive of a bacterial or parasitic process. Additionally, the presence of fecal leukocytes excludes viral infection, as it is suggestive of colonic inflammation. Otitis media, meningitis, and pneumonia may present with predominantly intestinal symptoms. Noninfectious processes, such as inflammatory bowel disease, toxic ingestions, medication side effects, celiac sprue, diabetes, dysmotility syndromes, and hyperthyroidism should also be considered.

Diagnostic Evaluation

Viral gastroenteritis is a clinical diagnosis, so an extensive diagnostic workup for specific viral pathogens is not recommended in most circumstances. However, screening for a specific virus should be done when evaluating hospital outbreaks, when considering cohorting admission groups, or when specific antiviral measures (immunoglobulin or colostrums) are being entertained. Patients presenting to the emergency department (ED) should be evaluated for signs and symptoms of dehydration. Febrile patients and those with moderate to severe dehydration (ie, who require intravenous rehydration) should have a complete blood count to assess for anemia and leukocytosis, as well as serum electrolytes to determine the need for repletion. Fecal leukocytes and stool pH may be considered in admitted patients. The absence of stool lactoferrin and a pH of < 6 are most suggestive of a viral process.

Organisms

Rotavirus

Rotavirus A is responsible the majority of gastroenteritis worldwide and is particularly severe in malnourished children in developing countries. Since the widespread use of the *Rotavirus* vaccine in the United States, positive laboratory testing for *Rotavirus* has decreased by 67%. The vast majority of unvaccinated children will contract rotavirus gastroenteritis by age 3. Although reinfection is possible, symptoms may be less severe or absent in older children and adults. Children aged 6 months to 2 years are the most commonly affected. Infection occurs 48 hours after exposure and is most frequently transmitted via the fecal–oral route. Although there is some supposition that rotavirus may also be transmitted through the respiratory route, this is less likely to cause acute gastroenteritis. Within a family unit, up to 50% of exposed children and 15% to 30% of exposed adults become infected. Infection peaks in the winter months, with reports of 25% of all pediatric admissions during the most prevalent time due to *Rotavirus* infection. Children hospitalized with *Rotavirus* are more likely to have vomiting in association with diarrhea and high fever (> 39°C) compared with other causes of viral gastroenteritis.

Norovirus

Norovirus, also known as the Norwalk virus, is a member of the *Caliciviridae* family and is the most common cause of epidemic viral gastroenteritis. It is also the most common virus affecting older children and adults. *Norovirus* is responsible for most epidemic outbreaks (93% of 234 outbreaks studied by the CDC between 1997 and 2000). Outbreaks occur in the following settings: restaurants or events with catered meals (39%); nursing homes or hospitals (25%); schools, day cares, or camps (13%); and vacation settings, including cruise ships (10%). Infection occurs most commonly via the fecal–oral route. *Norovirus* is highly transmissible, requiring only 10 to 100 viral particles to cause infection. Alternative routes of infection, such as aerosolized vomitus and persistence of viral particles on fomites, may play an important role in certain epidemics. Food-associated outbreaks can be directly traced back to contamination of food by infected food handlers, or food that has been irrigated or washed with fecally contaminated water. Contamination of oysters, raspberries, cold salads, and sandwich meat is commonly seen. Compared to *Rotavirus*, *Norovirus* tends to be less severe, have a shorter duration, and affect older children and adults more commonly. Vomiting is often the most prominent symptom.

Enteric *Adenovirus*

Enteric *Adenovirus* is thought to cause 3% to 15% of endemic gastroenteritis. It is most commonly seen in children less than 2 years old. Incubation lasts from 8 to 10 days, and infection can last 5 to 12 days. *Adenovirus* is less contagious than *Rotavirus*. Typically, those infected present with 1 to 2 days of vomiting and fever, followed by a prolonged course of watery diarrhea.

Astrovirus

Human Astrovirus is responsible for 3% to 9% of endemic gastroenteritis. It causes infection in both children and adults and is particularly prevalent in immunocompromised patients (eg, human immunodeficiency virus and bone marrow transplant) and the institutionalized elderly. *Human Astrovirus* is rarely the cause of epidemic outbreaks. Commonly linked to food or water contamination, outbreaks that infect a large portion of older children and adults are most likely caused by either *Norovirus* or *Human Astrovirus*.

Treatment

The primary goal of treatment for viral gastroenteritis is fluid repletion. Although commercially available oral rehydration can be used in patients tolerating oral intake, many patients who present to the ED require parenteral fluids. No specific antiviral agents are available. Bismuth subsalicylate is useful in treating abdominal cramping, but it has not been shown to reduce volume or frequency of diarrhea. Antiemetics can be used in patients with severe vomiting; specific antiemetic choice should be tailored to patient age and comorbidities. In contrast to acute bacterial colitis, antimotility and antisecretory agents, such as loperamide and diphenoxylate/atropine, can be used safely.

Other Key Issues

Infection control plays an important role in controlling the spread of viral gastroenteritis. Infections occurring in the hospital or in long-term care facilities can be managed with meticulous handwashing, the use of gloves with patient contact, and the proper disposal of soiled bedding and diapers. A meta-analysis suggests handwashing alone may reduce the spread of infection by 47%. The use of alcohol-based hand sanitizers and daily disinfection of surfaces with quaternary ammonium wipes has reduced the spread of *Norovirus* and was found superior to handwashing alone. *Norovirus*, in particular, is difficult to eradicate and may persist on surfaces despite extensive cleaning with chlorine-based wipes.

Disease prevention and control of spread are key issues for viral gastroenteritis. In 2009, the World Health Organization declared that the *Rotavirus* vaccine should be included in national immunization programs, and it is likely that the vaccine will have a major impact in countries with a high disease burden. It is recommended that the vaccine be administered at birth, 6 weeks, and 12 weeks of age. There is a higher risk of intussusception in infants given the vaccine after 12 months of life.

Suggested Readings and References

1. Blacklow NR, Greenberg HB. Viral gastroenteritis. *N Engl J Med*. 1991;325:252.

2. Parashar UD, Burton A, Lanata C, et al. Global mortality associated with rotavirus disease among children in 2004. *J Infect Dis*. 2009;200(suppl 1):S9.

3. Glass RI, Bresee J, Jiang B, et al. Gastroenteritis viruses: an overview. *Novartis Foundation Symp*. 2001;238:5–19.

4. Matson DO, Estes MK. Impact of Rotavirus infection at a large pediatric hospital. *J Infect Dis*. 1990;162:598–604.

5. Oh DY, Gaedicke G, Schreirer E. Viral agents of acute gastroenteritis in German children: prevalence and molecular diversity. *J Med Virol*. 2004;71:82.

6. Guerrat RL, Van Gilder T, Steiner TS, et al. Practice guidelines for the management of infectious diarrhea. *Clin Infect Dis*. 2001;32:331–351.

7. Widdowson, MA, Cramer EH, Hadley L, et al. Outbreaks of acute gastroenteritis on cruise ships and on land: identification of a predominant circulating strain of norovirus—United States, 2002. *J Infect Dis*. 2004;190:27.

8. Parashar UD, Glass RI. Rotavirus vaccines—early success, remaining questions. *N Engl J Med*. 2009;360:1063.

9. Blacklow NR, Greenberg HB. Viral gastroenteritis. *N Engl J Med*. 1991;325:252.

10. Musher DM, Musher BL. Contagious acute gastroenteritis infections. *N Engl J Med*. 2004;351:2417.

11. Staat MA, Azimi PH, Berke T, et al. Clinical presentations of rotavirus infection among hospitalized children. *Pediatr Infect Dis J*. 2002;21:221–227.

12. Fankauser RL, Monroe SS, Noel JS, et al. Epidemiologic and molecular trends of "Norwalk-like viruses" associated with outbreaks of gastroenteritis in the United States. *J Infect Dis*. 2002;186:1.

13. Bresee JS, Widdowson MA, Monroe SS, Glass RI. Foodborne viral gastroenteritis: challenges and opportunities. *Clin Infect Dis*. 2002;35:748.

14. Curtis V, Cairncross S. Effect of intensive handwashing promotion on childhood diarrhea in high-risk communities in Pakistan: a randomized controlled trial. *JAMA*. 2004;291:2457.

15. Cutis V, Cairncross. Effect of washing hands with soap on diarrhea risk in the community: a systemic review. *Lancet Infect Dis*. 2003;3:275.

16. Sandora TJ, Shih MC, Goldmann DA. Reducing absenteeism from gastrointestinal and respiratory illness in elementary school students: a randomized controlled trial of an infection-control intervention. *Pediatrics*. 2008;121:e1555.

17. Danchin MH, Bines JE. Defeating rotavirus? the global recommendation for rotavirus vaccination. *N Engl J Med*. 2009;361:1919–1921.

Infectious Colitis

David Scordino

Summary Box

Disease Description: Infectious colitis is defined as diarrhea with evidence of colonic inflammation by visualization (colonoscopy), history (blood or mucus in the stool), or laboratory evidence (high lactoferrin). It is most commonly associated with bacterial or bacterial toxin invasion of the colonic mucosa, leading to toxicity, volume loss, hemorrhage, and colonic inflammation.

Organisms: See Table 31.1.

Treatment: Ensure hydration. Mild to moderate cases do not require further therapy. Targeted antibiotics (see Table 31.1) should be reserved for those with high fevers, bloody stools, severe diarrhea, traveler's diarrhea, *Clostridium difficile*, or positive stool cultures.

Other Key Issues: Diarrhea is one of the leading causes of death in children worldwide.

Disease Description

Epidemiology

Diarrhea is formally defined as three or more loose stools per day due to increased water content of the stool from either impaired water absorption or active fluid secretion by the bowel. Patients with severe cases of infectious diarrhea may defecate more than two liters of stool daily, resulting in significant volume and electrolyte perturbations. Diarrhea is a common illness, with an estimated 211 to 375 million cases annually in the United States alone. Globally, infectious diarrhea is responsible for millions of deaths each year, averaging **greater than 3,000 deaths in children under the age of 5 each day**. Infectious colitis or dysentery is identified by the presence of diarrhea with evidence of colonic inflammation (eg, positive fecal inflammatory markers, gross blood or mucus in the stool, or visualization of inflamed mucosa via colonoscopy or sigmoidoscopy). Dysentery is of particular interest and concern because it is most commonly secondary to an infectious bacterial agent or its associated toxin rather than a viral etiology, which is the most common cause of diarrhea in general.

In 1996, the Centers for Disease Control and Prevention instituted a program called FoodNet to determine the prevalence of specific enteric bacterial and protozoal sources of infectious gastroenteritis. In 2010, the incidence of laboratory-confirmed cases per 100,000 persons (in parentheses) for each etiologic pathogen was as follows: *Salmonella* (17.55), *Campylobacter* (13.52), *Shigella* (3.77), *Cryptosporidium* (2.75), Shiga toxin producing *E. coli* O157 (0.95), Shiga toxin producing *E. coli* non-O157 (0.95), *Yersinia* (0.34), *Vibrio* (0.41), *Listeria* (0.28), and *Cyclospora* (0.06).

Presenting Features

Patients with dysentery present with bloody diarrhea, fever, and systemic symptoms. The incidence of bacterial colitis is increased by international travel, hospitalization, antibiotic use, nursing home care, and exposure to untreated water (eg, camping). Other common symptoms include nausea, vomiting, abdominal pain, and tenesmus. Evidence of hypovolemia and shock are also possible.

Diagnostic Considerations

The differential diagnosis for patients presenting with acute diarrhea (ie, less than 2 weeks duration) is extensive. Viruses are responsible for the vast majority of diarrhea, but they rarely cause colitis. A review by Guerrant et al. identified the low incidence of bacterial diarrhea and the consequent cost ineffectiveness of routine stool culture, which yields a positive result in only 1.5% to 5.8% of cultures. Highlighting the viral predominance and the low detection rates of testing stool in diarrhea cases, a study by Tamm et al. using polymerase chain reaction testing of stool sample identified no organism in 60.2% of stool samples, *Norovirus* in 16.5% of stool samples, *Sapovirus* in 9.2% identified, and *Rotavirus* in 4.1% of stool samples. *Campylobacter* (the most prevalent bacterial cause) accounted for only 4.6% of stool findings. The likelihood of isolating a specific bacterial enteropathogen increases with the presence of bloody diarrhea. In a review of 30,000 stool cultures in which 3% were grossly bloody, a pathogen was identified in 20% of the grossly bloody specimens. *E. coli* 0157:H7 was identified in 7.8% of all visibly bloody stool specimens and accounted for 39% of all cultured pathogens in this group.

Other etiologies of acute diarrheal illness include inflammatory bowel disease, diverticulitis, partial small bowel obstruction, constipation, medication, irritable bowel syndrome, lactose intolerance, celiac disease, and thyrotoxicosis. A careful history, physical exam, selective laboratory testing, and radiographic imaging may help distinguish these various etiologies.

Typical Disease Course

Disease course varies based on the infecting organism and the individual infected. Most patients experience a mild to moderate disease course that is self-limited and resolves within 1 to 2 weeks. Protracted courses may occur, so more subacute (ie, between 2 and 4 weeks) and chronic (ie, greater than 4 weeks) cases of diarrhea can still be the result of an underlying infectious etiology.

Complications

Hemorrhage and volume loss are the most common complications of infectious colitis. Perforation, toxic megacolon, hemolytic uremic syndrome (HUS), seizures, and sepsis are also serious but less common complications. The very young (less than 5 years), elderly, and immunocompromised are at the highest risk for serious complications.

Diagnostic Tests

Because most cases of infectious diarrhea are self-limited, very few patients need diagnostic workup with stool studies and cultures. Patients with profuse diarrhea, dehydration, bloody diarrhea, fever, severe abdominal pain, or systemic symptoms should be considered for diagnostic evaluation with stool studies and/or cultures. One should have a lower threshold for evaluating the elderly, immunocompromised, children under 5 years, and hospitalized patients. The presence of fecal inflammatory markers and occult blood support a bacterial etiology. The use of fecal leukocytes has been highly variable, with sensitivity and specificity ranging from 20% to 90%. Stool lactoferrin is a more precise measure of fecal white cells with less variation in specimen processing, and it should be used if available. Although fecal leukocytes can be seen in both infectious and inflammatory causes of colitis, their presence indicates a decreased likelihood of a viral etiology. Certain patients may warrant more specific testing, such as stool assessment for ova and parasites. These include patients with exposure to untreated water, patients who have traveled out of the country, men who have sex with men, patients exposed to day-care centers, and patients with AIDS. *C. difficile* toxin should be sent in patients with recent hospitalization or exposure to antibiotics.

Organisms

Table 31.1 Recommendations for Therapy Against Specific Pathogen[a]

Pathogen	Immunocompetent Patients	Immunocompromised Patients
Shigella species	TMP-SMZ, 160 and 8000 mg, respectively (pediatric dose, 5 and 25 mg/kg, respectively) BID × 3 days (if susceptible) or fluoroquinolone (eg, 300 mg ofloxacin, 400 mg norfloxacin, or 500 mg ciprofloxacin BID × 3 days) (A-I); nalidixic acid, 55 mg/kg per day (pediatric) or 1 g/day (adults) × 5 days; ceftriaxone; azithromycin	× 7–10 days
Non-typhi species of Salmonella	Not recommended routinely (E-I). If severe or patient is < 6 months or >50 years old or has prostheses, valvular heart disease, severe atherosclerosis, malignancy, or uremia: TMP-SMZ (if susceptible) or fluoroquinolone as previously BID × 5–7 days (B-III); ceftriaxone, 100 mg/kg per day in 1 or 2 divided doses	× 14 days (or longer if relapsing)
Campylobacter species	Erythromycin 500 mg BID × 5 days (B-II)	Same (but may require prolonged treatment)
Enterotoxigenic E. coli (ETEC)	TMP-SMZ, 160 and 800 mg, respectively BID × 3 days (if susceptible) or fluoroquinolonec (eg, 300 mg ofloxacin, 400 mg norfloxacin, or 500 mg ciprofloxacin BID × 3 days) (A-I)	Same (B-III)
Enteropathogenic E.Coli	As per ETEC (B-II)	Same (B-III)
Enteroinvasive E.coli	As per ETEC (B-II)	Same (B-III)
Enteroaggregative E. coli	Unknown (C-III)	Consider fluoroquinolone as for Enterotoxigenic *E. coli* (B-I)
Shigella Enterohemorrhagic E.coli (STEC)	Avoid antimotility drugs (E-II); role of antibiotics unclear, and administration should be avoided (C-II)	Same (C-III)
Aeromonas/Plesimonas	TMP-SM 160 and 800 mg, respectively, BID × 3 days (if susceptible), fluoroquinolone (eg, 300 mg ofloxacin, 400 mg norfloxacin, or 500 mg ciprofloxacin BID × 3 days (B-III)	Same (B-III)
Yersinia species	Antibiotics are not usually required (C-II); deferoxamine therapy should be withheld (B-II); for severe infections or associated bacteremia, treat as for immunocompromised hosts using combination therapy with doxycycline, aminoglycoside, TMP-SMZ, or fluoroquinolonec (B-III)	Doxycyclin, aminoglycoside (in combination), or TMP-SMZ or fluoroquinolonec (B-III)
Vibrio cholera O1 or O139	Doxycycline, 300 mg single dose, tetracycline,500 mg QID × 3 days, TMP-SMZ 160 and 800 mg, respectively, BID × 3 days, or single-dose fluoroquinolonec (A-I)	Same (B-III)

(continued)

Table 31.1 Continued

Pathogen	Immunocompetent Patients	Immunocompromised Patients
Toxigenic Clostridium difficile	Offending antibiotic should be withdrawn if possible (B-II)]; metronidazole 250 mg QID to 500 mg TID × 10 days (A-I)	Same (B-III)
Giardia	Metronidazole, 250–750 mg TID × 7–10 days (A-I); if severe, consider paromomycin, 500 mg TID × 7 days as with immunocompromised hosts (C-III)	Same (B-III) If needed, paromomycin 500 mg TID × 14–28 days then BID (B-I); highly active antiretroviral therapy including a protease inhibitor is warranted for patients with AIDS (A-II)
Cryptosporidium species	TMP-SMZ, 160 and 800 mg, respectively, BID × 7–10 days (B-III)	TMP-SMZ, 160 and 800 mg, respectively, QID × 10 days, followed by TMP-SMZ thrice weekly or weekly sulfadoxine (500 mg) and pyrimethamine (25 mg) indefinitely for patients with AIDS (A-I)
Isospora species	TMP-SMZ, 160 and 800 mg, respectively, BID × 7 days (A-I)	TMP-SMZ 160 and 800 mg, respectively, QID × 10 days, followed by TMP-SMZ thrice weekly indefinitely (A-II)
Cyclospora species	Not determined	Albenzadole, 400 mg BID × 3 weeks (B-I); highly active antiretroviral therapy including a protease inhibitor is warranted for patients with AIDS (A-II)
Microsporidium species	Metronidazole, 750 mg TID × 5–10 days plus diiodhy-droxyquin, 650 mg TID × 7 days (A-II)	Same
Entamoeba histolytica		

Abbreviations: TMP, trimethoprim; SMZ, sulfamethoxazole; BID, twice daily; TID, three times a day; QID, four times a day; Shiga toxin-producing E. coli.

[a]Adapted from Guerrant RL, Van Gilder T, Steiner TS, et al. Practice guidelines for the management of infectious diarrhea. *Clin Infect Dis.* 2001;32:331–351. Copyright 2001 NAME OF COPYRIGHT HOLDER. Reprinted with permission. Uppercase letters (A–E) indicate the strength of the recommendation, and Roman numerals (I–III) indicate the quality of evidence supporting it, respectively (eg, A-I, B-III, etc; see Table 31.2).

[b]Because up to 20% of isolates from foreign travelers are resistant to TMP-SMZ and resistance to quinolones is rare, a fluoroquinolone is preferred as initial therapy for travel-related shigellosis.

[c]Fluoroquinolones are not approved for treatment of children in the United States.

[d]Antibiotics are most effective if given early in course of illness.

[e]Fosfomycin, not licensed for this use in the United States in 1999, may be safer and possible effective but requires further study [44, 46, 47, 59].

Table 31.2 Categories Indicating the Strength of Recommendations and the Quality of Evidence on Which They Are Based[a]

Category	Definition
Strength of Evidence	
A	Good evidence to support a recommendation for use
B	Moderate evidence to support a recommendation for use
C	Poor evidence to support a recommendation for or against use
D	Moderate evidence to support a recommendation against use
E	Good evidence to support a recommendation against use
Quality of Evidence	
I	Evidence from at least one properly randomized, controlled trial
II	Evidence from at least one well-designed clinical trial without randomization, from cohort or case-controlled analytic studies (preferably from more than one center), from multiple time-series studies, or from dramatic results in uncontrolled experiments
III	Evidence from opinions of respected authorities, based on clinical experience, descriptive studies, or reports of expert committees

[a]Adapted with permission from Gross PA, Barrett TL, Patchen Dellinger E, et al. Purpose of quality standards for infectious diseases. *Clin Infect Dis.* 1994;18:421. Copyright 1994 NAME OF COPYRIGHT HOLDER.

Treatment

The most important component of treatment is adequate hydration. In the United States, intravenous (IV) fluid is grossly overutilized, whereas oral rehydration therapy (ORT) could prevent hospitalization in more than 100,000 children per year. There are many over-the-counter forms of ORT available, but patients can make a simple solution at home by adding one half teaspoon of salt, one half teaspoon of baking soda, and four tablespoons of sugar to one liter of water.

Infectious Diseases Society of America guidelines from 2001 conclude that the benefits of antibiotic treatment should be weighed against the risk of using them, such as prolonging *C. difficile* infection or increasing the risk of HUS in patients with Enterohemorrhagic *E. Coli* (EHEC). Randomized trials suggest that it is beneficial to treat diarrhea in patients with severe traveler's diarrhea with fever and blood, mucus, or pus in their stool. Patients with large volume stool output, dehydration, or compromised immunity should also be considered for empiric treatment.

Treatment options for symptomatic relief include loperamide (Imodium), which is useful in patients without fever and with nonbloody stools. Diphenoxylate (Lomotil) should be used with caution because it has central opioid and cholinergic side effects, which may slow diarrhea and allow pooling of infectious fluid within the intestine. Both loperamide and diphenoxylate have been shown to increase the risk of HUS in patients with EHEC. Probiotics and bismuth subsalicylate (Pepto-Bismol) may improve symptoms and reduce the volume of stool. Patients with diarrhea may develop secondary lactose malabsorption and should consider avoiding dairy products while symptomatic.

The treatment of infectious colitis in adults depends on the infecting organism. *Campylobacter, Shigella*, and *Salmonella* are the most common causes of infectious colitis in the United States. All can be successfully treated with a fluoroquinolone. Appropriate empiric therapy includes ciprofloxacin 500 mg or norfloxacin 400 mg oral administration twice a day for 3 to 5 days for adults. *Campylobacter* can be effectively treated with azithromycin 500 mg daily for 3 days, and this is a reasonable option for empiric therapy given the high prevalence of *Campylobacter*. Children are much less likely to have colitis, and empiric therapy is not recommended.

Alternatively, awaiting stool cultures for definitive management may be reasonable based on the clinical setting. Antibiotics are appropriate in individuals with evidence of colitis. However, they are **not recommended** in cases of mild to moderate diarrhea without evidence of colitis. Specific therapy based on organism is located in Table 31.1. Individuals with hypotension, severe dehydration, significant bleeding, sepsis, or severe electrolyte abnormalities should be admitted to the hospital for IV hydration and, potentially, antibiotic therapy. Discharge home with close follow-up is reasonable for those who have mild to moderate symptoms and who can tolerate oral hydration. Additionally, in countries or populations with a high incidence of zinc deficiency, oral zinc supplementation is both inexpensive and helpful in decreasing stool output.

Other Key Issues

In any individual with diarrhea, address recent travel history, possible immunosuppression, the presence of blood or mucus in the stool, and any history of vomiting or severe abdominal pain. The focus of therapy should be maintaining adequate hydration and not missing potentially dangerous etiologies. Oral hydration is the preferred method of rehydration for mild to moderate dehydration. IV hydration can be used for those with moderate to severe dehydration with supplemental oral hydration solutions if discharge is possible.

Suggested Readings and References

1. Wolfson AB. Diarrhea. In: *Harwood-Nuss' Clinical Practice of Emergency Medicine*. 5th ed. Philadelphia, PA: Lippincott, Williams and Wilkins; 2010:599–605.
2. *Harrison's Principles of Internal Medicine*. 17th ed. New York: McGraw-Hill Companies. 2008:247–253.
3. Lamberti LM, Walker CLF, Black RE. Systematic review of diarrhea duration and severity in children and adults in low- and middle-income countries. *BMC Public Health*. 2012;12:276.
4. Tam CC, O'Brien SJ, Tompkins DS, et al. Changes in causes of acute gastroenteritis in the United Kingdom over 15 years. *Clin Infect Dis*. 2012;54:1275–1286.
5. Huicho L, Sanchez D, Contreras M, et al. Occult blood and fecal leukocytes as screening tests in childhood infectious diarrhea: an old problem revisited. *Pediatr Infect Dis J*. 1993;12:474–477.
6. Slutsker L, Ries AA, Greene KD, et al. Escherichia coli O157:H7 diarrhea in the United States: clinical and epidemiological features. *Ann Intern Med*. 1997;126:505–513.

7. Santosham M, Keenan EM, Tulloch J, et al. Oral rehydration therapy for diarrhea: an example of reverse transfer of technology. *Pediatrics*. 1997;100:E10.

8. Guerrant RL, Van Gilder T, Steiner TS, et al. Practice guidelines for the management of infectious diarrhea. *Clin Infect Dis*. 2001;32:331–351.

9. CDC. Foodborne Diseases Active Surveillance Network (FoodNet): FoodNet Surveillance Report for 2010 (Final Report). Atlanta, Georgia: US Department of Health and Human Services, CDC. 2011.

10. Kollaritsch H, Paulke-Korinek M, Wiedermann U. Traveler's diarrhea. *Infect Dis Clin N Am*. 2012;26:691–706.

11. Pfeiffer ML, DuPont HL, Ochoa TJ. The patient presenting with acute dysentery - a systematic review. *J Infect*. 2012;64:374–386.

12. Gerding DN, Johnson S, Peterson LR, Mulligan ME, Silva J Jr. Clostridium difficile-associated diarrhea and colitis. *Infect Control Hosp Epidemiol*. 1995;16:459–477.

13. Costa AD, Silva GA. Oral rehydration therapy in emergency departments. *J Pediatr (Rio J)*. 2011;87:175–179.

14. Scrimgeour AG, Lukaski HC. Zinc and diarrheal disease: current status and future perspectives. *Curr Opin Clin Nutr Metab Care*. 2008;11:711–717.

Peritonitis

Elizabeth Rosenblatt

Summary Box

Disease Description: Peritonitis, or inflammation of the serosal membranes lining the abdominal cavity, is a term used predominately to describe primary peritonitis (spontaneous bacterial peritonitis) and secondary peritonitis—two conditions with distinct pathophysiologies requiring different diagnostic and therapeutic approaches.

Organisms:
  Primary Peritonitis: Monomicrobial
    Escherichia coli
    Klebsiella species
    Streptococcus pneumoniae and other streptococcal species
    Other Enterobacteriaceae
    Staphylococci species
  Secondary Peritonitis: Polymicrobial, organisms vary based on affected organ system
    Gram-negative bacilli (especially in distal small bowel and colonic sources)
    Anaerobes (especially in distal small bowel and colonic sources)
    Gram positives (especially in proximal bowel sources)
        Dialysis-Associated Peritonitis:
        Coagulase-negative Staphylococci
        Staphylococcus aureus
        Gram negative bacilli
        Candida

Diagnostic tests:
  Paracentesis
  Peritoneal lavage
  Consider abdominal and chest imaging
  Treatment:
  Primary Peritonitis:
    First-line Parenteral—cefotaxime 2 g q8 hours OR ceftriaxone 1 g q12 hours
    First-line Oral—ofloxacin 400 mg q12 hours
    Other Parenteral Options—amoxicillin/clavulanic acid, 1 g/0.2 g q6 to 8 hours; levofloxacin 750 mg q24 hours; ciprofloxacin 400 mg q12 hours; moxifloxacin 400 mg q24 hours; piperacillin/tazobactam, 3.375 to 4.5 mg q6 to 8 hours

Secondary Peritonitis:

Patients in intensive care unit—imipenem 500 mg q6 hours; OR meropenem 1 g q8 hours; OR combination of ampicillin 1 to 2 g q4 to 6 hours, ciprofloxacin 400 mg q8 hours, and metronidazole 500 mg q8 hours

Other hospitalized patients—third or fourth generation cephalosporin OR ampicillin-sulbactam 1.5 to 3 g q6 hours; OR ticarcillin/clavulanate 3.1 g q6 hours; OR aztreonam 1 to 2 g q8 hours; OR imipenem cilastatin 500 mg q6 hours; OR piperacillin tazobactam 3.375 to 4.5 g q6 to 8 hours PLUS metronidazole 500 mg q8 hours OR clindamycin, 600 mg q8 hours

Dialysis-Associated Peritonitis:

Intraperitoneal first-generation cephalosporin, such as cefazolin 15 mg/kg q24 hours PLUS fluoroquinolone OR third generation cephalosporin.

In areas with high prevalence of methicillin-resistant *Staphylococcus aureus*, use vancomycin instead of cefazolin.

Other Key Issues: One-third of patients with spontaneous bacterial peritonitis (SBP) develop renal dysfunction, which is an independent predictor of mortality.

Peritonitis is defined as inflammation of the peritoneum, the membrane that lines the abdominal cavity and its organs. This inflammation can be localized or diffuse, acute or chronic, and infectious or aseptic.(1) It can be further specified as primary peritonitis, secondary peritonitis, or tertiary peritonitis.

Primary peritonitis almost invariably occurs in patients with ascites and is thought to be caused by bacterial translocation into the peritoneal cavity in the setting of immune system dysfunction, altered portal circulation, and abnormal gut motility. In **secondary peritonitis**, a clear nidus of infection is identified, whether it be a perforated viscus, external penetrating injury, or presence of a foreign body, among others. The term **tertiary peritonitis** is used to describe persistent symptoms or signs of infection despite appropriate treatment of primary or secondary peritonitis. Patients undergoing peritoneal dialysis are at risk for **catheter associated peritonitis,** which is sometimes considered an additional category of peritonitis. Each of the previous conditions affects a distinct patient population and is characterized by a distinct pathophysiology, thus requiring different diagnostic and therapeutic approaches.

This chapter will focus on primary peritonitis as the management of secondary peritonitis varies widely depending on the underlying nidus of infection.

Disease Description

Primary peritonitis, otherwise known as spontaneous bacterial peritonitis (SBP), is most commonly defined as an infection of the peritoneal cavity without an identifiable intra-abdominal source of infection. The underlying pathophysiology of SBP is incompletely understood, but it is thought to occur by bacterial translocation from the gut to the bloodstream and subsequently to the ascitic fluid. This process likely takes place in the setting of altered gut motility, small bowel bacterial overgrowth, portal hypertension, and impaired host immune defenses.

Epidemiology

SBP almost invariably occurs in the presence of ascites, usually from ascites in the setting of liver cirrhosis. In this patient population, the prevalence is high—recent studies have suggested that 10% to 30% of patients with cirrhosis and ascites admitted to the hospital have evidence of SBP.(2) Of these patients, the vast majority have decompensated liver failure. In one review of patients with cirrhosis and SBP, 70% were Child Pugh class C (a classification of liver disease severity ranging from A to C, with C being more advanced disease).(3,17) SBP can more rarely occur in the setting of ascites secondary to congestive heart failure, systemic lupus erythematosus, lymphedema, hepatitis, or metastatic disease.

Presenting Features

The presenting features of SBP are nonspecific. The most common manifestation of SBP is fever, which occurs in up to 80% of affected patients. In addition, patients often endure abdominal pain, general malaise, fatigue, and hepatic encephalopathy. Other symptoms may include worsening ascites, decreased urine output, ileus, or diarrhea. Approximately 10% of patients are asymptomatic.(4, 17)

On physical examination, patients will invariably have ascites. Abdominal exam may range from lack of any abdominal tenderness to the presence of acute abdomen. Patients often have signs of decompensated liver failure, including gynecomastia, lower extremity edema, spider angiomata, jaundice, and asterixis.

Disease Course

Over the past several years, improvements in diagnostic testing and antibiotic therapy have resulted in a significant reduction of morbidity and mortality from SBP. In patients who receive early treatment, mortality rates have been reported at less than 10%. In patients with delayed treatment, mortality may exceed 30%.(6) Over a year, the mortality rate of patients diagnosed with SBP has been reported as high as 70%, likely reflecting the severity of the underlying liver disease that predisposes patients to peritonitis in the first place.(7)

Patients are at high risk for recurrence of SBP. Without antibiotic prophylaxis, 70% will have recurrence within 1 year. Prophylaxis with antibiotics may reduce recurrence in these patients to less than 20% per year and has also been shown to improve short-term survival.(4,17)

Complications

One-third of patients with SBP develop renal dysfunction, which is an independent predictor of mortality and thought to be secondary to decreased effective circulating volume.(18)

Other common complications of SBP include sepsis and hepatic encephalopathy.

Diagnostic Considerations

Because the clinical presentation of SBP is nonspecific, evaluation for SBP by ascitic fluid analysis is essential. All patients with suspected SBP should have consideration for diagnostic paracentesis with cell count, differential, and culture. The utility of paracentesis increases if performed prior to the administration of antibiotics, as even a single dose of antibiotic may lead to negative ascitic fluid culture in almost 90% of cases.(5) Primary sources of abdominal infection, such as perforated viscus or abscess should be excluded, so abdominal imaging with computed tomography (CT) can be useful.

Diagnostic Tests

The diagnosis of SBP is established by paracentesis with greater than 250 polymononuclear cells/uL; positive ascitic fluid bacterial culture; and lack of evidence of a surgically treatable, intra-abdominal source of infection.

Diagnostic Paracentesis: Diagnostic paracentesis with cell count, differential, and culture remains the test of choice for diagnosing SBP. Polymononuclear cells (PMNs) of > 250/uL has a sensitivity of 93% and specificity of 94% for the detection of SBP.(3) In peritoneal dialysis patients, the threshold for the diagnosis of peritonitis is lowered to PMNs of > 100/uL. In the case of traumatic paracentesis or hemorrhagic ascites, 1 polymononuclear cell should be subtracted for every 250 red blood cells in the cell count.(8) Total protein, glucose, lactate dehydrogenase, and albumin (both ascitic and serum) should also be measured. A serum-ascites albumin gradient greater than or equal to 1.1 g/dL is highly suggestive of portal hypertension, which is a key factor in the pathogenesis of SBP. The presence of thousands of polymononuclear cells on cell count, multiple organisms, total protein greater than 1 g/dL, glucose less than 50 mg/dL, or lactate dehydrogenase above the upper limit of normal for serum should raise suspicion for secondary bacterial peritonitis and should prompt urgent surgical evaluation(9,19) (see Table 32.1). A monocyte predominant cell count should raise suspicion for peritonitis related to tuberculosis or to peritoneal carcinomatosis.(19)

Blood cultures: Blood cultures should be drawn because patients are often bacteremic with the causative organism for SBP.

Abdominal imaging: Abdominal imaging is an important consideration in patients with suspected SBP and abdominal pain as it can aid in ruling out intra-abdominal source of infection. CT chest and abdomen

Table 32.1 Peritoneal Fluid Analysis in SBP and in Secondary Peritonitis

Peritoneal Fluid	Spontaneous Bacterial Peritonitis	Secondary Peritonitis
Lymphocytes PMNs	> 500 (> 250 PMNs)	Often in the thousands[a]
LDH	Less than upper limit of normal for serum LDH	Greater than upper limit of normal for serum LDH
Glucose	> 50	< 50
Protein	< 1 g/dL	> 1 g/dL
Culture	Single organism	Multiple organisms, including anaerobes, fungi, and enterococcus
Other		CEA > 5 or alk phos > 240 has sensitivity of 92% for perforating secondary peritonitis

Abbreviations: SBP, spontaneous bacterial peritonitis; PMN, polymorphonuclear leukocyte; LDH, lactate dehydrogenase; CEA, carcinoembryonic antigen; alk phos, alkaline phosphatase.

[a]In nonperforating secondary peritonitis, PMNs are often not as elevated as in perforating secondary peritonitis but will increase despite antibiotic management.

may reveal free fluid, abscess, or free air under the diaphragm. Abdominal films may also reveal dilatation of bowel with edema or free air suggestive of bowel perforation.

Organisms

SBP is almost always caused by a single organism. *Escherichia coli, Klebsiella pneumoniae*, and pneumococci comprise the majority of organisms; enterobacteriaceae, staphylococci, and pseudomonas are other potential causative organisms.(10,18)

Treatment

Antibiotic Therapy: In patients with ascites and high clinical suspicion for infection (ie, fever, abdominal pain, or encephalopathy), empiric antibiotic therapy should be started immediately following blood cultures and diagnostic paracentesis. Empiric therapy should cover gram-negative aerobic enterobacteriaceae and non-enterococcal streptococci.

First-line therapy for SBP is cefotaxime 2 g q8 hours, which has been shown to be more effective than ampicillin plus tobramycin in the treatment of SBP.(11) Other third-generation cephalosporins, such as ceftriaxone 1 g q12 hours, have been shown to be equally efficacious in some trials. Alternative regimens include amoxicillin plus clavulanic acid, fluoroquinolones, and piperacillin/tazobactam.(12,18) Fluoroquinolones should be avoided in those currently taking fluoroquinolones for prophylaxis (these patients are more likely to harbor resistant organisms).(3) In patients without severe underlying disease (defined as vomiting, shock, greater than grade 2 encephalopathy, or creatinine > 3), oral ofloxacin 400 mg q12 hours for 8 days has been shown to be as effective as parenteral cefotaxime in one randomized trial.(13)

Antibiotic coverage should be narrowed based on blood and ascitic fluid culture analysis. In patients without bacteremia, it is reasonable to treat for 5 days, as studies have shown similar mortality and cure rates in patients with SBP treated with a 5- versus 10-day course of cefotaxime.(14) After an episode of SBP, all patients should receive consideration for indefinite SBP prophylaxis with daily quinolone or trimethoprim-sulfamethoxazole therapy.

Supportive Therapy: Administration of 1.5 g/kg of intravenous albumin on day 1 and 1 g/kg on day 3 results in improved in-hospital survival as well as decreased incidence of renal impairment in patients with SBP.(15) However, the benefit of albumin may extend only to patients with significant underlying disease—in one trial, albumin resulted in improved survival and decreased morbidity only in patients with serum creatinine > 1, blood urea nitrogen > 30, or total bilirubin > 4.(16)

Treatment Response: In most cases of uncomplicated SBP, clinical improvement is demonstrated within 72 hours of antibiotic initiation. Patients who have typical symptoms, ascitic fluid analysis consistent with SBP, and symptom improvement following treatment do not need repeat paracentesis to gauge treatment response. In those patients with atypical findings, a repeat paracentesis is useful to monitor for a secondary causes of peritonitis.

Suggested Readings and References

1. Silen W. Acute appendicitis and peritonitis. In: Fauci A, ed. *Harrison's Principles of Internal Medicine*. 18th ed. New York: McGraw-Hill; 2012.

2. Lata J, Stiburek O, Kopacova M. Spontaneous bacterial peritonitis: a severe complication of liver cirrhosis. *World J Gastroenterol*. 2009;15:5505–5510.

3. Runyon BA. Management of adult patients with ascites due to cirrhosis. *Hepatology*. 2004;39:841–856.

4. Baron MJ, Kasper DL. Intraabdominal infections and abscesses. In: Fauci A, ed. *Harrison's Principles of Internal Medicine*. 18th ed. New York: McGraw-Hill; 2012.

5. Akriviadis EA, Runyon BA. The utility of an algorithm in differentiating spontaneous from secondary bacterial peritonitis. *Gastroenterology*. 1990;98:127–133.

6. Katz J, ed. Medscape: Peritonitis and Abdominal Sepsis. http://emedicine.medscape.com/article/180234-overview

7. Moore KP, Aithal GP. Guidelines on the management of ascites in cirrhosis. *Gut*. 2006;55(suppl 6):vi1–v12.

8. Rimola A, Garcia-Tsao G, Navasa M, et al. Diagnosis, treatment, and prophylaxis of spontaneous bacterial peritonitis: a consensus document. International Ascites Club. *J Hepatol*. 2000;32:142–153.

9. Cohen J, ed. *Infectious Diseases*. 3rd ed. Philadelphia, PA: Elsevier; 2010: Chapter 37.

10. In: Surawicz CM, Owen RL, eds. *Gastrointestinal and Hepatic Infections*. Philadelphia, PA: WB Saunders; 1995:455.

11. Felisart J, Rimola A, Arroyo V, et al. Cefotaxime is more effective than is ampicillin-tobramycin in cirrhotics with severe infections. *Hepatology*. 1985;5:457–462.

12. Parsi MA, Atreja A, Zein NN. Spontaneous bacterial peritonitis: recent data on incidence and treatment. *Cleve Clin J Med*. 2004;71;569–576.

13. Navasa M, Follo A, Llovet JM, et al. Randomized, comparative study of oral ofloxacin versus intravenous cefotaxime in spontaneous bacterial peritonitis. *Gastroenterology*. 1996;111:1011–1017.

14. Runyon BA, McHutchison JG, Antillon MR, et al. Short-course vs long course antibiotic treatment of spontaneous bacterial peritonitis: a randomized controlled study of 100 patients. *Gastroenterology*. 1991;100:1737–1742.

15. Sort P, Navasa M, Arroyo V, et al. Effect of intravenous albumin on renal impairment and mortality in patients with cirrhosis and spontaneous bacterial peritonitis. *N Engl J Med*. 1999;341:403–409.

16. Sigal SH, Stanca CM, Fernandez J, Arroyo V, Navasa M. Restricted use of albumin for spontaneous bacterial peritonitis. *Gut*. 2007;56:597–599.

17. Such J, Runyon BA. Spontaneous bacterial peritonitis. *Clin Infect Dis*. 1998;27:669–676.

18. Xia HH. Spontaneous bacterial peritonitis. *World J Gastroenterol* 2009;15(9):1042–1049.

19. Levinson ME, Bush, LM. Peritonitis and intraperitoneal abscesses. In: Mandel GL, ed. *Principles and Practice of Infectious Diseases*. 7th ed. Philadelphia, PA: Churchill and Livingstone; 2010:1011–1034.

Chapter 33

Diverticulitis

Bharati Kocher

Summary Box

Disease Description: Diverticulitis is acute inflammation of diverticula, which are saclike protrusions of the mucosal and submucosal walls of the colon.

Treatment:
Antibiotics:
- Metronidazole and a quinolone or third-generation cephalosporin
- Beta lactam with beta lactamase inhibitors
- Typically 7 to 10 day course

Pursue surgical intervention as needed.

Other Key Issues: The incidence of diverticular disease increases with age. 80% of people who present with diverticulitis are older than age 50.

Computed tomography (CT) is the gold standard for diagnosis; it additionally rules out other abdominal pathology and detects any other complications of diverticulitis.

A high fiber diet is recommended to prevent recurrent attacks.

Disease Description

Terminology and Presenting Features

Diverticular disease is an umbrella term for two conditions, diverticulosis and diverticulitis, which both involve saclike protrusions of the mucosal and submucosal walls (typically in the colon). Diverticulosis is the presence of multiple diverticula, which may or may not be symptomatic. Symptomatic diverticulosis can present with indistinct symptoms (eg, cramping, bloating, flatulence, and changes in bowel movements) and, less commonly, with more severe symptoms, such as bleeding that can be slow (causing anemia) or rapid (causing frank hematochezia and even hemodynamic instability).

Diverticulitis is acute or chronic inflammation of the diverticula, which can lead to the development of abscesses and even perforation. The classic triad for diverticulitis includes fever, leukocytosis, and left-sided abdominal pain with localized tenderness and guarding. However, the presentation of diverticulitis varies with the extent of disease progression and can be seen with abdominal pain alone. Scant blood per rectum or guaiac-positive stool may also be observed.

Epidemiology

The incidence of diverticulosis increases with age. In the United States, approximately 10% of adults under the age of 40 and 70% of people older than 70 have diverticulosis. In fact, diverticulosis is the most commonly reported finding on screening colonoscopies. Nearly 80% of people who present with diverticulitis are older than 50 years. Diverticulitis accounts for approximately 300,000 hospitalizations annually. The annual mortality is about 2.5 per 100,000 cases. In Western societies, diverticular disease tends to primarily affect the distal descending and sigmoid colon. In Asia, it more commonly occurs in the cecum and ascending colon. The reason for this difference is not well established.

Risk Factors

Exact risk factors for diverticulitis have yet to be elucidated. However, as with diverticulosis, there is thought to be an association with diets low in fiber and high in refined carbohydrates. Increased intra-colonic pressures, such as that from constipation, have been observed in patients with diverticulosis. Other risk factors noted in the literature include physical inactivity, obesity, smoking, and nonsteroidal anti-inflammatory drug use.

Pathogenesis

In gastrointestinal diverticula, the submucosa and mucosa herniate, but the surrounding muscle layers and adventitia do not. Diverticula herniate through the mucosal layer of the colonic wall at sites of weakness created by the penetration of the vasa recta vessels, typically at the margins of the taenium coli. Although it is not clearly elucidated, the pathogenesis is thought to be due to increased intraluminal pressures, which result in abnormal colonic motility and outpouching. Stasis and obstruction in a diverticulum may lead to bacterial overgrowth and local tissue ischemia, which can cause diverticulitis. The pathophysiology may be similar to appendicitis.

Diagnosis

Ultrasonography and CT are equally accurate in the diagnosis of diverticulitis. However, CT more accurately detects other etiologies of abdominal pain. Therefore, CT is the gold standard for diagnosis of diverticulitis. CT has a sensitivity of approximately 95% and a specificity of nearly 100% for the diagnosis of diverticulitis. Typical CT findings for diverticulitis include the presence of diverticula, pericolic inflammation, bowel thickness > 4 mm, and peridiverticular abscesses. CT is helpful in the staging of the disease as well.

Staging

The severity of diverticulitis is most commonly graded by Hinchey's criteria:
- Stage 1: small (< 4 cm), confined pericolic or mesenteric abscesses without peritonitis
- Stage 2: large abscesses
- Stage 3: perforated diverticulitis
- Stage 4: free rupture or rupture of the uninflamed or unobstructed diverticulum, resulting in peritonitis

Stage 1 and 2 disease have less than a 5% mortality, whereas mortality is approximately 13% for those with stage 3 disease and 43% for those with stage 4 disease.

Differential Diagnosis

The differential diagnosis for diverticulitis is broad and encompasses most abdominal pathologies, including the following:

- Appendicitis
- Infectious Colitis
- Inflammatory Bowel Disease (IBD)
- Advanced colon cancer
- Cystitis
- Pelvic Inflammatory Disease
- Ectopic pregnancy

Complications

Abscesses are common in diverticular disease; even uncomplicated diverticulitis may present with microperforations. Large abscesses may cause worsening symptoms and major perforation. Thankfully, major perforation only occurs in 1% to 2% of cases. When it does occur, peritonitis and fistulas with other peritoneal organs may occur. Severe peridiverticular disease and recurrent diverticulitis may result in strictures, which can, at times, result in high grade bowel obstruction.

Treatment

A 7- to 10-day outpatient course of oral antibiotics can be prescribed for uncomplicated diverticulitis in an immunocompetent patient who can tolerate oral intake. The most commonly used regimen is ciprofloxacin and metronidazole. A low residue liquid diet is recommended during the course of treatment, although the utility of this recommendation has not been studied.

In hospitalized patients, parenteral antibiotics targeting anaerobes and gram-negative organisms are indicated. Typical combinations include a beta lactam with a beta lactamase inhibitor or metronidazole with a quinolone or third-generation cephalosporin. If there is no clinical improvement after 3 days of treatment, repeat imaging is indicated to evaluate for the development of complications. Bowel rest and parenteral antibiotics are indicated when patients are unable to tolerate oral intake or in advanced stages of diverticulitis.

Notably, a Cochrane review of the use of antibiotics in **uncomplicated** diverticulitis concludes that there is no difference in the mode of administration or the length of antibiotics. The only study to evaluate the use of antibiotics versus no antibiotics demonstrated a nonsignificant trend toward greater abscess formation in the no antibiotics group. Fewer than 10% of patients admitted for diverticulitis require surgical intervention during the same admission. However, patients with Hinchey stage 2 disease should undergo percutaneous drainage of their abscesses before discharge. Indications for surgery are generalized peritonitis or large abscesses that cannot be drained, typically Hinchey stage 3 or 4 disease. Current surgical management involves a one-step sigmoid resection with primary anastomosis. In rare cases, a traditional three-stage sigmoid drainage with diverting colostomy, interval sigmoid resection with primary anastomosis, and ostomy reversal has to be performed. Currently, laparoscopic colectomy is not the standard; however, there is a move toward laparoscopic procedures, especially in milder cases.

After an episode of diverticulitis, an interval colonoscopy or sigmoidoscopy is recommended to rule out malignancy and to evaluate for other etiologies, such as IBDs. Retrospective cohort studies reveal that is there a 10% to 30% risk of recurrence within the first decade after an episode of diverticulitis. Young age (< 50 years), multiple comorbidities, and obesity are risk factors for recurrence.

A high-fiber diet is recommended for those with diverticular disease; however, there is little evidence supporting this recommendation. There is anecdotal evidence that mesalamine use after an episode of acute diverticulitis decreases inflammation via an unknown mechanism. In general, there is a paucity of literature on preventing the occurrence or recurrence of acute diverticulitis.

Suggested Readings and References

1. Jacobs DO. Diverticulitis. *N Engl J Med*. 2007;357:2057–2066.
2. Maconi G, Barbara G, Bosetti C, Cuomo R, Annibale B. Treatment of diverticular disease of the colon and prevention of acute diverticulitis: a systematic review. *Dis Colon Rectum*. 2011;54:1326–1338.

3. Shabanzadeh DM, Wille-Jorgensen P. Antibiotics for uncomplicated diverticulitis. *Cochrane Database Syst Rev.* 2012;11:CD009092.

4. Strate LL, Modi R, Cohen E, Spiegel BMR. Diverticular disease as a chronic illness: evolving epidemiologic and clinical insights. *Am J Gastroenterol.* 2012;107:1486–1493.

5. Wolff BG, Boostrom SY. Prophylactic resection, uncomplicated diverticulitis and recurrent diverticulitis. *Dig Dis.* 2012;30:108–113.

Chapter 34

Cholecystitis and Cholangitis

Sarah Carle

Summary Box

Disease Description: At least 10% of Americans are affected by biliary disease. Presenting complaints include right upper quadrant (RUQ) pain, nausea, vomiting, and fever.

Organisms: *Escherichia coli* and *Klebsiella, Enterobacter*, and *Enterococcus* species are commonly seen. *Pseudomonas* and anaerobes are seen in elderly patients and in nosocomial infections

Treatment: Pursue early surgical consult for cholecystostomy or cholecystectomy. Gastroenterology should be consulted in cases of suspected or confirmed common bile duct (CBD) stones and in ascending cholangitis, as endoscopic retrograde cholangiopancreatography (ERCP) with sphincterotomy or dilation is the initial procedure of choice.

Suggested antibiotic regimens include Beta-lactamase inhibitors: ampicillin-sulbactam 3 g IV q6 hours, piperacillin-tazobactam 3.375 g IV q6 hours, or ticarcillin-clavulanate 3.1 g IV q4 hours.

Gastrointestinal Infections

Disease Description

Epidemiology

At least 10% of Americans are affected by gallstones, accounting for approximately 1.8 million ambulatory visits per year and an estimated six billion dollars in annual medical costs. Mortality from biliary disease has decreased with advancements in diagnostic and treatment modalities. The current death rate is low at 0.7 per 100 000, but morbidity is abundant with more than 500,000 patients undergoing cholecystectomy annually. The female to male ratio in biliary disease is roughly three to one, but this narrows after age 50.[1]

Pathogenesis

The gallbladder stores, concentrates, and secretes bile to aid in fat digestion and absorption. During the concentration process, components of bile may become supersaturated, precipitate out of solution, and form crystals. Up to 80% of gallstones in the United States result from the crystallization of cholesterol. Risk factors for cholesterol stones include hyperlipidemia, advancing age, female gender, pregnancy, obesity, European or Native American ethnicity, prolonged total parenteral nutrition, rapid weight loss, Crohn's disease, and ileal resection.

Less commonly, gallstones are composed of supersaturated calcium bilirubinate. Known as pigment stones, these form as a result of high heme turnover, which is seen in patients with hemolytic anemia, cirrhosis, structural gallbladder abnormalities, or infection.

The pathogenesis of acute cholecystitis requires both mechanical obstruction (generally from a stone lodged in the cystic duct) and the release of inflammatory mediators, generally due to trauma to the gallbladder wall. Although secondary bacterial infection plays a role in some patients, it is not necessary for the development of acute cholecystitis. Bile cultures taken at the time of surgery are positive in only 32% to 37% of patients.[2]

Disease Course

Cholelithiasis

Most patients with gallstones remain asymptomatic. Those who develop symptoms often present with RUQ or epigastric pain, which is typically postprandial and associated with nausea. As the disease progresses, pain may radiate to the back or to the right shoulder and may be associated with vomiting.

Acute Cholecystitis

Patients with acute cholecystitis appear ill on exam and often have fever and tachycardia. Abdominal examination generally shows RUQ tenderness and a positive *Murphy's sign* (pain and inspiratory arrest when the examiner's hand is applying pressure to the gallbladder fossa, which resides at the intersection of the inferior costal margin and the right midclavicular line). Patients with acute cholecystitis pause during inspiration due to peritoneal irritation experienced as the inflamed gallbladder moves inferiorly during inspiration and comes into contact with the examiner's hand. A positive Murphy's sign has a sensitivity of 97% and specificity of 48% when compared with cholescintigraphy.[3]

Up to 10% of acute cholecystitis cases are due to biliary disease without gallstones, a condition termed acalculous cholecystitis. Classically, acalculous cholecystitis occurs as a complication of major surgery, trauma, burns, or sepsis due to resulting bile stasis and poor gallbladder perfusion. Ambulatory cases are increasingly recognized, typically in elderly males with underlying major medical disease such as diabetes, congestive heart failure, atherosclerosis, vasculitis, and end-stage renal disease. Patients with acalculous cholecystitis may present with classic features of acute cholecystitis or with fever and sepsis alone. Generally, acalculous cholecystitis is associated with a higher degree of morbidity and mortality.

Choledocholithiasis

Choledocholithiasis results from gallstone obstruction of the CBD. Presentation is similar to that of acute cholecystitis but may also be associated with jaundice or acute pancreatitis.

Cholangitis

Cholangitis is a bacterial infection of the biliary system that is commonly associated with mechanical obstruction of the cystic or common bile duct. Obstruction is usually caused by choledocholithiasis but may also be seen with biliary stricture, malignancy, or cyst. Biliary obstructions cause increased intraluminal pressure, which favors the migration of bacteria from the portal system into the biliary tract and leads to bacterial colonization and proliferation. Cholangitis can also occur in patients with recent biliary manipulation or stenting, which disrupts the normal protective barrier and sterile biliary environment. The classic presentation of cholangitis consists of RUQ pain, jaundice, and fever (*Charcot's triad*); however, this triad is only seen in half of patients with cholangitis. The eponym *Reynold's pentad* is applied to the symptom complex that includes mental status changes and shock in addition to Charcot's triad. Reynold's pentad carries significant morbidity and mortality.

Complications

Bacterial proliferation may lead to gangrenous cholecystitis, gallbladder perforation (with potential for cholecystoenteric fistula creation), and/or sepsis. Passage of a gallstone into the bowel may cause a gallstone ileus, which is a mechanical obstruction of the bowel that typically occurs in the relatively narrow terminal ileum. Secondary infection of the gallbladder wall by gas-forming organisms, such as *Clostridium*, *E. coli*, *Pseudomonas*, and *Klebsiella*, may lead to emphysematous cholecystitis. Patients with emphysematous cholecystitis may have crepitus on exam. Ultrasound may misidentify bacterially formed gas as normal bowel gas overlying the gallbladder. Patients with emphysematous cholecystitis are at higher risk of perforation, abscess formation, and peritonitis.

Differential Diagnosis

A high degree of clinical suspicion is necessary because patients often present atypically with symptoms that may mimic other causes of intra-abdominal, cardiac, and pulmonary pathology. Other sources of RUQ pain include acute hepatitis, early appendicitis, pancreatitis, right-sided pneumonia, pathology of the right kidney or ovary, and Fitz-Hugh-Curtis syndrome (inflammation of the liver surface due to gonococcal infection).

Diagnostic Tests

Laboratory Evaluation

Laboratory studies are generally adjunctive as the diagnosis of cholecystitis is often made based on history, risk factors, and examination followed by confirmation with radiography. Leukocytosis may be present in acute cholecystitis and cholangitis. Elevations of aspartate aminotransferase, alanine aminotransferase, total bilirubin, and alkaline phosphate are not common with simple cholecystitis and should raise concern for cholangitis, choledocholithiasis, or Mirizzi syndrome (extrinsic compression of the CBD due to a stone in the distal cystic duct). Elevation of lipase indicates concomitant pancreatitis or CBD stone. Blood cultures should be drawn from all febrile patients.

Imaging

Ultrasound is the first-line imaging study in the diagnosis of cholecystitis and cholangitis. Ultrasound may show gallbladder wall thickening (greater than 4–5 mm), pericholecystic fluid, gallbladder sludge or stones, or a sonographic Murphy's sign (pain and inspiratory arrest on inhalation while the ultrasound examiner applies pressure over the gallbladder with the ultrasound probe). Dilation of the CBD indicates choledocholithiasis. The sensitivity and specific of ultrasound findings is widely variable among studies, with sensitivity ranging from 48% to 95% and specificity ranging from 48% to 100%.[4] Sensitivity and specificity is highest in studies showing stones greater than 2 mm, a positive Murphy's sign, and multiple abnormal findings suggestive of cholecystitis.

Radionuclide cholescintigraphy (hepatobiliary iminodiacetic acid scan) is 90% to 100% sensitive and 85% to 95% specific and is used when clinical suspicion is high for acute cholecystitis but ultrasound is equivocal or negative.[5] This nuclear medicine study involves administering IV iminodiacetic acid labeled with technetium, which is selectively taken up by the liver and secreted into the bile. The test is considered positive for cholecystitis if the gallbladder is not visualized after 60 minutes, as this suggests cystic duct obstruction. Computed tomography (CT) scan may show gallbladder wall edema, pericholecystic stranding, and gallbladder perforation; but CT often fails to detect gallstones, which are isodense with bile. CT is most useful when trying to rule out alternative intra-abdominal pathology. Magnetic resonance cholangiography is a noninvasive way of assessing intrahepatic and extrahepatic bile ducts and is used most commonly when the surgeon is concerned about a stone in the common bile duct.

Organisms

The sterility of bile is maintained by the sphincter of Oddi, which prevents reflux from the duodenum, as well as the bacteriostatic activity of bile salts, secretory immunoglobulin A, and bile mucous. Bile is thought to be secondarily infected after biliary obstruction when normal defenses are impaired and bile stasis promotes colonization. The exact mechanism of infection is unknown, but possibilities include direct spread of bacteria from the small bowel, hematogenous spread from the portal vein, and lymphatic spread. Despite acute cholecystitis typically being considered an infectious process, bile cultures are positive in only 30% to 70% of cases.

Table 34.1 Suggested Antibiotic Regimens for Suspected Bacterial infections of the Biliary System

Regimen	Dose
Monotherapy	
Beta-lactamase inhibitors:	
• Ampicillin-sulbactam	3 g IV q6 h
or	
• Piperacillin-tazobactam	3.375 g IV q6 h
or	
• Ticarcillin-clavulanate	3.1 g IV q4 h
Carbapenems:	
• Ertapenem[a] or	1 g IV daily
• Meropenem or	1 g IV q8 h
• Doripenem or	500 mg IV q8 h
• Imipenem-cilastin	500 mg IV q6 h
Combination Therapy	
Third- or Fourth-Generation Cephalosporins:	
• Ceftriaxone or	2 g IV q12 h
• Cefepime	2 g IV q12 h
Fluoroquinolones:	
• Ciprofloxacin or	400 mg IV q12 h
• Levofloxacin	750 mg IV daily
Monobactam	
• Aztreonam	1 g IV q8 h
Plus	
Flagyl	500 mg IV q8 h

Abbreviations: IV, intravenous; h, hours.

[a]Ertapenem does not have antipseudomonal activity and is not recommended in patients with severe or hospital-acquired infection.

When positive, bile cultures typically consist of mixed gram-negative and gram-positive species.

The most common isolated gram-negative enteric pathogens include *E. coli* (22%–50% of isolates) in addition to *Klebsiella* (15%–20%) and *Enterobacter* (5%–10%) species. *Enterococcus* species are the most commonly isolated gram-positive species (10%–20% of isolates). *Pseudomonas* and anaerobes, including *Clostridium* and *Bacteroides fragilis*, are found in up to 15% of cases, most commonly in elderly patients and those with repeated infections or biliary procedures.[6]

Treatment

Patients should be managed based on clinical severity and symptoms with attention paid to volume and electrolyte status. General surgery should be consulted early in the diagnosis of acute cholecystitis and cholangitis. Early cholecystectomy, via either laparoscopic or open approach, is generally preferred in acute cholecystitis. The benefit of early surgery has been demonstrated in multiple studies. In one study of 29,818 Medicare patients with acute cholecystitis, patients who were discharged without surgery were more likely to require readmission than those who underwent surgery (38% vs 4%) and had a higher mortality rate than those who had surgery (hazard ratio of 1.56).[7]

Patients with significant comorbidities may benefit from percutaneous cholecystostomy with delayed cholecystectomy. Gastroenterology should be consulted in cases of suspected or confirmed CBD stones and in ascending cholangitis, as ERCP with sphincterotomy or dilation is the initial procedure of choice. These patients may undergo subsequent cholecystectomy.

Many patients with acute cholangitis respond to antibiotic therapy and supportive treatments. Those with hypotension, altered mental status, high fever, or persistent abdominal pain necessitate further evaluation by general surgery and gastroenterology and may require urgent biliary drainage, usually accomplished by ERCP or percutaneous cholecystostomy.

The Infectious Disease Society of America recommends empiric broad-spectrum antibiotics in patients suspected of having an infectious component, including those who are febrile, have an elevated white blood cell count (> 12,500), have air in the gallbladder wall, or are elderly or immunocompromised.[8] There is little consensus on a single best treatment for biliary infection. Although certain antibiotics, such as fluoroquinolones, have better biliary penetration, they have not been widely shown to improve outcomes. Multiple appropriate regimens exist (see Table 34.1), and antibiotic regimens should be selected based on the patient's history, the likelihood of anaerobic infection, local bacterial sensitivities, and antibiotic toxicity.

Disposition decisions should be made in conjunction with consultants, but patients with acute cholecystitis and cholangitis generally require admission and prompt surgical intervention.

Suggested Readings and References

1. Peery AF, Dellon ES, Lund J, et al. Burden of gastrointestinal disease in the United States: 2012 update. *Gastroenterology*. 2012;143:1179–1187.
2. Ohdan H, Oshiro H, Yamamoto Y, et al. Bacteriological investigation of bile in patients with cholelithiasis. *Surg Today*. 1993;23:390–395.
3. Singer AJ, McCracken G, Henry MC, et al. Correlation among clinical, laboratory, and hepatobiliary scanning findings in patients with suspected acute cholecystitis. *Ann Emerg Med*. 1996;28:267–272.
4. Martinez A, Bona X, Velasco M, Martin J. Diagnostic accuracy of ultrasound in acute cholecystitis. *Gastrointest Radiol*. 1986;11:334–338.
5. Shea JA, Berlin JA, Escarce JJ, et al. Revised estimates of diagnostic test sensitivity and specificity in suspected biliary tract disease. *Arch Intern Med*. 1994;154:2573–2581.
6. Csendes A, Becerra M, Burdiles P, et al. Bacteriological studies of bile from the gallbladder in patients with carcinoma of the gallbladder, cholelithiasis, common bile duct stones and no gallstones disease. *Eur J Surg*.1994;160:363.
7. Riall TS, Zhang D, Townsend CM Jr, et al. Failure to perform cholecystectomy for acute cholecystitis in elderly patients is associated with increased morbidity, mortality, and cost. *J Am Coll Surg*. 2010;210:668.
8. Solomkin JS, Mazuski JE, Bradley JS, et al. Diagnosis and management of complicated intra-abdominal infection in adults and children: guidelines by the Surgical Infection Society and the Infectious Diseases Society of America. *Clin Infect Dis*. 2010;50:133–164.

Chapter 35

Hepatitis

Deanna Wilson

Summary Box

Disease Description: Viral hepatitis causes significant morbidity and mortality globally. Patients with acute hepatitis present initially with vague constitutional symptoms during the prodromal period and then go on to develop abdominal pain, hepatomegaly, and jaundice during the icteric phase. Serum transaminases peak during the prodromal period with elevated serum bilirubin and with varying levels of hepatic protein synthesis impairment. There is limited therapy for acute hepatitis; however, the majority of adults with hepatitis A, B, D, and E will spontaneously clear the virus during the acute phase. In contrast, the majority of individuals with Hepatitis C will develop chronic hepatitis. Chronic hepatitis is associated with an increased risk of cirrhosis, liver failure, and hepatocellular carcinoma.

Organisms: Hepatitis A, B, C, D with concomitant B, and E.

Treatment: Predominantly supportive therapies during the acute phase: IV fluids, management of symptoms (pruritis can be treated with antihistamines or cholestyramine), close monitoring for liver failure.
- Oral first line: Lamivudine 100 mg/day for severe, acute hepatitis B treatment
- Parenteral: Consider interferon for severe hepatitis D
- Promising Therapies: Multiple promising therapies (in particular protease inhibitors and interferon-free regimens for hepatitis C) are in varying stages of development.
- Fulminant Hepatic Failure: Definitive treatment is liver transplant

Other Key Issues: Patients with known hepatitis A, B, or E exposures may be eligible for post-exposure prophylaxis.

Diseases Description

Epidemiology

The vast majority of viral hepatitis is caused by the following hepatitis viruses: A, B, C, E, and D with concomitant B. Hepatitis A virus (HAV) and hepatitis E virus (HEV) are spread via the fecal-oral route, often through the contamination of food and water.[1] Whereas the developing world continues to have nearly universal HAV infection in childhood, HEV is primarily found in Asia, Africa, and Central America.[2] Prior to routine vaccination, nearly one-third of the adults in the United States also showed evidence of prior HAV infection. Due to improved sanitation, most HAV and HEV infection in the United States today is a result of recent travel to an endemic area.[3]

Over 350 million people have hepatitis B virus (HBV) worldwide.[4] Universal vaccination of newborns has sharply decreased the rates of HBV in the United States; the highest incidence now occurs in adolescents and young adults, 25 to 44 years of age, who are exposed via occupational exposures or recreational activities (eg, sexual activity or IV drug use).[4] In contrast to the developing world, vertical transmission (from mothers to newborns) is a significant contributor.[1] Of individuals with chronic HBV, 5% are also infected with hepatitis D virus (HDV), a virus that can only coinfect with HBV or superinfect those with chronic HBV.[5] HDV is also spread parentally. Outbreaks of severe hepatitis can occur in nonendemic areas with populations that have high rates of chronic HBV.[5]

Hepatitis C virus (HCV) is the leading contributor to hepatitis-associated morbidity and mortality in the United States. Adults between 30 and 49 years of age have the highest rates of infection.[6] The predominant route of transmission is parenteral exposure, and the highest risk group is injection drug users. However, about 10% to 15% of patients with new infection have sexual transmission as a risk factor.[1]

Clinical Presentation

Acute viral hepatitis has a broad range of clinical presentations based on the causative organism and on patient age and comorbidities. Not all individuals with acute hepatitis will be symptomatic. For example, less than a third of individuals with acute HCV develop symptoms compared to approximately 50% of teens and adults with acute HBV.[7]

The hepatitis viruses' incubation periods vary. Incubation is followed by a prodromal period in which patients endorse nonspecific symptoms such as fatigue, malaise, nausea, vomiting, and anorexia.[1] Patients may report dark-colored urine or clay-colored stools.[7] These symptoms often persist for less than a week before the development of jaundice. Patients often endorse right upper quadrant pain with liver enlargement on exam.[1] Patients with HAV and HEV may develop low-grade fevers; 5% to 20% of patients with HBV develop a serum sickness-like syndrome with arthralgias, rash, and angioedema.[1] There are numerous other extrahepatic manifestations. These range from renal complications, such as glomerulonephritis, to cutaneous manifestations, such as porphyria cutanea tarda or lichen planus. Essential mixed cryoglobulinemia is seen in nearly a third of individuals with HCV.[6]

Laboratory Studies

At the time of presentation, individuals often have alanine transaminase and aspartate transaminase (ALT and AST, respectively) 10 to 50 times the upper limit of normal, except in HCV, when they rarely go above 800 IU/L (international unit per liter). AST and ALT rise during the prodromal phase, peak during the icteric phase, and decline during the recovery phase; both the peak and recovery in bilirubin lags slightly behind.[1] The rate of rise may be slower in HBV than in HAV.[4] A bilirubin level that rises to greater than 20 mg/dl and persists late in the clinical course indicates high severity. Both the direct and indirect components of bilirubin are often elevated.[1]

Laboratory tests that measure synthetic function of the liver provide insight into the severity of the hepatocellular damage. Prolonged prothrombin time, low serum albumin, hypoglycemia, and very high serum bilirubin are all markers of severe hepatitis. There can be a range of hematologic abnormalities, including a leukocytosis with a predominance of atypical lymphocytes.[1,10]

Diagnostic Considerations

The differential for markedly elevated transaminases (> 10–20 times the upper limit of normal) is limited to infectious hepatitis, drug-induced liver injury, toxic ingestion, and hypoperfusion. Patients with mild transaminitis and symptoms, such as high fever or splenomegaly, should be tested for Epstein-Barr virus and cytomegalovirus. Various bacteria, in particular *Rickettsia rickettsii* (ie, Rocky Mountain spotted fever) and *Leptospira* spp. (ie, leptospirosis) can all present with transaminitis, although rarely in isolation of their more classic clinical syndromes.[1,7]

Typical Disease Course
The vast majority of individuals with acute viral hepatitis recover from the acute stage of the illness without difficulty. Most will have resolution of the acute phase of their illness within 6 months.[1] A significant portion of the morbidity and mortality associated with hepatitis is a result of chronic infection. Chronic hepatitis increases the risk for cirrhosis, liver failure, and hepatocellular carcinoma.[1] Individuals with HAV and HEV rarely develop chronic hepatitis[10]; 5% of adults with HBV will develop chronic disease compared to nearly 80% of patients with HCV.[7] Among subsets of the population, rates are even higher: 90% of neonates who acquire HBV from perinatal exposure are unable to clear the virus[7] (see Table 35.1).

Complications
Patients with acute hepatitis can develop ascites, pancreatitis, encephalopathy, and impaired hepatic synthetic function.[1] Elderly patients and those with comorbid liver disease have more frequent complications and more severe presentations.[8,9] Fulminant hepatic failure (FHF) is a potentially lethal complication associated with massive hepatocellular necrosis.[1] HBV is responsible for greater than 50% of the cases of FHF. Individuals with FHF have impaired synthetic function. They are at increased risk for cerebral edema, coma, and death. Both the mortality and the rate of FHF vary by virus type. The definitive treatment is liver transplant.[1,8,9]

Diagnostic Tests
If acute hepatitis is suspected, initial laboratory studies should include serum transaminases (ALT and AST); direct and indirect bilirubin; a complete blood count; and markers of liver function, including serum albumin and prothrombin time.[1] In addition, the following serologies should be obtained: immunoglobulin M (IgM) antibodies to HAV, a marker of acute HAV infection; HAB surface antigen, a marker of HBV infection (could be acute or chronic); IgM antibodies to HBcAg (HBV core antigen; anti-HBcAg) that develop at the onset of infection; and antibodies to HCV (anti-HCV).[1,4,7] If there is concern for bacterial infection, blood cultures should be obtained. If HBV is the likely causative agent, HBV envelope antigen, a marker of active viral replication and high transmissibility, should be obtained.[4] If there is clinical concern, patients should be screened for other causes for elevated transaminitis.

Organisms

There is rich diversity among the five viral hepatitides. The viral life cycles are similar: each enters the blood stream and travels to the liver where they infect hepatocytes. Viral replication occurs predominantly in the liver, although the virus is often found in extrahepatic locations. The virus binds to the hepatocyte via virus-specific receptors that are not yet well understood. Once HBV enters the cell, its nuclear material is taken into the nucleus where it forms covalently closed circular DNA. This eventually forms pre-genomic RNA, which uses reverse transcriptase for replication and virion assembly. For RNA viruses like HCV, the viral RNA is both directly translated into vesicles and also amplified and expressed to form new progeny virions that are secreted by the cell.[1]

Treatment

The treatment for acute hepatitis is predominantly supportive.[1] Individuals may require IV hydration and parenteral nutrition if unable to tolerate oral intake.[4,7] All potentially hepatotoxic agents, such as alcohol, should be avoided. Individuals with FHF require intensive care; definitive treatment is liver transplant.[8,9]

There is no role for treatment of acute HCV immediately following infection.[11] Nearly one-third of patients will spontaneously clear the infection. However, earlier treatment is associated with a better response to therapy and higher rates of cure for those with chronic HCV.[12] Current consensus suggests waiting at least 8 to 12 weeks prior to initiating therapy.[6]

Acute HBV is treated only in those with severe liver disease. Lamivudine (100 mg orally daily) in those with severe acute HBV or FHF from HBV improves survival.[9] There are no clear criteria for when to initiate therapy, although outcomes are better if given earlier in the treatment course. There is limited evidence at this time to support using the new protease inhibitors, entecavir and tenofovir, in place of lamivudine. However, they appear promising and may be more potent.[9]

Table 35.1 Typical Disease Course for Hepatitis[1]

Virus	Transmission	Presentation	Prevention	Course	Diagnosis	Treatment	Other
Hepatitis A	Fecal contamination of food or water	Usually mild, often asymptomatic in children; chronic HAV does not occur. Dark urine, clay-colored stool, and jaundice peaks within 1 to 2 weeks and resolves in another 2 to 4 weeks. Tender hepatomegaly, splenomegaly, cervical lymphadenopathy; Extrahepatic manifestations are rare but might include evidence of vasculitis, arthritis, mononeuritis multiplex, hemolytic anemia, or cholecystitis.	Both passive and active vaccinations available. Lifelong immunity after exposure.	Spontaneously resolves in most cases. Fulminant hepatitis can rarely occur, seen primarily when HAV occurs with underlying chronic liver disease or in pregnancy.	History of likely exposure, clinical presentation, and results of liver function tests as well as hepatitis serologic markers; IgM-acute Infection IgG reflects past infection, or postimmunization	Mainly supportive, postexposure prophylaxis following acute exposure to HAV.	
Hepatitis B	Transmitted parenterally, usually sexual contact or IV drug use or in the perinatal period	Usually self-limited condition that is treated supportively.	Three injection vaccine series	Usually self-limited, 5% of cases become chronic; these patients are at increased risk of liver cirrhosis, liver failure, and hepatocellular carcinoma	HBsAg, antibodies to HBcAg, HBeAg	Supportive care, chronic HBV treated with interferon and nucleoside analogs; liver transplant may be needed for individuals with end-stage liver disease	
Hepatitis C	IV drug use primarily Less commonly, blood transfusion before 1992; sexual contact with infected person; needlestick injury; perinatal transmission from mother	Acute HCV is rarely diagnosed; acutely infected patients are rarely symptomatic until decades later.	No vaccine, no current postexposure prophylaxis	15% to 45% of patients with acute infection will experience spontaneous resolution of viremia. A high percentage will develop chronic disease. Can progress to cirrhosis, hepatic failure, hepatocellular carcinoma.	Anti-HCV antibodies and HCV RNA indicates infection. HCV RNA used to measure viral load. HCV genotyping guides therapy	Treatment varies by a number of factors, including degree of hepatic damage, genotype, viral load, and past treatment. Meds include pegalyted interferon, nucleoside analogs, and protease inhibitors	

Type	Transmission	Clinical Features	Clinical Course	Diagnosis	Prevention	Treatment
Hepatitis D	The dependent HDV virus is parenterally transmitted	Coinfection with HBV	Clinical course ranges from self-limited to fulminant hepatic failure	HDV antigen, HDV RNA, anti-HDV	Associated with HBV prevention	No current pharmacologic approved treatment
Hepatitis E	Usually waterborne (fecal contamination) More common in developing countries No clear evidence of sexual transmission, rare reports of parenteral transmission	Usually presents with jaundice, often mild; can be asymptomatic in children; often highly virulent in pregnant women; chronic HEV does not occur	Can progress to fulminant hepatitis, which can occur in up to 30% of women during the third trimester of pregnancy; Patients can develop hepatic encephalopathy, coagulopathy.	Clinical diagnosis based on exposure to endemic areas, LFTs, HEV IgM acute infection, HEV IgG indicates past infection	No vaccine available.	Acute infection, mainly supportive and may be life-saving in cases of severe hepatitis and fulminant hepatic failure. Transplantation is sometimes required as a last resort. Often requires immediate attention to stabilize the metabolic and coagulopathic state.

Abbreviations: HAV, hepatitis A virus; IgM, immunoglobulin M; IgG, immunoglobulin G; IV, intravenous; HBsAg, hepatitis B surface antigen; HBcAg, hepatitis B core antigen; HBeAg, hepatitis B envelope antigen; HBV, hepatitis B virus; HCV, hepatitis C virus; HDV, hepatitis D virus; HEV, hepatitis E virus; LFT, liver function test; FDA, [US] Food and Drug Administration.

Other Issues To Consider

Individuals with known exposures to HAV, HBV, and potentially HEV can receive post-exposure prophylaxis to reduce their risk of infection.[7]

Suggested Readings and References

1. Dienstag JL. Acute viral hepatitis. In: Longo DL, Fauci AS, Kasper DL, Hauser SL, Jameson JL, Loscalzo J, eds. *Harrison's Principles of Internal Medicine*. 18th ed. New York, NY: McGraw-Hill; 2012. http://www.accessmedicine.com/content.aspx?aID=9133433. Accessed October 23, 2012.

2. Kuniholm MH, Purcell RH, McQuillan GM, Engle RE, Wasley A, Nelson KE. Epidemiology of hepatitis E virus in the United States: results from the Third National Health and Nutrition Examination Survey, 1988–1994. *J Infect Dis*. 2009;200:48–56.

3. Wasley A, Samandari T, Bell B. Incidence of hepatitis A in the United States in the era of vaccination. *JAMA*. 2005;294:194–201.

4. Shiffman MS. Management of acute hepatitis B. *Clin Liver Dis*. 2010;14:75–91

5. Farci P, Niro GA. Clinical features of hepatitis D. *Semin Liver Dis*. 2012;32:228–236.

6. Kamal, SM. Acute hepatitis C: a systemic review. *Am J Gastroenterol*. 2008;103:1283–1297.

7. Viral hepatitis. Centers for Disease Control; 2012. http://www.cdc.gov/hepatitis/. Accessed October 23, 2012.

8. Rezende G, Roque-Afonso AM, Samuel D, et al. Viral and clinical factors associated with the fulminant course of hepatitis A infection. *Hepatology*. 2003;38:613–618.

9. Tillman HL, Zachou K, Dalekos GN. Management of severe acute to fulminant hepatitis B: to treat or not to treat or when to treat? Liver International. 2011;32:544–553.

10. Patra S, Kumar A, Trivedi SS, Puri M, Sarin SK. Maternal and fetal outcomes in pregnant women with acute hepatitis E virus infection. *Ann Intern Med*. 2007;147:28–33.

11. Ghany MG, Nelson DR, Strader DB, Thomas DL, Seeff LB; American Association for Study of Liver Diseases. An update on treatment of genotype 1 chronic hepatitis C virus infection: 2011 practice guideline by the American Association for the Study of Liver Diseases. *Hepatology*. 2011;54:1433–1444.

12. Klenerman P, Gupta PK. Hepatitis C virus: current concepts and future challenges. *QJM*. 2012;105:29–32.

Appendicitis

David Scordino

Summary Box

Disease Description: Acute appendicitis remains the most common abdominal surgical emergency in the United States. Lifetime risk is 8.6% in males and 6.7% in females. It is caused by acute inflammation of the appendix, most frequently secondary to obstruction. This inflammation can result in perforation, leading to peritonitis, sepsis, and/or abscess formation.

Organisms: Gram-negative anaerobic and aerobic gut flora, including *Escherichia coli, Peptostreptococcus, Bacteriodes fragilis, Pseudomonas* species, *Fusobacterium nucleatum,* and *Fusobacterium necrophorum.*

Treatment:
    Nonperforated: single dose of cefoxitin 1 to 2 g IV; ampicillin/sulbactam 3 g IV; or cefazolin 1 to 2 g IV plus metronidazole, 500 mg IV
    Penicillin allergy: clindamycin (1.2 to 1.8 g/day IV in divided doses q6 to 12 hours) plus fluoroquinolone (moxifloxacin 400 mg IV q day)
    Perforated: Pipercillin-tazobactam 3.375g IV q6 hours or Ertapenam 1 g IV daily

Other Key Issues: Patients at the extremes of age and pregnant women may have atypical presentations and higher rates of perforation and complications.

Disease Description

Epidemiology

Appendicitis is the most common acute abdominal surgical emergency in the United States. Appendicitis is listed as the final diagnosis for nearly one in every 1,000 hospitalizations.[1] There is a slight male predominance (1.4 to 1 male to female ratio) with a lifetime risk of 8.6% in males and 6.7% in females.[2,3,4] The peak age of diagnosis is between 10 and 14 years in males and 14 and 19 years in females. Of all cases, 45% occur between 15 and 44 years of age.[1,2,3,5,6]

Presenting Features

The presenting manifestations of appendicitis vary based on the anatomical location of the appendix. Classic symptomatology includes anorexia, nausea, vomiting, and periumbilical pain that later localizes to the right lower quadrant (RLQ). This "classic" migrating pain is seen in 50% to 60% of patients.[4,7,8,] Low-grade fever may be present, but high fever (> 38.3°C) is typically not seen on presentation. Physical examination may identify maximal tenderness at McBurney's point, rebound tenderness, guarding, Rovsing's sign, obturator sign, and/or psoas sign. These tests must be put in context, as no single maneuver is definitive for appendicitis (see Box 36.1).

The classic presentation is less common in pediatric patients less than 3 years old, geriatric patients older than 60 years, and pregnant women in their second or third trimesters.[1,2,4,5,9] These patients have higher rates of appendiceal perforation because the diagnosis is often delayed secondary to atypical history or unremarkable physical examination. Pediatric patients are more likely to present with diarrhea. Elderly patients may have a diminished inflammatory response, leading to less pronounced symptomatology and physical exam findings. Pregnant women often have a superiorly displaced appendix, leading to pain above the RLQ. Additionally, pregnant women may not mount classic peritoneal signs due to a diminished inflammatory response.[4] A high index of suspicion should always be maintained in these groups to prevent unnecessary delay in diagnosis and treatment.

Diagnostic Considerations

The differential diagnosis of RLQ pain is broad and includes cecal diverticulitis, Meckel's diverticulitis, acute infectious ileitis (from *Yersinia, Campylobacter*, or *Salmonella*), and Crohn's disease. In women, pelvic inflammatory disease, tubo-ovarian abscess, or a ruptured ovarian cyst should also be considered. Endometriosis, ovarian torsion, ovulation, and ectopic pregnancy are also possible sources of acute abdominal pain in women. Similarly, testicular torsion in men may cause acute RLQ pain. Additionally, renal colic and pyelonephritis may mimic appendicitis.[4] Select laboratory testing and a discriminating physical examination can help distinguish between these diagnoses.

Perforation of the appendix must be considered in patients at the extremes of age, with a prolonged course (more than 24 hours), with fever higher than 38.3°C, with toxic appearance, or who have evidence of peritonitis on exam.[4] Time to perforation varies; 20% of patients develop perforation in less than 24 hours of symptom onset. Overall, 65% of patients with perforation have had symptoms for more than 48 hours.[10]

Box 36.1 Physical Examination Findings (Eponyms) in Appendicitis

McBurney's point: Pain at the point in the RLQ that is one-third of the distance from the anterior superior iliac spine to the umbilicus (sensitivity 50%–94%; specificity 75%–86%).[16–18,22]

Aaron's sign: Pain referring to the epigastrium with palpation over McBurney's point.

Rovsing's sign: Increased RLQ pain on palpation of the left lower quadrant (sensitivity 22%–68%; specificity 58%–96%).[17,18–22]

Obturator sign (Cope sign): Increased RLQ pain on internal rotation of the right hip with both the right hip and right knee flexed to 90 degrees (sensitivity 8%; specificity 94%).[22–23]

Psoas Sign: With the patient on his side, both passive flexion and passive extension of the right hip (with an extended knee) elicit increased RLQ pain (sensitivity 13%–42%; specificity 79%–97%).[19,22–24]

Markle sign (Jar tenderness): Dropping from the toes to the heel while standing, causing a jarring action, elicits pain in the RLQ. A modified version involves the physician striking the right heel to create a jarring motion and elicit pain in the RLQ.

Dunphy's sign: Abdominal pain with coughing.

Typical Disease Course

Appendiceal obstruction is thought to be the cause of the majority of cases of appendicitis with occlusion of the lumen by fecaliths, calculi, lymphatic tissue, infection, or benign or malignant neoplasms.[2,4,5] Following obstruction, mucus formed within the lumen continues to accumulate, leading to increased intraluminal pressure, decreased venous and arterial flow, necrosis, and potentially perforation.[2,4,5] In the diseased appendix, bacterial overgrowth occurs with invasion of the appendiceal wall, leading predominantly to a neutrophilic response causing localized inflammation.[4]

Disease course is as variable as the presentation. Patients identified prior to perforation may undergo laparoscopic removal of the appendix and be discharged the following day. However, those who experience perforation with or without abscess will have longer hospitalization, requiring parenteral antibiotics and possibly a percutaneous drain.

Complications

The most common complication following appendicitis is infection, including intra-abdominal abscess formation and surgical wound infection. Although both occur more frequently in patients with perforation, broad-spectrum antibiotics and intraoperative irrigation have reduced their incidence. Patients who undergo laparoscopic appendectomy have a lower risk (1.7%) of incisional infection than those who have an open appendectomy (5.2%), but they have a higher risk of intra-abdominal infection (odds ratio: 1:44).[11]

Diagnostic Tests

A careful history and physical exam is imperative, as the diagnosis is still clinical and **not** based on radiographic imaging. Testicular exam in men and a pelvic exam (with few exceptions) in women are critical to making a correct diagnosis. Rectal exam should be performed on patients with atypical presentations.

Most patients should have a comprehensive metabolic panel, complete blood count with differential, and urinalysis. Women of childbearing age should have a urine pregnancy test. Coagulation factors and a type and screen should be obtained on patients with a high likelihood of needing urgent surgical intervention.

Most patients with acute appendicitis have a total white cell count of greater than 10,000 cell/μL, generally with a left shift (sensitivity of 80% and specificity 55%).[12] A normal white cell count dramatically decreases the likelihood of acute appendicitis except early in the disease course or when the patient is immunocompromised. The white cell count may be useful to follow along with serial abdominal examinations in equivocal patients.

Clinical decision tools, such as the Alvarado score, are available to help determine the need to obtain radiographic imaging (see Table 36.1). A recent systematic review by Ohle et al. identified that the Alvarado score is well calibrated for men; however, it overestimates disease in women and is inconclusive in children.[13] This review identified that 99% of patients with appendicitis had an Alvarado score ≥ 5.[4,13] An Alvarado score ≥ 7 only had a sensitivity of 82% and specificity of 81%, making a low score better at "ruling out" appendicitis rather than a high score "ruling it in."[4,13] Clinical decision tools must be considered in the context of the clinical judgment of an experienced physician, which is 75% to 90% accurate in diagnosing appendicitis without imaging.[14,15,16,17]

Patients with score ≤ 3 are at low risk for appendicitis and are appropriate, given the ability to return, to be discharged with strict precautions. Alvarado scores of 4 to 6 should have additional testing, including imaging or observation with serial abdominal exams. Alvarado ≥ 7 should have emergent surgical consultation with appendectomy.[4,13]

Table 36.1 Alvarado Score of Acute Appendicitis	
Migratory right iliac fossa pain	1 point
Anorexia	1 point
Nausea/Vomiting	1 point
Tenderness in the right iliac fossa	2 points
Rebound tenderness in the right iliac fossa	1 point
Fever > 37.5°C	1 point
Leukocytosis	2 points

Ultrasound is the imaging modality of choice in children and pregnant women. The most specific finding for acute appendicitis is an appendiceal diameter of greater than 6 mm. Sensitivity ranges from 35% to 98% and specificity from 71% to 98% with accuracy limited by operator skill, patient body habitus, and overlying bowel gas.[2]

Computed tomography (CT) scan is commonly used to evaluate patients with acute abdominal symptoms. A non-contrast CT scan is 90% sensitive in diagnosing acute appendicitis. The following radiographic findings are suggestive: dilated appendiceal diameter to greater than 6 mm with an occluded lumen, wall thickening of greater than 2 mm, fat stranding around the appendix, wall enhancement, and the presence of an appendicolith (seen in 25% of patients). The addition of oral, IV, and/or rectal contrast increases the sensitivity to 97% to 98%. Because women are more likely to have a nontherapeutic appendectomy rate (twice the rate of men), preoperative CT scan may be particularly useful in their evaluation. A retrospective review of 1,425 patients undergoing appendectomy found that adult women with a preoperative CT had a nontherapeutic appendectomy rate of 8% compared with 21% of those who did not have imaging.[18]

Organism

Gram-negative anaerobic and aerobic gut flora, including *Escherichia coli, Peptostreptococcus, Bacteriodes fragilis, Pseudomonas* species, *Fusobacterium nucleatum, Fusobacterium necrophorum, Eubacterium rectale, Clostridium, Faecalibacterium prausnitzii,* and *Akkermansia.*

Treatment

The vast majority of patients suspected of having appendicitis are treated with prompt surgical intervention. Most surgeons prefer a relatively aggressive approach and are willing to tolerate a low rate of nontherapeutic appendectomies to avoid missing true cases of appendicitis. With modern imaging, an acceptable rate is generally less than 10%. A review of three randomized trials comparing appendectomy to medical management with antibiotics alone found that a third of patients treated medically failed and required an appendectomy in the acute setting, and another 16% required surgery within 1 year.[19]

The majority of patients today undergo laparoscopic surgery. A recent meta-analysis of 56 trials and 11 studies comparing the outcomes of 6,000 adults and children with possible appendicitis who underwent open or laparoscopic surgery found the following: patients undergoing laparoscopic surgery had lower rates of wound infection, lower postoperative pain, shorter hospital stay, and quicker return of bowel function. Patients undergoing laparoscopic procedures did, however, have higher rates of intra-abdominal abscess, longer operative time, and a higher total hospital cost.[20] In particular, patients with an unclear source of their pain benefit from laparoscopic intervention, as it permits inspection for alternative pelvic pathology. Obese patients may also benefit from laparoscopic surgery, as they are predisposed to incisional wound dehiscence and infection. Finally, geriatric patients have better outcomes with laparoscopic procedures due to shortened hospital stays and fewer surgical complications.

Antibiotic therapy should be initiated preoperatively, often in the emergency department, and it varies for perforated versus nonperforated appendicitis. For nonperforated appendicitis, a single dose of cefoxitin 1 to 2 g IV, ampicillin/sulbactam 3 g IV, or cefazolin, 1 to 2 g IV plus metronidazole 500 mg IV are reasonable options. In those with penicillin allergy, clindamycin can be considered (1.2 to 1.8 g/day IV in divided doses q6 to 12 hours) plus fluoroquinolone (moxifloxacin 400 mg IV q day) is the preferred treatment. If no perforation is identified intraoperatively, antibiotics may be discontinued; however, some surgeons may choose to give additional dosing for 24 hours. In the event perforation is identified, broad coverage with piperacillin-tazobactam 3.375 g IV every 6 hours or Ertapenam 1 g IV daily should be utilized. Cultures should be obtained intraoperatively with targeted therapy for 5 to 7 days following the operation.[21]

Other Key Issues

Geriatric, pediatric, and pregnant populations may be particularly difficult to diagnose and may have a higher rate of perforation.

In patients with evidence of a contained abscess, consideration of nonoperative therapy is reasonable. These individuals generally have a prolonged course (more than 5 days) prior to presentation and have a well-circumscribed abscess or phlegmon that appears to be walled off. If immediate surgical intervention is attempted, there is the risk of significant morbidity due to adhesions to adjacent tissues.[21] If the patient clinically appears well, then a CT-guided percutaneous drainage may be attempted. Parenteral antibiotics, IV fluids, and bowel rest are important aspects of management. If the patient improves over days, then he or she may be discharged with IV antibiotics via a peripherally inserted central catheter line or oral antibiotics based on susceptibility. Interval appendectomy is recommended to prevent recurrent appendicitis and to exclude neoplasm as the inciting event.[21]

Suggested Readings and References

1. Christensen BV, Colomb-Lippa D. Acute appendicitis: can antibiotics ever take the place of surgery. *J Am Acad Physician Assist.* 2012;25:32–36.

2. Snyder BK. Appendicitis. *Harwood & Nuss' Clinical Practice of Emergency Medicine.* 5th ed. Philadelphia, PA: Lippincott, Williams and Wilkins; 2010:586–590.

3. Addiss DG, Shaffer N, Fowler BS, Tauxe RV. The epidemiology of appendicitis and appendectomy in the United States. *Am J Epidemiol.* 1990;132:910–925.

4. Black CE, Martin RF. Acute appendicitis in adults: clinical manifestations and diagnosis. http://www.uptodate.com/contents/acute-appendicitis-in-adults-clinical-manifestations-and-differential-diagnosis. UpToDate website. 2013. Updated September 13, 2012. Accessed March 31, 2013.

5. Gearhart SL, Silen W. Acute appendicitis and peritonitis. *Harrison's Principles of Internal Medicine.* 17th ed. New York, NY: McGraw-Hill; 2008:1914–1917.

6. Swidsinski A, Dorffel Y, Loening-Baucke V, et al. Acute appendicitis is characterised by local invasion with *Fusobacterium nucleatum/necrophorum. Gut.* 2011;60:34–40.

7. Birnbaum BA, Wilson SR. Appendicitis at the millennium. *Radiology.* 2000;215:337–348.

8. Chung CH, Ng CP, Lai KK. Delays by patients, emergency physicians, and surgeons in the management of acute appendicitis: retrospective study. *Hong Kong Med J.* 2000;6:254–259.

9. Hardin DM Jr. Acute appendicitis: review and update. *Am Fam Physician.* 1999;60:2027–2034.

10. Temple CL, Huchcroft SA, Temple WJ. The natural history of appendicitis in adults: a prospective study. *Ann Surg.* 1995;221:278–281.

11. Fleming FJ, Kim MJ, Messing S, Gunzler D, Salloum R, Monson JR. Balancing the risk of postoperative surgical infections: a multivariate analysis of factors associated with laparoscopic appendectomy from the NSQIP database. *Ann Surg.* 2010; 252:895–900.

12. Thompson MM, Underwood MJ, Dookeran KA, Lloyd DM, Bell PR. Role of sequential leukocyte counts and C-reactive protein measurements in acute appendicitis. *Br J Surg.* 1992;79(8):822–824.

13. Ohle R, O'Reilly F, O'Brien KK, Fahey T, Dimitrov BD. The Alvarado score for predicting acute appendicitis: a systematic review. *BMC Medicine.* 2011;9:139–151.

14. Berry J Jr, Malt RA. Appendicitis near its centenary. *Ann Surg.* 1984;200:567–575.

15. Lee SL, Walsh AJ, Ho HS. Computed tomography and ultrasonography do not improve and may delay the diagnosis and treatment of acute appendicitis. *Arch Surg.* 2001;136:556–562.

16. Andersson RE. Meta-analysis of the clinical and laboratory diagnosis of appendicitis. *Br J Surg.* 2004;91:28–37.

17. Hong JJ, Cohn SM, Ekeh AP, et al. A prospective randomized study of clinical assessment versus computed tomography for the diagnosis of acute appendicitis. *Surg Infect (Larchmt).* 2003;4:231–239.

18. Wagner PL, Eachempati SR, Soe K, Pieracci FM, Shou J, Barie PS. Defining the current negative appendectomy rate for whom is preoperative computed tomography making an impact? *Surgery.* 2008;144:276–282.

19. Varadhan KK, Humes DJ, Neal KR, Lobo DN. Antibiotic therapy versus appendectomy for acute appendicitis: a meta-analysis. *World J Surg.* 2010;34:199–209.

20. Sauerland S, Jaschinski T, Neugebauer EA. Laparoscopic versus open surgery for suspected appendicitis. *Cochrane Database Syst Rev.* 2010;10:CD00156.

21. Smink D, Soybel DI. http://www.uptodate.com/contents/management-of-acute-appendicitis-in-adults. Acute appendicitis in adults: management. UpToDate website. 2013. Updated February 14, 2013. Accessed March 31, 2013.

22. Golledge J, Toms AP, Franklin IJ, Scriven MW, Galland RB. Assessment of peritonism in appendicitis. *Ann R Coll Surg Engl.* 1996;78:11–14.

23. Andersson RE, Hugander AP, Ghazi SH, et al. Diagnostic value of disease history, clinical presentation, and inflammatory parameters in appendicitis. *World Surg.* 1999;23:133–140.

24. Lane R, Grabham J. A useful sign for the diagnosis of peritoneal rupture in the right iliac fossa. *Ann R Coll Surg Engl.* 1997;79:128–129.

25. Izbicki JR, Knoefel WT, Wilker DK, et al. Accurate diagnosis of acute appendicitis: a retrospective and prospective analysis of 686 patients. *Eur J Surg.* 1992;158:227–231.

26. Alshehri MY, Ibrahim A, Abuaisha N, et al. Value of rebound tenderness in acute appendicitis. *East Afr Med J.* 1995;72:504–506.

27. Jahn H, Mathiesen FK, Neckelmann K, Hovendal CP, Bellstrom, Gottrup F. Comparison of clinical judgment and diagnostic ultrasonography in the diagnosis of acute appendicitis: experience with a score aided diagnosis. *Eur J Surg.* 1997;163(6).433–443.

28. John H, Neff U, Keleman M. Appendicitis diagnosis today: clinical and ultrasonic deductions. *World J Surg.* 1993;17:243–249.

Genitourinary Infections

Chapter 37

Urinary Tract Infections in Women

Arjun S. Chanmugam and Gino Scalabrini

Disease Description: Urinary tract infections (UTIs) are common infections most frequently caused by *E. coli* and other bacteria. Uncomplicated UTIs refer to those infections that occur in healthy premenopausal, non-pregnant women with a normal urinary tract and who have a high likelihood to respond favorably to treatment. Complicated UTIs are found in men or in women with coexisting pathology, anatomical abnormality, underlying comorbidity, or women who may be immunocompromised in some way. If untreated, UTIs can progress to more severe disease including pyelonephritis and urosepsis.

Diagnostic Tests: Urine analysis and urine dipstick are helpful for diagnosis; urine culture can definitively identify the organism.

Organisms: Most common organisms are *E. coli* and other gram-negative bacteria.

Treatment: Empiric antibiotic treatment includes trimethoprim-sulfamethoxazole (160 mg to 800 mg PO twice BID) for 3 days or a 5-day course of nitrofurantoin (100 mg po BID) or fosfomycin trometamol 3 g orally in single dose.

   Complicated UTI can be treated with ciprofloxacin (500 mg PO BID or 400 mg intravenous IV BID) or levofloxacin (500 mg PO or IV q day). More serious infections can be treated with cefepime 2 g IV every 12 hours or ceftazidime 2 g IV every 8 hours. Other options for ill patients include piperacillin-tazobactam 3.375 to 4.5 g IV every 6 hours.

Other Key Issues: Bacteriuria in pregnancy should be treated even if asymptomatic.

Disease Description

UTIs refer to the range of clinical entities that result in a urine culture yielding a minimum of 100 to 100,000 bacteria colony forming units per millimeter of urine, usually from a clean catch midstream urine sample. This can result from infection of the lower urinary tract involving the bladder (cystitis) or from an infection of the upper urinary tract involving the kidneys (pyelonephritis). Although a variety of bacteria, virus, and fungi can cause these infections, the most common organism is *E. coli*, a gram-negative bacterium.

UTI's are often divided into two basic categories, uncomplicated and complicated. Uncomplicated UTI's refer to those infections that occur in healthy premenopausal, non-pregnant women with a normal urinary tract and who have a high likelihood to respond favorably to appropriately targeted antibiotics with complete recovery. Complicated UTIs are found in women with coexisting pathology, anatomical abnormality, underlying comorbidity, or those who may be immunocompromised in some way.

Recurrent UTIs are comprised of two types of infections that occur after an initial infection. The first type of recurrent infection is called relapse and refers to infections that occur within 2 weeks after treatment caused by the same organism. The second type of recurrent infection is called reinfection and signifies an infection that occurs at least 2 weeks after the initial infection.

Epidemiology

UTIs are one of the most common infections seen in outpatient settings, accounting for nearly 9 million visits. Adult women have a higher incidence of UTI than men, presumably because of anatomical differences. Specifically, in women there is a shorter distance from urethra to bladder, from anus to urethral opening, and a periurethral orifice environment that retains a higher degree of moisture. By the age of 32, nearly half of all women report having had at least one UTI. However, above the age of 65, the rates of infection equalize between men and women, with some estimates of asymptomatic bacteriuria in this population at nearly 40%.

Risk Factors

Any significant obstruction to the free flow of urine can potentially lead to UTI. Common risk factors for UTIs include recent instrumentation, diabetes mellitus, pregnancy, vesicoureteral reflux, incomplete bladder emptying as a result of other disease process, recent sexual intercourse, previous urinary tract infections, and inadequate hygiene. Advanced age, female sex, anatomic urological abnormalities, and immunocompromised states further increase a patient's predisposition toward UTI.

Presenting Features

Classically, UTIs present initially with urinary frequency, urgency, hesitancy, hematuria, nocturia, dysuria, and or suprapubic pain. Cloudy urine or urine with a strong odor is often found with UTIs.

More advanced disease can include fever, malaise, flank pain, or costovertebral tenderness as it progresses toward pyelonephritis.

Complications

If allowed to progress, complicated UTIs can ultimately become serious infections with significant systematic findings, including multiorgan system dysfunction resulting in hypoperfusion and hypotension. Urosepsis accounts for nearly 5% of severe sepsis cases and has a significant mortality in certain groups.

Diagnosis

The diagnosis of UTI can most reliably be made on the basis of urine bacterial culture results. These are considered positive if 100 to 100,000 colony-forming units are found. Urine culture is advantageous as is it allows for identification of the organism causing infection. Other diagnostic interventions include urine microscopy, which can reveal pyuria (greater than five white blood cells in the urine), hematuria (red cells in the urine), or bacteria, all of which alone or in combination can indicate a UTI. Urine dipstick readings can also be helpful, as they can indicate the presence of leukocyte esterase as a marker of white blood cells and hemoglobin as a marker of red blood cells. Nitrates can also be detected and are most often caused by any number of the uropathogenic gram-negative rods (Enterobacteriaceae family), which convert nitrates to nitrites.

In many cases of both uncomplicated and complicated UTIs, history and physical examination will provide significant clues. Imaging is usually unwarranted.

Organisms

Uropathogenic *E. Coli* are the most commonly found pathogens, accounting for nearly 80% of community-acquired uncomplicated UTIs, and nearly 50% of UTIs among hospitalized patients or patients with diabetes. Interestingly, uropathogenic *E. coli* are unique in the fact that they express genes that may be associated with increased virulence, including fimbrial adhesin, hemolysin, and aerobactin. Unfortunately, at this time, there is no way to easily differentiate the uropathogenic *E. Coli* with the nonuropathogenic variety.

Other organisms can infect the urinary tract, but bacteria remain the most common cause, with *E. Coli* responsible for up to 95% of uncomplicated UTIs. Other bacterial species besides *E. coli* include *Proteus mirabilis, Staphylococcus saprophyticus, Streptococcus agalactiae, Pseudomonas,* and *Enteroccocus faecalis.*

Treatment

For uncomplicated UTI, resistance patterns in local communities should be considered. In many cases of uncomplicated UTI and in areas where resistance is low, empiric therapy against the most common offender (*E. coli*) using a 3-day course of trimethoprim-sulfamethoxazole (160–800 mg PO BID) is an acceptable choice, as is a 5-day course of nitrofurantoin (100 mg PO BID). Fosfomycin trometamol, 3 g orally in single dose, has also been recommended as a first-line dose.

Depending on antibiotic resistance patterns, empiric therapy for complicated cystitis can be accomplished with a fluoroquinolone (ciprofloxacin 500 mg PO BID or 400 mg IV BID; or levofloxacin, 500 mg PO or IV q day). More serious infections can be treated with cefepime 2 g IV every 12 hours or ceftazidime 2 g IV every 8 hours. Other options for ill patients include piperacillin-tazobactam 3.375 to 4.5 g IV every 6 hours, imipenem 500 mg IV every 6 hours, or meropenem 1 g IV every 8 hours. In patients who may have a gram-positive infection, especially with methicillin resistant staphylococci or enterococci, the addition of vancomycin (1 g IV q12 hours) should be considered.

Other Considerations

Asymptomatic bacteriuria (ABU) in pregnant women can progress very quickly. Pyelonephritis can threaten the pregnancy in multiple ways, including premature delivery. Pregnant patients with ABU should be treated with cephalexin, amoxicillin, or amoxicillin-clavulanic acid. Fluoroquinolones should be avoided in pregnancy. Nitrofurantoin and trimethoprim-sulfamethoxazole have been reported to be safe in the first trimester, but there are some concerns regarding use in the second or third trimester. The American College of Obstetricians and Gynecologists recommended in a committee opinion in 2011 that both sulfonamides and nitrofurantoin may be used in pregnancy.

Chapter 38

Cervicitis and Vulvovaginitis

Shannon B. Putman

Summary Box

Disease Description:
- Cervicitis: inflammation and irritation of the cervix, often caused by sexually transmitted infection (STI).
- Vulvovaginitis: inflammation of the vagina and/or vulva with itching, erythema, and mucopurulent discharge; it may or may not be related to STI.

Organisms:
- *Chlamydia trachomatis* is most common STI, followed by *Neisseria gonorrhea*, *Trichomonas vaginalis*, bacterial vaginosis (principally, *Gardnerella vaginalis*), HSV, *Mycoplasma genitalium*, *Candida* spp.

Diagnostic tests:
- Wet prep, nucleic acid amplification testing (NAAT) for *Chlamydia* and *N. gonorrhea*, *herpes simplex virus* (HSV) culture in appropriate setting

Treatment:
- *C. trachomatis*: azithromycin 1 g PO single dose or doxycycline 100 mg PO BID for 7 days plus ceftriaxone 250 mg IM once*
- *N. gonorrhea*: ceftriaxone 250 mg IM once plus azithromycin 1 g PO single dose**; doxycycline 100 mg PO BID for 7 days may be substituted for azithromycin allergy
- *T. vaginalis*: metronidazole 2 g PO single dose or 500 mg PO BID for 7 days
- HSV: valacyclovir 1000 mg PO BID for 7 to 10 days
- Bacterial vaginosis: metronidazole 500 mg PO BID for 7 days or metronidazole cream 5 g intravaginally for 5 days
- *M. genitalium*: azithromycin 1 g PO single dose.

Other Key Issues:
- Prophylaxis, vaccination, high degree of suspicion, and early intervention can help improve morbidity and mortality.

*Empiric treatment of *N. gonorrhea* should be considered in all who test positive for *C. trachomatis*.
**Co-treatment with ceftriaxone and azithromycin is thought to decrease the development of *N. gonorrhea* resistance to ceftriaxone and additionally will treat for possible *C. trachomatis* coinfection.

Disease Description

Cervicitis is characterized by inflammation of the cervix, often with mucopurulent discharge, friability, and bleeding or irritation upon cervical manipulation. It may be asymptomatic and only identified with specific screening studies. It is clinically important, as it can lead to pelvic inflammatory disease (PID), endometritis, and pregnancy complications. In turn, PID is associated with chronic pelvic pain, infertility, and ectopic pregnancy. Cervicitis and PID can be caused by a polymicrobial infection often involving N. gonnorhea and C. trachomatis as well as endogenous, non-sexually transmitted pathogens.

Vulvovaginitis is characterized by irritation, erythema, and mild discharge from vaginal mucosa. It is most commonly caused by infection (bacterial vaginosis, Candida spp., and T. vaginalis).

Epidemiology

The prevalence of cervicitis and vulvovaginitis is difficult to assess given the lack of diagnostic and clinical standards, proportion of asymptomatic cases, and underreporting of positive test results. The Centers for Disease Control (CDC) estimates that there are more than 19 million new sexually transmitted infections annually, with more than 50% occurring in the 15- to 24-year-old age group.[1] This was estimated to have a financial impact of 14.7 billion dollars in 2006.[2] One estimate found 8% of patients presenting to a university health clinic and up to 40% of patients evaluated in community STI clinics had an STI .[3] Another study that vigorously evaluated sexually active, non-pregnant, premenopausal women in the military with endocervical, urine, and vaginal swabs found a 14% prevalence of STI.[4,5] Notably, this group was not specifically seeking care for symptoms or concern about STI exposure.

C. trachomatis is the most common sexually transmitted infection, with 347.8 cases per 100 000 patients and 1 030 911 new cases in 2006. Because it is likely dramatically underdiagnosed, this likely represents 2.8 million cases per year.[1] Disease is most common in the 15- to 19-year-old age group, followed by 20- to 24-year-old group. African Americans are seven times more likely than their white counterparts and two times more likely than Hispanics to be diagnosed with chlamydial genital infections.

The majority of patients have neither signs nor symptoms of infection; only 10% to 20% of patients testing positive for Chlamydia were found to have purulent discharge on exam (5). This provides the rational for empiric testing for all sexually active women on an annual basis. Although the incubation period for symptomatic infection is 1 to 2 weeks, it is not clear how long patients with asymptomatic infection remain infected. In one review of untreated infection, C. trachomatis was detected in weeks to months in 56% to 89% and for at least 1 year in 46% to 57%, serving as a reservoir for ongoing infection in the community (6). Symptomatic patients can have cervicitis, urethritis, PID, perihepatitis (Fitz-Hugh–Curtis syndrome), and proctitis.

There were 358,366 new cases of Gonorrhea in 2006. Although there was a 75% decline in cases from 1975–1997, followed by a plateau in incidence, cases increased by 5.5% between 2004 and 2006.[1] Because it is underdiagnosed, it is estimated that there are more than 600,000 cases of gonorrhea annually in the United States.

Disease Description

Many patients with cervicitis or vulvovaginitis are asymptomatic, and infection is only apparent on physical exam or with specific testing. All patients with symptoms complain of purulent vaginal discharge. Other symptoms include vaginal irritation, dyspareunia, dysuria, urinary frequency, and post-coital bleeding or spotting. On physical exam, purulent discharge can be seen draining from the endocervical canal. The cervix may appear erythematous, edematous, and may be friable with manipulation. Cervical motion tenderness, uterine fullness or pain, or unilateral ovarian tenderness on bimanual exam is suggestive of an ascending infection, such as PID or tubo-ovarian abscess. Diffuse shallow tender ulceration of the vagina and cervix is consistent with HSV infection. Punctate hemorrhage of the cervix, also known as "strawberry cervix," is suggestive of T. vaginalis. The physical exam does not distinguish well between infectious and noninfectious causes of cervicitis.

Differential Diagnosis

Infectious causes of cervicitis and vaginitis include C. trachomatis, N. gonorrhoeae, T. vaginalis, HSV (most commonly HSV-2 but also HSV-1), M. genitalium, Streptococcus species, Candida species, and bacterial vaginosis (principally, *G. vaginalis*). Risk factors for infection include women who fall in the 15- to 24-year-old age range, history of multiple sexual partners, and prior STI.

The noninfectious causes of cervical inflammation with discharge are cervical dysplasia or malignancy, chemical irritation (secondary to douches, vaginal sprays, and latex), mechanical irritation from an intra-uterine device, and systemic inflammatory disease, such as Bechet's syndrome (systemic vasculitis).

Diagnostic Evaluation

Patients at risk for cervicitis should have routine surveillance testing for chlamydia and gonorrhea. Microscopy of the vaginal swab, also known as a wet prep, may provide timely information about the presence of yeast, clue cells (cervical epithelial cells lined with bacteria), or trichomonads. The presence of more than 10 white blood cells per high powered field is abnormal and suggestive of cervical inflammation. Chlamydia and gonorrhea are most frequently assessed with NAAT from vaginal swabs or urine specimens (sensitivity and specificity of 97%–99% for vaginal swabs).[6] Because microscopy lacks sensitivity for trichomonal infection, vaginal swabs can be sent for specific rapid antigen testing or NAAT. Routine testing for infections other than *T. vaginalis*, gonorrhea, Chlamydia, and bacterial vaginosis is not useful or cost effective. HSV testing with viral culture should be sent for patients with tender shallow punctuate ulcers. Any woman who tests positive for cervicitis caused by a STI should be offered HIV, syphilis, and Hepatitis B and C testing.

Organism and Treatment

Treatment of *C. trachomatis* cervicitis is with azithromycin 1 g PO once or doxycycline 100 mg PO twice daily for 7 days. Women who test positive for *N. gonorrhea* should empirically be treated for *C. trachomatis* given the risk of coinfection, which is noted to be as high as 46% in some studies.[8] Treatment for gonorrhea should be considered for anyone who is being treated for chlamydia.

Gonorrhea treatment has become more complex in the recent decades due to rapid antibiotic resistance. Fluoroquinolones are no longer appropriate given resistance rates of 10% to 100% throughout the world.[9] Additionally, there is well-documented resistance to sulfonamides, penicillins, tetracyclines, and some cephalosporins. For uncomplicated urogenital gonococcal infections, the CDC recommends Ceftriaxone 250 mg IM once as a single dose plus Azithromycin 1 g PO once for possible additional coverage against *N. gonorrhoeae* and treatment of possible chlamydial coinfection. Although ceftriaxone is thought to cure 98% to 99% of current infection, dual coverage may help prevent the emergence of cephalosporin resistance.[10]

T. vaginalis can be treated most effectively with metronidazole 2 g PO as a single dose, or, alternatively, metronidazole 500 mg OP twice daily for 7 days.

Bacterial vaginosis is incredibly common, identified in close to 30% of women by surveillance cultures.[11] It is caused by shifts in normal healthy vaginal flora from a predominance of hydrogen producing *Lactobacilli* to more pathological anaerobic gram-negative rods. *G. vaginalis* plays a prominent role, in addition to *Prevotella, bacteroides*, and *peptostreptococci*. Although it is not considered a sexually transmitted infection and male partners do not need to be treated, sexual activity is a risk factor. Patients can be treated with metronidazole 500 mg twice daily for 7 days, metronidazole 0.75% gel 5 g intravaginally for 5 days, or clindamycin 2% gel 5 g intravaginally for 7 days.

Primary HSV infection can be treated with acyclovir 400 mg orally three times daily or 200 mg orally five times daily, valacyclovir 1000 mg orally twice daily, or famciclovir 240 mg orally three times daily.

M. genitalium is an emerging cause of cervicitis and PID and is found more frequently in vaginal specimens from patients with documented mucopurulent discharge. It can be treated with azithromycin 1 g orally as a single dose, or, alternatively, doxycycline 100 mg orally twice daily for 7 days.

Other Issues

Given the prevalence of STI in sexually active women less than 25 years old, they should be offered empiric treatment for gonorrhea and chlamydia at the time of presentation and prior to NAAT testing results. Patients testing positive for STI should be offered counseling regarding safe sex and testing for syphilis, HIV, and viral hepatitis. Sexual partners of women testing positive for gonorrhea, chlamydia, or trichomoniasis should be informed and treated to prevent reinfection. Patients and their partners should abstain for intercourse until the course of treatment is complete and symptoms resolve. Test of cure is not necessary, but patients with STI should be retested at 6 months given high rates of recurrent infection in high-risk populations.

Suggested Readings and References

1. Centers for Disease Control and Prevention (CDC). Trends in reportable sexually transmitted diseases in the United States 2006. STD surveillance 2006. November 2007. http://www.cdc.gov/std/stats06/trends2006.htm Accessed April 3, 2013).

2. HW Chesson, JW Blandfort, TL Gift, G Toa, KL Erwin. The estimated direct cost of STD's among American youth 2000–2004. National STD Prevention Conference, Philadelphia, PA, March 8–11, 2000, abstract P075.

3. Boyer CB, Shafer MB, Pollack LM, et al. Sociodemographic markers and behavioral correlates of STIs in a non-clinical sample of adolescent and young adult women. *J Infect Dis.* 2006:194:307–315.

4. Groetsch S. Cervicitis. *Clin Fam Pract.* 2005;7:43–56.

5. Gaydos, CA, Howel MR, Pare B, et al. Chlamydia trachomatis infections in female military recruits. *N Engl J Med.* 1998; 339:739–744.

6. Cook RL, Hutchison SL, Ostergaard L, et al. Systemic review: noninvasive testing for Chlamydial trachomatis and Neisseria gonorrhoeae. *Ann Intern Med.* 2005;142:914.

7. Geisler WM. Duration of untreated, uncomplicated Chlamydia tranomattis genital infection and factors associated with Chlamydia resolution: a review of human studies. *J Infect Dis.* 2010;201(suppl 2):S104.

8. Datta DS, Sternberg M, Johnson RE, et al. Gonorrhea and chlamydia in the United States among persons 14 to 39 years of age, 1999 to 2002. *Ann Intern Med.* 2007;147:89.

9. Workowski KA, Berman SM, Douglas JM Jr. Emerging antimicrobial resistance in Neisseria gonorrhoeae: urgent need to strengthen prevention strategies. *Ann Intern Med.* 2008;148:606.

10. Newman LM, Moran JS, Workowski KA. Update on the management of gonorrhea in adults in the United States. *Clin Infect Dis.* 2007;44(suppl 3):S84.

11. Allsworth JE, Peipert JF. Prevalence of bacterial vaginosis: 2001–2004 National Health and Nutrition Examination Survey. *Obstet Gynecol.* 2007;109:114–120.

Chapter 39

Urethritis, Prostatitis, and Epididymitis

Shannon B. Putman and Arjun S. Chanmugam

Disease Description: Urethritis, prostatitis, and epididymitis are a constellation of diseases that can result in dysuria, pain, urethral discharge, and fever. These diseases can result from urinary pathogens or sexually transmitted infections (STIs).

Organisms: Chlamydia, *Neisseria gonorrhoeae* (GC), and *Trichomonas* are common sexually transmitted infections; *E. Coli* is the most common urinary pathogen.

Diagnostic Tests: Urethral swabs, culture, urine analysis and culture, ultrasound

Treatment
    Targeted antibiotics based on lab and culture results.

Urethritis
    Chlamydia: doxycycline 100 mg PO BID for 7 days or azithromycin 1 g PO single dose plus ceftriaxone 250 IM once (CDC recommends also empirically treating gonorrhea)
    Gonorrhea: ceftriaxone 250 IM once plus doxycycline 100 mg PO BID for 7 days or azithromycin 1 g PO single dose (CDC recommends also empirically treating Chlamydia)
    Trichomonas: metronidazole 2 g PO single dose or 500 mg PO BID for 7 days

Prostatitis
    STI suspected: ceftriaxone 250 IM once plus doxycycline 100 mg PO BID or ciprofloxacin 500 mg PO BID for at least 28 days (avoid in quinolone-resistant gonorrhea).
    STI not suspected: ciprofloxacin 500 mg PO BID, levofloxacin 500 mg PO once daily, or trimethoprim/sulfamethoxazole 160 mg/800 mg PO twice daily for at least 28 days.
    Serious infections (involving hospitalization): ceftriaxone 1 to 2 g IV q24 hours.
    Epididymitis (if associated with prostatitis, continue treatment for at least 28 days)

STI suspected: ceftriaxone 250 mg IM once and doxycycline 100 mg PO BID for 10 days. Azithromycin 2 g PO once if penicillin allergic.
    STI not suspected: ofloxacin 300 mg PO BID or levofloxacin 500 mg PO q day for 10 days.

Dysuria in men can be the presenting complaint in patients with urethritis, prostatitis, epididymitis, or cystitis. Urethritis is most frequently secondary to a sexually transmitted infection and is most commonly diagnosed in young men. Prostatitis can be acute or chronic and is diagnosed in both older men with prostatic hypertrophy and young men without genitourinary anatomical abnormalities. Acute cystitis is rare in young men but is frequently diagnosed in men with prostatic hypertrophy with urethral obstruction. Acute epididymitis can be diagnosed in young men due to a sexually transmitted infection or in older men with underlying prostatic obstruction.

History and physical examination will help distinguish between the various causes of dysuria. Men with urethritis often complain of penile discharge in addition to painful urination. In general, the acute onset of frankly purulent discharge is most consistent with gonorrheal infection. Dysuria in a young man with scant or no penile discharge is more likely to be secondary to chlamydial infection. Dysuria with painful genital ulcers is often due to genital herpes infection. Patients with acute bacterial prostatitis complain of systemic symptoms such as fever, chills, malaise, and dysuria with cloudy urine. They may complain of urinary hesitancy or dribbling as well as perineal pain or pain with ejaculation. Patients with epididymitis complain of urinary frequency, urgency, dysuria, and testicular pain. They may also have systemic symptoms, such as fever and rigors.

Urethritis

STI in young men is very common. In a study evaluating the incidence of reinfection over one year, 1,183 men seen in an urban STI clinic following the diagnosis of a STI had a reinfection rate of 15%. Notably, 66% of these new infections were asymptomatic.[1]

Gonorrhea

In 2008, there were 336 742 new cases of gonorrhea diagnosed. Women were more frequently diagnosed (119.4 per 100 000) compared with men (103 per 100 000), with the greatest number of cases seen in 13- to 19-year-old women (636.8 per 100 000) and 20- to 24-year-old men (433.6 per 100 000). African Americans were more than 20 times more likely to be diagnosed with gonorrhea. Most male patients with gonorrhea are symptomatic with purulent penile discharge and dysuria and present to medical care for evaluation. Diagnosis can be made with a urethral swab using a narrow cotton applicator inserted 2 to 3 cm into the urethral meatus or with a first voided urine sample. Routine culture is not commonly performed because Neisseria gonorrhoeae requires a carbon-dioxide-rich transport media and is difficult to grow in culture. Nucleic acid amplification testing (NAAT) is the recommended testing method for diagnosis of genital tract infections from gonorrhea, with a sensitivity of 98% to 100%.[2] Both urine and urethral swabs are equally sensitive.

The treatment of suspected or confirmed urogenital gonorrhea is a single IM dose of ceftriaxone 250 mg IM once. Azithromycin 1 g PO as a single dose is added to cover possible Chlamydial pathogens in addition to N. gonorrhoeae. Patients who are allergic to cephalosporins can be treated with a single dose of Azithromycin 2 g orally. Repeat testing after treatment is not routinely recommended, but patients with recurrent symptoms or who have received suboptimal therapy should be retested. Patients should be advised to inform their sexual partners and to use barrier protection until symptoms resolve and their partner has received adequate treatment.

Chlamydia

Chlamydia trachomatis is the most common sexually transmitted disease in both men and women. A prospective cohort study of 14,322 individuals ages 18 to 26 in the United States found a prevalence of 3.7% in men, with the highest prevalence in African American men at 11%.[3] The Centers for Disease Control recommends routinely screening men in high-risk populations, such as those presenting to STI clinics, inmates of correctional facilities, and men who have sex with men and who have had receptive anal intercourse within the last year.[4] From 40% to 96% of men with Chlamydia urethritis are asymptomatic and serve as a reservoir for ongoing infection in the community.[5] Typically, patients with symptoms complain of dysuria and scant mucoid to clear penile discharge. The incubation period after exposure is 5 to 10 days. The preferred method to diagnose chlamydial infection is the NAAT, which amplifies C. trachomatis DNA sequences and has a sensitivity of 83% to 93%, depending on the specific technique used.[6] First voided urine (from the first 10 mL of stream) without precleaning of urethral meatus is the ideal specimen and is comparable to urethral swabs in terms of sensitivity.

Patients with Chlamydial urethritis should be treated with Azithromycin 1 g orally as a single dose or doxycycline 100 mg by PO BID for 7 days. Erythromycin 500 mg orally four times per day for 7 days or levofloxacin 500 mg daily for 7 days are appropriate alternative regimens. Ceftriaxone 250 mg IM once should be added for possible gonorrheal co-infection. As above, azithromycin 2 g PO once can be used in patients allergic to penicillin.

Mycoplasma Genitalium

Mycoplasma genitalium is recognized as an emerging cause of nongonococcal urethritis in men. In the United States, it has a 1% prevalence among young sexually active adults, placing it between *Neisseria gonorrhoeae* (0.4% prevalence) and *Chlamydia trachomatis* (2.3% prevalence) in frequency of diagnosis.[7] The majority of patients with *M. genitalium* urethritis are symptomatic with dysuria and purulent penile discharge. Commercial testing is not widely available, but some labs can process NAATs on first voided urine or vaginal swabs. Optimal treatment is Azithromycin 1 g orally as a single dose, which has consistently been shown superior to doxycycline in randomized trials.[8]

Trichomonas

Trichomonas vaginalis, a flagellated motile organism, is one of the most common sexually transmitted diseases and affects nearly 6 million people. Although it is one of the most common causes of vulvovaginitis in women, it can cause symptoms in men as well.

Trichomonas has been cited as a possible cause of both male and female infertility. This infection can be asymptomatic in up to 70% of male patients (range 15%–70%), with the more common symptoms being dysuria, urethral irritation, urinary frequency, and urethral discharge. It can also lead to epididymitis and prostatitis. Physical findings can be minimal but often include some urethral discharge. Risk factors include multiple sex partners as well as other sexually transmitted diseases.

Diagnosis is usually made by a wet mount examination of secretions or urine microscopy and identifying the motile *T. vaginalis*; in men, culture from a urethral swab, urine or semen, polymerase chain reaction, or transcription mediated amplification tests are important diagnostic tools. Prostatic message before urethral swab may improve sensitivity.

Treatment consists of metronidazole 2 g orally or 500 mg orally twice a day for 7 days.

Prostatitis

The National Institutes of Health consensus classifies prostatitis into four categories: acute bacterial, chronic bacterial, chronic prostatitis/chronic pelvic pain, and asymptomatic inflammatory prostatitis. It is estimated that prostatitis results in about 2 million visits per year and that there is a 14% lifetime prevalence of prostatitis in men aged 20 to 59 years of age.

Acute bacterial prostatitis (ABP) is usually due to the common gram-negative uropathogens, the most common being *E. coli* (87% in one study), followed by *Klebsiella, Pseudomonas*, and others.[1] Both *N. gonorrhea* and Chlamydia are other less common causes of ABP and must be considered in men who are sexually active. In immunodeficient states, other opportunistic organisms, including *Mycobacterium tuberculosis* and candida, should also be considered.

ABP is often associated with fever, chills, and malaise as well as dysuria and increased urinary frequency, urgency, and nocturia. A tender, warm, and sometimes swollen prostate is found on physical examination. Risk factors include recent urinary instrumentation, sexual activity, prostatic biopsy, and anatomical abnormalities, including benign prostatic hypertrophy. Other related infections such as cystitis and epididymitis are also risk factors.

Diagnosis is usually made on the basis of clinical findings confirmed by urine analysis (greater than 10 white blood cells and bacteria) and urine culture. Other laboratory findings may be helpful, including inflammatory markers. Prostatic massage may be uncomfortable for the patient with ABP and is generally not indicated.

Treatment for ABP depends on the etiology of the infection but should include agents that have good prostatic penetration and should be targeted to the culture results and their sensitivities. Empiric treatment depends on whether or not STI is suspected. A general guideline for suspecting STI is age less than 35. Treatment of prostatitis due to suspected STI includes ceftriaxone 250 IM once plus doxycycline 100 mg BID or ciprofloxacin 500 mg PO BID for at least 28 days (avoid in quinolone-resistant gonorrhea). Treatment of prostatitis not suspected to be due to STI includes ciprofloxacin 500 mg BID, levofloxacin 500 mg once daily, or trimethoprim/sulfamethoxazole 160 mg/800 mg twice daily for at least 28 days. Serious infections (involving hospitalization) should be treated with IV antibiotics, such as ceftriaxone 1 to 2 g IV q24 hours.

Chronic prostatitis is generally diagnosed after symptoms have persisted for at least 3 months, and has symptoms similar to ABP and should be treated with fluoroquinolones. Diagnostic imaging may be necessary to rule out abscess.

Epididymitis

Epididymitis is an inflammation of the epididymis, with or without infection, lasting less than 6 weeks. Acute epididymitis usually involves the testicles, resulting in an epididymo-orchitis. Although trauma is one example of a noninfectious cause of epididymitis, infectious causes must be considere: especially GC and Chlamydia in younger, sexually active males and gram-negative uropathogens in men older than 35 years old and prepubertal boys.

Symptoms include the gradual onset of testicular pain and swelling, which can radiate to the abdomen and is sometimes accompanied by fever. Urinary tract symptoms can present as well, including dysuria, urgency, frequency, and hematuria and sometimes urethral discharge.

Diagnosis can be made based on clinical findings, but urine analysis and culture, urethral swabs for gram stain and culture, and testicular ultrasound are important diagnostic tools. First void urine testing (NAAT) for Chlamydia and GC should be considered in any sexually active male.

In patients for whom sexually transmitted diseases are the suspected source, treatment should include ceftriaxone 250 mg IM once and doxycycline 100 mg PO BID for 10 days or azithromycin 2 g PO once if the patient is allergic to penicillin. In those whom STI is not suspected, ofloxacin 300 mg PO BID or levofloxacin 500 mg PO q day for 10 days are recommended.

Prepubertal boys often have self-limited disease, but additional testing for urinary reflux should be considered.

Suggested Readings and References

1. Peterman TA, Tian LH, Metcalf CA, et al. High incidence of new sexually transmitted infections in the year following a sexually transmitted infection: a case for rescreening. *Ann Intern Med.* 2006;145:564–572.

2. Stary A, Bilina A, Kerschbaumer M, et al. Performance of Aptima Combo 2 assay for chlamydial and gonococcal diagnosis from invasive and non-invasive specimens in men and women. In: Schachter J, Christiansen G, Clarke IN, et al., eds. *Chlamydial Infections 2002: Proceedings of the 10th International Symposium on Human Chlamydial Infections.* Antalya, Turkey.

3. Miller WC, Ford CA, Morris M, et al. Prevalence of chlamydial and gonococcal infections among young adults in the United States. *JAMA.* 2004;291:2229.

4. http://www.cdc.gov/std/treatment/2010/default.htm. Accessed June 22, 2013.

5. Detels R, Green AM, Klausner JD, et al. The incidence and correlates of symptomatic and asymptomatic Chlamydia trachomatis and Neisseria gonorrhoeae infections in selected populations in five countries. *Sex Transm Dis.* 2011;38:503–509.

6. Cook RL, Hutchinson SL, Ostergaard L, et al. Systemic review: noninvasive testing for Chlamydia trachomatis and Neisseria gonorrhoeae. *Ann Intern Med.* 2005;142:914–925.

7. Anagrius C, Lore B, Jensen JS. Mycoplasma genitalium:prevalence, clinical significance, and transmission. *Sex Transm Infec.* 2005;81:458–462.

8. Mena LA, Mroczkowski TF, Nsuami M, et al. A dandomized comparison of azithromycin and doxycycline for the treatment of Mydcoplasma genitalium-positive urethritis in men. *Clin Infec Dis* 2009;48:1649.

Chapter 40

Pelvic Inflammatory Disease and Tubo-Ovarian Abscess

John Holst

Summary Box

Disease Description: Pelvic inflammatory disease (PID) consists of inflammation, typically caused by a polymicrobial infection, in various parts of the upper genital tract. PID usually occurs in sexually active women and includes endometritis, salpingitis, tubo-ovarian abscess (TOA), and/or pelvic peritonitis.

Organisms: The most common causative organisms include *Neisseria gonorrhoeae*, *Chlamydia trachomatis*, and *Mycoplasma genitalium* as well as other anaerobic and aerobic bacteria.

Treatment:
   Oral First line: Ceftriaxone 250 mg IM once plus doxycycline 100 mg PO for 14 days with or without metronidazole 500 mg BID for 14 days
   Second line: Cefoxitin 2 g IM once plus probenecid 1 g PO once plus doxycycline 100 mg PO BID for 14 days with or without metronidazole 500 mg BID for 14 days
   Parenteral: Cefoxitin 2 g IV q6 hours plus doxycycline 100 mg IV q12 hours

Other Key Issues: Human immunodeficiency virus (HIV) patients are treated like immunocompetent patients. Mandatory reporting to local health departments is required for cases of *N. gonorrhoeae* and *C. trachomatis*. It is imperative to treat sexual partners to prevent re-infection.

Disease Description:

PID consists of inflammation, which typically results from a polymicrobial infection, in various parts of the upper genital tract in sexually active women. PID includes endometritis, salpingitis, tubo-ovarian abscess (TOA), and/or pelvic peritonitis.

Epidemiology

The incidence of PID and TOA has been steadily declining since their peak in 1982. It was estimated that one million PID diagnoses were made that year, with 14.2% of reproductive-aged women in the United States receiving treatment for PID. Currently, an estimated 770,000 cases of PID are diagnosed in the United States annually with decreasing numbers of ambulatory and hospitalized cases of PID. Still, PID represents a substantial national health care cost, estimated at over two billion dollars annually for the treatment of PID and its complications.

Presenting Features

PID can present along a spectrum of disease severity, including acute, subclinical, and "silent" infections. Overt acute PID with severe symptomatology typically presents with an ill-appearing patient, pelvic pain, fever, chills, purulent vaginal discharge, nausea, vomiting, and elevated white blood cell (WBC) count. This presentation is usually not a diagnostic dilemma but represents only 4% of PID patient encounters. "Silent" PID is a more typical presentation, accounting for approximately 60% of PID cases. "Silent" PID presents with complaints of dyspareunia and irregular bleeding as well as urinary and gastrointestinal complaints in addition to other poorly defined abdominal or pelvic complaints.

For these reasons, many episodes of PID go undiagnosed, leading to the long-term sequelae of tubal factor infertility, ectopic pregnancy, and chronic pelvic pain. For this reason, the Centers for Disease Control (CDC) has recommended a liberal treatment regimen (see Box 40.1). No study to date has clearly demonstrated a single subjective complaint (see Box 40.2), physical finding, or laboratory value to identify PID with high sensitivity or specificity. The CDC notes that a clinical diagnosis of PID in a symptomatic patient has a positive predictive value of 65% to 90% for salpingitis when compared to laparoscopy as the gold standard. This highlights the imprecision of clinically diagnosing PID. Thus, clinicians should carefully consider their clinical impressions, exams, labs, and imaging when attempting to diagnose PID.

Diagnostic Tests

Laboratory tests can be of some assistance in the diagnosis of PID. Leukocytosis occurs in 44% of PID patients. Nonspecific markers of inflammation, such as erythrocyte sedimentation rate and C-reactive protein, demonstrate a sensitivity of 74% to 93% and a specificity of 25% to 90% in the diagnosis PID. Vaginal wet prep may further aid in the diagnosis of PID. Three or more WBCs per high power field, for example, correlate to a sensitivity of 87% to 91% for upper genital tract infection. The negative predictive value for a wet prep noting zero WBCs per high power field is 94.5%.

Although imaging is not required to diagnose PID in all cases, particularly in less symptomatic patients, ultrasound should be the initial modality if the diagnosis is unclear or the patient requires inpatient treatment (see Box 40.3). Transvaginal ultrasound has excellent specificity (97%–100%) but poor sensitivity (32%–85%) in the diagnosis of PID. Magnetic resonance imaging has a higher sensitivity (95%) for PID compared to ultrasound. Still, ultrasound remains the initial modality of choice due to its ease of access

---

Box 40.1 Empiric Treatment for Pelvic Inflammatory Disease

- Any at-risk sexually active female
- Lower abdominal or pelvic pain
- At least one clinical sign (see the following) without another etiology for her pain

  Cervical Motion Tenderness

  Or

  Uterine Tenderness

  Or

  Adnexal Tenderness

Data from (1)

Box 40.2 Symptoms Concerning for PID
Abdominal pain or pelvic pain
Abnormal vaginal discharge
Intermenstrual bleeding or postcoital bleeding
Fever
Lower back pain
Nausea/vomiting
Data from (1)

and low cost. Although ultrasound can be of benefit, the clinician must always remember that PID is a clinical diagnosis. A normal ultrasound should not halt investigation or treatment in an ill-appearing patient or in a patient for whom there is high clinical suspicion for PID.

In patients who meet criteria to be hospitalized with a diagnosis of PID, studies have identified that nearly one-third of these patients have a TOA. Computed tomography (CT) appears to have a better sensitivity (78%–100%) than ultrasound (75%–90%) for diagnosing TOA. However, ultrasound likely has better specificity (as high as 98.6%) versus CT (85%–100%). CT is also more costly and exposes the patient to radiation. If CT is utilized in a patient, IV and oral contrast are recommended for improved imaging.

Endometrial biopsies have demonstrated sensitivities that range from 70% to 90% and specificities that range from 67% to 90% for the diagnosis of PID. However, due to the processing time of this test, its utility in an acute or emergent setting is limited. Last, laparoscopic evaluation has been considered the gold standard for diagnosing PID in the past, but its utility in an emergent setting in the absence of a gynecologist remains limited.

Organisms

PID is often a polymicrobial infection. The organisms most often cultured include *N. gonorrhoeae, C. trachomatis*, and genital tract *Mycoplasma* species (most notably *M. genitalium*) as well as other anaerobic and aerobic bacteria comprising the endogenous vaginal flora (eg, *Prevotella* species, *Peptostreptococcus* species, *Garnerella vaginalis, Escherlichia coli, Haemophilus influenza*, and aerobic streptococci). In the largest treatment study to date for mild to moderate PID in the United States, the Pelvic Inflammatory Disease Evaluation and Clinical Health (PEACH) study noted that *N. gonorrhoeae* or *C. trachomatis* were recovered in less than one-third of the patients, highlighting the polymicrobial nature of PID.

A study by Jossens and colleagues noted that non-sexually transmitted disease (STD) organisms and endogenous organisms, including anaerobes and facultative bacteria, accounted for 30% of PID cases. Some of the most common anaerobes isolated from PID cases are *Prevotella, Bacteroides*, and *Peptostreptococcus*.

In PID complicated by TOA, the microbial etiology is generally polymicrobial with a mixture of anaerobic, aerobic, and facultative organisms on culture. The organisms most likely to be cultured from a TOA are *Prevotella, Bacteroides*, and *Peptostreptococcus* species in addition to *Escherichia coli*. Interestingly, *N. gonorrhea*, although rarely cultured from the abdominal abscess, is recovered from the endocervix

Box 40.3 Criteria for Hospitalization in Women with PID
Surgical emergencies (eg, appendicitis) cannot be excluded
Pregnancy
Failed outpatient therapy
Unable to follow or tolerate outpatient regimen
Clinically unstable
TOA on exam or imaging
Data from (1)

in nearly 31% of cases with a TOA. Additionally, in vivo studies show that *N. gonorrhea* may help lower genital tract flora to invade the upper genital tract. In this way, *N. gonorrhea* is implicated in TOA formation without ever entering the TOA itself, accounting for the lack of TOAs that are culture positive for *N. gonorrhea*.

Treatment

Multiple studies have demonstrated that bacterial vaginosis (BV) and associated microorganisms are present in patients with acute PID, leading some authors to believe that treatment should cover BV and anaerobes in addition to the pathogens noted previously. Concern for mandatory anaerobic or BV coverage in mild to moderate PID patients has definitely been raised in the literature, most recently by the PEACH trial. The PEACH trial compared inpatient treatment regimens (cefoxitin and doxycycline) versus traditional outpatient oral therapy (single dose of cefoxitin and 14 days of doxycycline) and found no superiority in therapies for acute or chronic symptoms in the inpatient group. The PEACH trial also demonstrated no difference on long-term outcomes, such as PID recurrence, chronic pelvic pain, infertility, ectopic pregnancy, and tubal obstruction after 3 years. These results call into question the need to cover for anaerobes in mild to moderate PID cases despite their presence in cultures in prior studies. This controversy is demonstrated in the CDC recommendations for the treatment of PID, which advise the clinician to "consider" anaerobic coverage with metronidazole.

Despite the controversy regarding the mandatory coverage of anaerobes and BV in PID, it is clearly established in the literature that PID coverage is focused on a polymicrobial infection. All guidelines recommend effective coverage against *N. gonorrhea* and *C. trachomatis* even in the presence of negative cultures. The 2010 CDC recommendations for parenteral and enteral PID therapy are formatted in Boxes 40.4 and 40.5. The recommended parenteral therapy can be discontinued 24 hours after clinical improvement, whereas doxycycline should be continued for 10 to 14 days. Due to similar bioavailability between oral and parenteral doxycycline, transition to the oral form is recommended as soon as the patient can tolerate enteral administration. The overall clinical cure rates when following the recommended regimens have been found to be over 90%. For patients that do not improve or fail outpatient therapy after 72 hours of observation, imaging should be obtained to help identify a possible TOA or to elucidate another possible diagnosis that may have been missed initially.

Historically, the surgical treatment of ruptured TOAs in the 1950s had a mortality rate as high as 85% to 100%. However, with the subsequent utilization of aggressive broad-spectrum antibiotics and surgical

---

Box 40.4 Parenteral Recommendations for PID

Regimen A:

Cefotetan 2 g IV q12 hours

Or

Cefoxitin 2 g IV q6 hours

Plus

Doxycycline 100 mg PO/IV q12 hours

Regimen B:

Clindamycin 900 mg IV q8 hours

Plus

Gentamicin loading dose IV/IM (2mg/kg), then maintenance dose (1–5 mg/kg) q8 hours

Or

Gentamicin daily dosing (3–5 mg/kg) can be substituted

Alternative:

Ampicillin/Sulbactam 3 g IV q6 hours

Plus

Doxycycline 100 mg IV/PO q12 hours

Data from (1)

Box 40.5 Oral Recommendations for PID
Regimen A:
Ceftriaxone 250 mg IM once
Plus
Doxycycline 100 mg PO for 10 to 14 days
With or without
Metronidazole 500 mg PO BID for 10 to 14 days
Regimen B:
Cefoxitin 2 g IM once and probenecid 1 g PO as a single dose
Plus
Doxycycline 100 mg PO for 10 to 14 days
With or without
Metronidazole 500 mg PO BID for 10 to 14 days
Regimen C:
Other parenteral third-generation cephalosporins (ceftizoxime or cefotaxime) in a single dose
Plus
Doxycycline 100 mg PO for 10 to 14 days
With or without
Metronidazole 500 mg PO BID for 10 to 14 days
Data from (1)

management, mortality has dropped to 3%. Current studies show that conservative, broad-spectrum, antibiotic management has success rates of 70% or greater; and conservative management only requires additional surgical intervention when patients have a ruptured TOA or if there is a poor response to antibiotic therapy. Recent studies have demonstrated that the size of the TOA may be inversely proportional to the success of medical management. TOAs greater than 10 cm have a 60% chance of requiring surgical intervention, whereas a TOA of 4 cm to 6 cm has a 20% chance of needing surgery. Most authors agree that clindamycin or flagyl should be added to the standard PID treatment regimen for increased anaerobic coverage in patients that require admission or present with a TOA.

Other Key Issues
Although patients with HIV typically have more severe symptoms and are more likely to have a TOA than an immunocompetent patient, studies have demonstrated that HIV alone does not mandate admission nor does parenteral therapy improve outcomes when compared to non-HIV patients. Male sex partners with a woman recently diagnosed with PID should be treated if contact was within the last 60 days preceding the patient's clinical symptoms. If it has been beyond 60 days since the last sexual contact, the patient's most recent sex partner should be treated. It is mandated that gonorrhea and chlamydia cases be reported to the local health department. If the patient has an intrauterine device in place at the time of diagnosis of PID, it is not mandatory to remove the device. There is insufficient evidence to recommend the immediate removal, but close medical follow-up is needed in these patients. If the prevalence of gonococcal resistance is low, patients allergic to cephalosporins may use fluoroquinolones, such as levofloxacin 500 mg PO daily or ofloxacin 400 mg BID for 14 days with or without metronidazole. Before pursuing this alternate treatment, however, it is recommended that cultures are drawn. Close follow-up is encouraged.

Suggested Readings and References

1. Centers for Disease Control and Prevention. *Sexually Transmitted Diseases Treatment Guidelines, 2010.* MMWR Morb Mortal Wkly Rep. 2010;59:1–116.
2. Washington AE, Cates W, Zadi AA. Hospitalization for pelvic inflammatory disease: epidemiology and trends in the United States, 1975 to 1981. *JAMA.* 1984;251:2529–2533.

3. Aral SO, Mosher WD, Cates W Jr. Self-reported pelvic inflammatory disease and its consequences in the industrialized countries. *Am J Obstet Gynecol*. 1980;138:880–892.

4. Sweet RL. Treatment of acute pelvic inflammatory disease. In: *Infectious Diseases in Obstetrics and Gynecology*, vol. 2011. Article ID 561909; 2011:13 pages. doi:10.1155/2011/561909.

5. Rein DB, Kassler WJ, Irwin KL, and Rabiee L. Direct medical cost of pelvic inflammatory disease and its sequelae: decreasing, but still substantial. *Obstet Gynecol*. 2000;95:397–402.

6. CDC. Pelvic inflammatory disease: STD curriculum for clinical providers. National Network of STD/HI Prevention Training Centers. http://www2a.cdc.gov/stdtraining/self-study/pid/pid4.asp Accessed

7. Wolner-Hanssen P, Kiviat NB, Holmes KK. Atypical pelvic inflammatory disease: subacute, chronic, or subclinical upper genital tract infection in women. In: Holmes KK, Mardh P-A, Sparling PF, et al., eds. *Sexually Transmitted Diseases*. 2nd ed. New York: McGraw-Hill; 1990:615–620.

8. Peipert JF, Ness RB, Blume J, et al. Clinical predictors of endometritis in women with symptoms and signs of pelvic inflammatory disease. *Am J Obstet Gynecol*. 2001;184:856–863.

9. Wolner-Hanssen P. Diagnosis of pelvic inflammatory disease. In: Landers DV, Sweet RL, eds. *Pelvic Inflammatory Disease*. New York: Springer-Verlag; 1997:60–75.

10. Eschenbach DA. Epidemiology and diagnosis of acute pelvic inflammatory disease. *Obstet Gynecol*. 1980;55:142S–153S.

11. Kahn JG, Walker CK, Washington AE, et al. Diagnosing pelvic inflammatory disease: a comprehensive analysis and considerations for developing a new model. *JAMA*. 1991;226:2594–2604.

12. Lehtinen M, Laine S, Heinonen PK, et al. Serum C-reactive protein determination in acute pelvic inflammatory disease. *Am J Obstet Gynecol*. 1986;154:158–159.

13. Hemila M, Henrikson L, Ylikorkala O, et al. Serum CRP in the diagnosis and treatment of pelvic inflammatory disease. *Arch Gynecol Obstet*. 1987;241:177–182.

14. Yudin MH, Hillier SL, Wiesenfeld HC, et al. Vaginal polymorphonuclear leukocytes and bacterial vaginosis as markers for histologic endometritis among women without symptoms of pelvic inflammatory disease. *Am J Obstet Gynecol*. 2003;188:318–323.

15. Peipert JF, Boardman L, Hogan JW, et al. Laboratory evaluation of acute upper genital tract infection. *Obstet Gynecol*. 1996;87:730–736.

16. Cacciatore B, Leminem A, Ingman-Friberg S, et al. Transvaginal sonographic markers of tubal inflammatory disease. *Obstet Gynecol*. 1992;80:912–916.

17. Boardman LA, Peipert JF, Brody JM, et al. Endovaginal sonography for the diagnosis of upper genital tract infections. *Obstet Gynecol*. 1997;90:54–57.

18. Sweet RL. Pelvic inflammatory disease: current concepts of diagnosis and management. *Curr Infect Dis Rep*. 2012;14:194–203.

19. Wiesenfeld HC, Sweet RL. Progress in the management of tubo-ovarian abscess. *Clin Obstet Gynecol*. 1993;36:433–444.

20. Landers DV, Sweet RL. Tubo-ovarian abscess: contemporary approach to management. *Rev Infect Dis*. 1983;5:876–884.

21. Sweet RL. Anaerobic-aerobic pelvic infection and pelvic abscess. In: Sweet RL, Gibbs RS, eds. *Infectious Diseases of the Female Genital Tract*. 4th ed. Philadelphia, PA: Lippincott Williams & Wilkins; 2001:189–206.

22. McClean KL, Sheehan GJ, Harding GK. Intra-abdominal infection: a review. *Clin Infect Dis*. 1994;19:100–116.

23. Gagliardi PD, Hoffer PB, Rosenfeld AT. Correlative imaging in abdominal infection: an algorithmic approach using nuclear medicine, ultrasound, and computed tomography. *Semin Nucl Med*. 1988;18:320–334.

24. Taylor KJ, Wasson JF, DE Graaff C, et al. Accuracy of grey-scale ultrasound diagnosis of abdominal and pelvic abscesses in 220 patients. *Lancet*. 1978;1:83–84.

25. Sellors J, Mahoney J, Goldsmith C et al. The diagnosis of pelvic inflammatory disease: the accuracy of clinical and laparoscopic findings. *Am J Obstet Gynecol*. 1991;164:113–120.

26. Sweet RL. Treatment of acute pelvic inflammatory disease. In: *Infectious Diseases in Obstetrics and Gynecology*. Vol. 2011. Article ID 561909; 2011:13 pages. doi:10.1155/2011/561909.

27. Ness RB, Soper DE, Holley RL, et al. Effectiveness of inpatient and outpatient treatment strategies for women with pelvic inflammatory disease: results from the pelvic inflammatory disease evaluation and clinical health (PEACH) randomized trial. *Am J Obstet Gynecol*. 2002;186:929–937.

28. Jossens MO, Schachter J, Sweet RL. Risk factors associated with pelvic inflammatory disease of differing microbial etiologies. *Obstet Gynecol*. 1994;83:989–997.

29. Sweet RL. Role of bacterial vaginosis in pelvic inflammatory disease. *Clin Infect Dis*. 1995;20(suppl 2):S271–275.

30. Ness RB, Hillier SL, Kip KE, et al. Bacterial vaginosis and risk of pelvic inflammatory disease. *Obstet Gynecol*. 2004;104:761–769.

31. Ness RB, Kip KE, Hillier SL, et al. A cluster analysis of bacterial vaginosis-associated microflora and pelvic inflammatory disease. *Am J Epidemiol*. 2005;162:585–590.

32. Workowski KA, Berman S. Sexually transmitted diseases treatment guidelines. *MMWR Morb Mortal Wkly Rep.* 2010;59:63–67.

33. Ross J, Judlin P, Nilas L. European guideline for the management of pelvic inflammatory disease. *Int J STD AIDS.* 2007;18:662–666.

34. Onderdonk AB, Kasper DL, Cisneros RL, et al. The capsular polysaccharide of Bacterioides fragilis as a virulence factor: comparison of the pathogenic potential of encapsulated and unencapsulated strains. *J Infect Dis.* 1977;136:82–89.

35. Beige RH, Wiesenfeld HC. Pelvic inflammatory disease: new diagnostic criteria and treatment. *Obstet Gynecol Clin North Am.* 2003;30:777–793.

36. Lareau SM, Beigi RH. Pelvic inflammatory disease and tubo-ovarian abscess. *Infect Dis Clin North Am.* 2008;22:693–708.

37. Reed SD, Landers DV, Sweet RL. Antibiotic treatment of tubo-ovarian abscess: comparison of broad-spectrum beta-lactam agent agents versus clindamycin-containing regimens. *Am J Obstet Gynecol.* 1991;164:1556–1561.

Skin and Soft Tissue Infections

Soft Tissue Infections

Michael Ehmann

Summary Box

Disease Description: Cellulitis is an acute, spreading infection of the deep dermis and subcutaneous fat characterized by erythema, warmth, swelling, and pain. Erysipelas is an infection of the more superficial cutaneous lymphatics and skin, including the epidermis and upper reticular and papillary dermal layers. It is commonly located on the lower extremities, face, and ears. Cutaneous abscesses are purulent collections that occupy the dermis and deeper soft tissues.

Organisms:
Cellulitis:
Adults: group A β-hemolytic Streptococci (GABHS) and *Staphylococcus aureus*
Children (under 3): *Haemophilus influenzae* type B
Erysipelas: GABS or less commonly methicillin-resistant *S. aureus* (MRSA)
Abscesses: S. aureus or, less commonly, *Escherichia coli, Pseudomonas aeruginosa, Streptococcus faecalis, Bacteroides, Lactobacillus, Peptococcus,* and *Peptostreptococcus*

Treatment:
Oral:
Cellulitis: Cephalexin 500 mg PO q6 hours or dicloxacillin 500 mg PO q6 hours
Erysipelas: Penicillin 500 mg PO q6 hours or amoxicillin 500 mg PO q8 hours
Oral for MRSA suspicion: Clindamycin 300 mg PO three to four times daily or trimethoprim/sulfamethoxazole double strength 1 to 2 tablets PO twice daily.

Parenteral:
Cellulitis: Cefazolin 1 g IV q8 hours, oxacillin 1 to 2 g IV q6 hours, nafcillin 1 to 2 g IV q6 hours
Erysipelas: Ceftriaxone 1 g IV daily, cefazolin 1 to 2 g IV q8 hours, or cefuroxime 750 mg to 1.5 g IV q6 hours
Parenteral for MRSA Suspicion: Clindamycin 600 to 900 mg IV q8 hours or vancomycin 1 g IV q12 hours ± meropenem 500 to 1000 mg IV q8 hours or piperacillin/tazobactam 4.5 g IV q6 hours.

Other Key Issues: The first-line treatment for abscess is incision and drainage (I&D). In an otherwise healthy, immunocompetent patient without valvular heart disease, there are no data that definitively demonstrate the utility of antibiotic therapy in conjunction with I&D of an uncomplicated cutaneous abscess.

Disease Description

Skin consists of two layers: the superficial epidermis and the deeper dermis, which is further divided into the more superficial papillary dermis and the deeper reticular dermis. The hypodermis or subcutis is a loose connective tissue containing various amounts of fat that lies directly beneath the skin.

Cellulitis

Cellulitis is an acute, spreading infection of the deep dermis and subcutaneous fat characterized by erythema, warmth, swelling, and pain. In the United States in 2010, more than 600,000 hospitalizations due to cellulitis were recorded, representing 3.7% of all Emergency Department (ED) admissions. The first sign of cellulitis is localized discomfort, followed by worsening tenderness, erythema, swelling, and expansion without distinct margins from uninvolved skin. Despite progression, systemic signs, including fever and chills, occur in fewer than 10% of cases. Lymphangitic "streaking" that extends proximally from the primary site of infection is a reliable diagnostic sign, and perifollicular edematous dimpling that leads to a *peau d'orange* appearance of the skin is common. Recurrent cellulitis is often associated with local anatomic abnormalities that compromise the venous or lymphatic circulation, such as prior episodes of cellulitis, surgery with lymphadenectomy, and radiation therapy.

Erysipelas

Erysipelas is an infection of the more superficial cutaneous lymphatics and skin, including the epidermis and upper reticular and papillary dermal layers. It is commonly located on the lower extremities, face, and ears. Erysipelas is caused almost exclusively by GABS, although occasionally more severe cases are due to MRSA. A prodrome of malaise, chills, and fever lasting from 4 to 48 hours is followed by one or more red, tender, and firm spots at the site of infection. The spots rapidly grow in size and form a tense, red, hot, shiny, and uniformly elevated plaque with an irregular outline, which is sharply defined with a raised border unlike in cellulitis. Without treatment, the rash peaks in approximately 1 week and subsequently subsides over 1 to 2 weeks. Erysipelas is especially common in infants and young children, but it also occurs in adults. Predisposing factors may include minor skin trauma, surgical intervention, or a preexisting skin condition.

Abscess

A cutaneous abscess (ie, furuncle) is a purulent collection that occupies the dermis and deeper soft tissues. Abscesses commonly begin as a localized, superficial cellulitis with microbial skin colonizers that cause necrosis and liquefaction, leading to accumulation of leukocytes and cellular debris. As these products are subsequently walled off, an abscess forms. Cutaneous abscesses accounted for 2.3% of all ED visits in the United States in 2009, and MRSA has recently been reported to be responsible for over 50% of these cases in an urban ED.

Diagnostic Considerations

Cellulitis and Erysipelas

Diagnosis of cellulitis and erysipelas is clinical. Clinical suspicion should be high in patients with predisposing conditions, such as tinea pedis, lymphedema, and chronic venous insufficiency. When involving a small area in an otherwise healthy patient, diagnosis does not require invasive diagnostics or laboratory testing. More extensive involvement may be associated with a leukocytosis with a left shift or a mildly increased sedimentation rate. Needle aspiration of the advancing margin of a cellulitic area for culture is relatively low yield and produces organisms in fewer than 10% of cases. Punch biopsy reveals an organism in only 20% of cases, and blood cultures are positive in only 5% of cases.

Radiographic evaluation is rarely necessary, unless osteomyelitis or a necrotizing soft tissue infection is suspected. However, doppler ultrasound studies may be useful in differentiating deep vein thrombosis (DVT) from cellulitis in a patient presenting with an unclear clinical picture. In general, a more extensive workup is warranted in those patients with underlying comorbidity (eg, diabetes mellitus, malignancy, chemotherapy, intravenous drug abuse, and human immunodeficiency virus), systemic toxicity, extensive skin involvement, or a high clinical suspicion for *H. influenzae* infection, as the incidence of bacteremia in *H. influenzae* cellulitis approaches 90%. Outlining the margins of an affected area with a marker aids in the follow-up of patients with cellulitis by clearly delineating lesion progression or regression.

Abscess

Diagnosis of a skin abscess is also clinical. Cutaneous abscesses are fluctuant, tender, and erythematous nodules, often with surrounding erythema. In general, patients experience discomfort and swelling for several days prior to presenting for care. Systemic symptoms, such as fever, chills, and tachycardia, are unusual but may occur if the abscess is extensive, surrounded by significant cellulitis, or located along a mucous membrane, such as the rectum or oral cavity. The differential diagnosis may include folliculitis, hidradenitis suppurativa, sporotrichosis, leishmaniasis, tularemia, and blastomycosis. *Nocardia* and *Cryptococcus* infections should also be considered in immunocompromised patients. Risk factors for abscess formation are intravenous drug use, insulin-dependent diabetes, hemodialysis, and cancer. Diagnostic bedside ultrasonography is critical in helping to differentiate cellulitis (characterized by "cobblestoning" or obliteration of the interface between the thickened echogenic subcutaneous fat and dermis) from an abscess (characterized by a heterogenic, anechoic or hypoechoic fluid collection with poorly defined borders).

Organisms

Cellulitis
The most common causal organisms of cellulitis are GABS and *S. aureus* (including MRSA) in adults. *Haemophilus influenzae* type B is the most common cause of cellulitis in children younger than 3 years of age.

Erysipelas
The most frequent organism causing erysipelas is GABS. Less commonly, MRSA is the source.

Abscess
The most common pathogenic organism of abscess formation is *S. aureus* (either methicillin-sensitive *Staphylococcus aureus* or MRSA) Other organisms include the aerobes *E. coli, P. aeruginosa,* and *S. faecalis* as well as the anaerobes *Bacteroides, Lactobacillus,* and *Peptococcus,* and *Peptostreptococcus.*

225

Treatment

Treatment of simple cellulitis and erysipelas includes antibiotics, elevation of the affected area to assist in lymphatic drainage, and treatment of any underlying conditions. In most cases, effective treatment may be accomplished in the outpatient setting. Antibiotic therapy should target *S. aureus* and GABS. Depending on local resistance patterns, a 5-day course of oral antibiotics is usually sufficient for effective treatment with close follow-up within 48 to 72 hours. Hospitalization and parenteral therapy is indicated for severely ill patients and for those unable to tolerate oral medications.

Cellulitis
Oral antibiotic therapy for the treatment of simple cellulitis should include cephalexin 500 mg PO every 6 hours or dicloxacillin 500 mg PO every 6 hours. For those with β-lactam allergy, clindamycin 150 to 450 mg PO every 6 hours, is an acceptable alternative. Parenteral therapeutic options include cefazolin 1 g IV every 8 hours, oxacillin 1 to 2 g IV every 6 hours, or nafcillin 1 to 2 g IV every 6 hours.

Erysipelas
Oral therapy of erysipelas should include penicillin 500 mg PO every 6 hours or amoxicillin 500 mg PO every 8 hours. For those with a β-lactam allergy, cephalexin, clindamycin, or linezolid may be used. Erysipelas parenteral therapy may include ceftriaxone 1g IV daily, cefazolin 1 to 2 g IV every 8 hours, or cefuroxime 750 mg to 1.5 g IV every 6 hours.

MRSA
MRSA infection should be considered in all patients with cellulitis or erysipelas who have failed initial therapy, who have a history of or risk factors for MRSA, or who have severe infection or systemic toxicity. In these cases, clindamycin 300 mg PO three to four times daily for 7 to 10 days or trimethoprim/sulfamethoxazol double strength 1 to 2 tablets PO twice daily for 7 to 10 days is appropriate. In more severe cases of MRSA infection, parenteral therapeutic options include clindamycin 600 to 900 mg IV every 8 hours, vancomycin 1 g IV every 12 hours, linezolid 600 mg IV every 12 hours, or daptomycin 4 mg/kg IV once daily.

Abscess
The first-line treatment for abscess is I&D. In an otherwise healthy, immunocompetent patient without valvular heart disease, there are no data that definitively demonstrate the utility of antibiotic therapy in conjunction with I&D of an uncomplicated cutaneous abscess. I&D may be performed in either the ED or the operating room. Abscesses that are large, deep, or proximal to neurovascular structures may

need drainage in the operating room. Although sterility is impossible to maintain during I&D, one should practice universal precautions, including eye protection and proper positioning of the patient to avoid contamination of surrounding tissue.

Anesthesia should be achieved with local anesthetics or a regional block. Procedural sedation may be necessary in the extremely anxious or uncomfortable patient. A number 11 or 15 scalpel, held perpendicular to the skin, is used to make a simple linear incision, which is made over the length of the abscess cavity. The abscess is then probed with a hemostat that is wrapped in gauze to assess the depth of the pocket and to lyse any loculations that would otherwise prevent proper drainage. The wound is then packed with gauze and dressed with an absorbent gauze pad. Reevaluation of the packed wound should occur within 1 to 3 days, and the first packing change should occur at that time.

Suggested Readings and References

1. Butler KH. Incision and drainage. In: Roberts JR, Hedges JR, eds. *Clinical Procedures in Emergency Medicine*. 5th ed. Philadelphia, PA: Saunders Elsevier; 2010:657–691.

2. Dong SL, Kelly KD, Oland RC, Holroyd BR, Rowe BH. ED management of cellulitis: a review of five urban centers. *Am J Emerg Med*. 2001;19:535–540.

3. Frazee BW, Lynn J, Charlebois ED, Lambert L, Lowery D, Perdreau-Remington F. High prevalence of methicillin-resistant Staphylococcus aureus in emergency department skin and soft tissue infections. *Ann Emerg Med*. 2005;45:311–320.

4. Habif, TP. Bacterial infections. In: *Clinical Dermatology: A Color Guide to Diagnosis and Treatment*. 5th ed. New York, NY: Elsevier; 2010:335–381.

5. Kelly EW, Magilner D. Soft tissue infections. In: Tintinalli JE, ed. *Tintinalli's Emergency Medicine: A Comprehensive Study Guide*. 7th ed. New York, NY: McGraw-Hill; 2011:1014–1024.

6. Krasagakis K, Samonis G, Maniatakis P, Georgala S, Tosca A. Bullous erysipelas: clinical presentation, staphylococcal involvement and methicillin resistance. *Dermatology*. 2006;212:31–35.

7. National Center for Health Statistics. *National Hospital Ambulatory Medical Care Survey: 2009 Emergency Department Summary Tables*. Hyattsville, MD. http://www.cdc.gov/nchs/data/ahcd/nhamcs_emergency/ 2009_ed_web_tables.pdf Accessed October 18, 2012.

8. Phoenix G, Das S, Joshi M. Diagnosis and management of cellulitis. *BMJ*. 2012;345:e4955.

9. Trott AT, Krupp S. Skin and soft-tissue infections. In: Wolfson AB, ed. *Harwood-Nuss' Clinical Practice of Emergency Medicine*. 5th ed. Philadelphia, PA: Lippincott, Williams & Wilkins; 2010:875–881.

Chapter 42

Necrotizing Soft Tissue Infections

Michael Ehmann

Disease Description: Necrotizing soft tissue infections (NSTIs) are a category of infectious disease characterized by extensive and rapidly progressive necrosis that may involve the skin, subcutaneous tissue, fascia, or muscle, and are associated with a high degree of morbidity and mortality.

Organisms: Streptococci, *Clostridium*, methicillin-resistant *Staphylococcus aureus* (MRSA), Enterobacteriaceae, *Bacteroides*, Peptostreptococci, Anaerobes

Treatment:
  Oral first line: N/A
  Oral second line: N/A
  Parenteral:
  Non-*Clostridial* NSTI: imipenem 1.5 to 3 g IV q6 hours, ticarcillin/clavulanate 3.0 g IV q4 to 6 hours, or clindamycin 300 to 900mg IV q8 hours plus gentamicin 1 to 1.7 mg/ kg q8 hours
  Clostridial NSTI: penicillin 4 million units IV q4 hours or clindamycin 900 mg q8 hours

Other Key Issues: Early stabilization, including antibiotics and supportive measures, should be considered. Early consultation with a surgeon is a key initial step. Management must include aggressive resuscitative measures and hemodynamic support.

Diease Description

Epidemiology

Necrotizing soft tissue infections (NSTIs) are a category of infectious disease characterized by extensive and rapidly progressive necrosis. The skin, subcutaneous tissue, fascia, or muscle are all often involved and are associated with a high degree of morbidity and mortality (Malangoni, 2001). NSTI are classified by anatomy, depth of infection, or microbial source (Table 42.1) (Sarani, 2009). NSTI has an incidence of 1,000 cases per year in the United States or 0.04 cases per 1,000 person-years (Ellis Simonsen, 2006). Patients with advanced age, diabetes mellitus, alcoholism, peripheral vascular disease, heart disease, renal disease, human immunodeficiency virus, cancer, nonsteroidal anti-inflammatory drug use, decubitus ulcers, chronic skin infections, IV drug abuse, and immune system impairment are at risk for these infections, which are most commonly polymicrobial in etiology (Elliott, 2000; Kelly, 2011). Although a relatively uncommon disease that may appear deceptively benign, NSTI has a mortality of 25% to 35% and demands early recognition and aggressive treatment (Malangoni, 2001; Sarani, 2009).

Disease Presentation

Recognition of certain characteristics should alert the physician team to potential NSTI. Preceding trauma, foreign body penetration, wound contamination, surgical intervention, and the medical conditions listed previously are all risk factors for development of NSTI. Clinical examination often reveals extensive tissue involvement with pain out of proportion to exam often without the classic signs of common cellulitis (warmth, erythema, and induration). As the soft tissue infection progresses, blebs, maceration, and exudate may appear, followed by crepitance secondary to gas formation. The lack of any of these clinical signs, however, does not exclude the diagnosis of NSTI (Trott, 2010). The diagnosis of NSTI may be confused with dry ischemic vascular gangrene, pressure necrosis of a limb, acute deep venous thrombosis, and preexisting changes of venous insufficiency. Additionally, subcutaneous air may be entrained by traumatic laceration and occasionally cause misplaced diagnostic concern (Trott, 2010). Nonetheless, the presence of subcutaneous air is an important clinical finding in NSTI. If subcutaneous air is discovered on clinical examination, NSTI must be considered.

Diagnostic Evaluation

Suspicion of NSTI demands an extensive and aggressive clinical evaluation that must be initiated promptly and maintained while resuscitative and stabilizing interventions are in progress (Trott, 2010). In addition to routine laboratory tests, wound culture and Gram stain must be performed immediately. Radiographs of anatomic areas of concern are obtained to evaluate for the presence and extent of subcutaneous emphysema. Finally, as NSTI can advance as rapidly as 2.5 cm per hour, the area of involvement should be outlined in ink and checked at frequent intervals (Kelly, 2011). Early consultation with the surgical team is a critical step.

Organisms

Crepitant cellulitis, or non-*Clostridial* anaerobic cellulitis, is one of the more superficial NSTIs and occurs most commonly in patients with preexisting lower extremity peripheral arterial disease, decubitus ulcer, or a traumatic wound. Synergistic infection with anaerobic *Bacteroides, Peptostreptococci,* and enteric Gram-negative bacteria occurs with gradual onset of mild local tenderness and low likelihood of systemic toxicity. Skin overlying the infected area is minimally discolored with a grayish brown appearance, depending on local vascularity. Exudate, when present, is dark and malodorous. This infection is always characterized by crepitance and radiographic evidence of abundant subcutaneous gas formation. The infection remains localized to the skin and subcutaneous tissues without extending deeper to muscle.

Synergistic necrotizing cellulitis, or non-*Clostridial* gangrene or non-*Clostridial* anaerobic myonecrosis, in contrast to crepitant cellulitis does involve deeper tissues. It occurs most often in elderly patients with significant comorbidity, including diabetes, congestive heart failure, renal failure, or obesity.

Fournier gangrene of the genitalia and perineum is one type of synergistic necrotizing cellulitis. Although first described in 1883 in young men, the disease is not limited to males or to young people. Trauma, host immunity, and perirectal infection are all risk factors for the development of Fournier's gangrene. The causative organisms of synergistic necrotizing cellulitis are Gram-positive *Streptococci*, Gram-negative enteric bacilli, and anaerobic *B. fragilis* (Stone, 1997). The onset may be acute or subacute, with rapid progression of the infection to severe local tissue destruction and systemic toxicity and high fever. Pain at the site of infection is often severe, affected skin is blue-gray in appearance, and exudate is thin and malodorous and has the appearance of dishwater. The infection spreads rapidly as

Table 42.1 Necrotizing Soft Tissue Infections[a]

Characteristics	Crepitant Cellulitis	Synergistic Necrotizing Cellulitis	Necrotizing Fasciitis	Clostridial Cellulitis	Clostridial Myonecrosis
Predisposing Conditions	Wounds, decubiti, peripheral vascular disease, DM	DM, obesity, advanced age	Postoperative wounds, perianal infection, chronic cutaneous ulcers, IVDU	Contaminated wound	Devitalized tissue, focal contamination
Onset	Gradual	Subacute (several days)	Variable: indolent to fulminant	Gradual, 4–5 days	Acute, 1–3 days
Pain	Mild	Severe	Minimal, sometimes hypesthesia	Mild	Severe, early
Systemic Toxicity	Mild to moderate	Moderate to severe	Marked	Mild to moderate	Marked, early
Overlying Skin	Minimal, brown to gray discoloration	Blue-gray, necrosis	Initially spared, then pale followed by gangrene	Minimal change, occasional blebs	Initially normal, then pale bronze discoloration followed by necrosis
Exudate	Minimal, dark	Thin, reddish brown ("dishwater pus")	Rare, serous	Thin, dark	Serosanguinous
Odor	Foul	Foul	Foul	Rarely foul	"Mousy," slightly sweet
Gas Formation	Abundant	Mild, up to 25%	Little	Abundant	Initially minimal, eventually moderate
Muscle Involvement	No	Prominent feature, moderate spread	Rare, late	No	Prominent
Common Pathogens	Anaerobes, Enterobacteriacea	Bacteriodes fragilis, Streptococci, Enterobacteriaceae	Enterobacteriaceae, Streptococci, Bacteroides, Peptostreptococci, MRSA	C. perfringens, C. septicum, C. novyi	C. perfingens, C. septicum, C. novyi

Abbreviations: DM, diabetes mellitus; IVDU, intravenous drug use; MRSA, methicillin-resistant Staphylococcus aureus.

[a]Adapted from Trott AT, Krupp S. Skin and soft-tissue infections. In: Wolfson AB, ed. Harwood-Nuss' Clinical Practice Of Emergency Medicine. 5th ed. Philadelphia, PA: Lippincott, Williams & Wilkins; 2010:875–881. Copyright 2010 NAME OF COPYRIGHT HOLDER. Reprinted with permission.

necrosis of the fascia and muscle occurs. Bacteremia occurs in 50% of cases, and mortality has been reported to be as high as 75% (Trott, 2010).

Necrotizing fasciitis is predominantly a disease of the subcutaneous tissue and fascia, with early sparing of the skin and late involvement of the muscle. Predisposing risk factors include trauma, surgery, perirectal infections, cutaneous ulcers, intravenous drug abuse, and infections of the head and neck. A wide range of organisms, including Gram-negative enteric bacilli, aerobic and anaerobic Gram-positive *Streptococci*, and other anaerobes have been implicated (Elliott, 2000). Although the microbiologic etiology of necrotizing fasciitis is most often polymicrobial, recent studies have suggested that monomicrobial infections with group A *Streptococcus* or MRSA are becoming more common (Tsitsilonis, 2012; Miller, 2005; Cheng, 2011). Acute onset of symptoms with rapid development of severe systemic toxicity is common, especially when infection is caused by streptococcal organisms capable of producing scarlatina pyrogenic exotoxins types A, B, and C, and streptococcal superantigen (Elliott, 2000). In the early stages, the skin appears erythematous with minimal tenderness, followed by more extensive subcutaneous involvement leading to mottling, discoloration, marked edema, and bleb formation. Exudate is scant, malodorous, and purulent. Although gas may be evident radiographically, clinical crepitance is unusual.

Clostridial cellulitis is most commonly a result of trauma. The presence of foreign debris, soil, and necrotic tissue allows rapid growth of *Clostridial* organisms, including *C. perfringens* and *C. septicum*. It is distinguished from *Clostridial* myonecrosis (gas gangrene) by the lack of muscle involvement. Unlike gas gangrene, the onset is gradual, and systemic toxicity is only mild to moderate. Skin changes are minimal, but often there is a thin, dark, occasionally foul-smelling exudate at the wound. The most prominent features of the wound site are subcutaneous emphysema appearing radiographically as aggregates of bubbles and crepitance often well beyond the actual area of cellulitis (Trott, 2010). *Clostridial* infection should be suspected when Gram stain reveals Gram-positive bacilli with few leukocytes, compared to synergistic or polymicrobial infection wherein there will be numerous leukocytes on the smear (Trott, 2010).

Clostridial myonecrosis, or gas gangrene, almost always results from a deep injury to skeletal muscle leading to ischemia and tissue necrosis. The incubation period of *Clostridial* myonecrosis ranges from 7 hours to 6 weeks, but, once symptoms begin, severe deterioration and death can occur within hours (Trott, 2010). Myositis and severe pain are the primary clinical features. Systemic toxicity resulting from *Clostridial* exotoxins is profound, leading to hemodynamic instability and an altered sensorium, often without fever. The overlying skin has a yellow or bronze appearance, progressing to bullae and green or black necrotic patches. A serosanguinous discharge can develop with a characteristic "mousy" odor. Gas formation is initially minimal but eventually extends throughout the muscle in a feathery pattern. Intravascular hemolysis with thrombocytopenia is often present.

Treatment

Close consultation with a surgeon should occur as an early intervention for necrotizing soft tissue infection. Initial management must include aggressive resuscitative measures and hemodynamic support without the use of vasoconstrictors, which may decrease perfusion to already ischemic tissue. Aggressive resuscitation, early empiric antibiotic coverage, and prompt surgical intervention are the mainstays of optimal therapy. Antibiotic choices for non-*Clostridial* NSTI include imipenem 1.5 to 3 g IV q6 hours, ticarcillin/clavulanate 3.0 g IV q4 to 6 hours, or clindamycin 300 to 900 mg IV q8 hours plus gentamicin 1 to 1.7 mg/kg q8 hours. *Clostridial* infections should be treated with penicillin 4 million units IV q4 hours or clindamycin 900 mg q8 hours in β-lactam–sensitive patients. Antitoxin therapy has not been shown to be effective.

Operative debridement of all necrotic tissue is vital and allows for Gram stain and culture specimens for appropriate tailoring of antibiotic therapy. Further debridements should be repeated every 24 to 48 hours until the infection is controlled. The use of hyperbaric oxygen (HBO) has been shown to arrest the advance of the hemolytic, necrotizing, and potentially lethal tissue toxins produced by multiple *Clostridium* species by producing suprabacteriostatic oxygen at the tissue level (Trott, 2010). In limited clinical data, HBO has been shown to reduce the need for extensive debridement and amputation, but prospective study is still required (Jallali, 2005).

Suggested Readings and References

1. Cheng NC, Wang JT, Chang SC, Tai HC, Tang YB. Necrotizing fasciitis caused by Staphylococcus aureus: the emergence of methicillin-resistant strains. *Ann Plast Surg*. 2011;67:632–636.
2. Elliott D, Kufera JA, Myers RAM. The microbiology of necrotizing soft tissue infections. *Am J Surg*. 2000;179:361–366.

3. Ellis Simonsen SM, van Orman ER, Hatch BE, et al. Cellulitis incidence in a defined population. *Epidemiol Infect.* 2006;134:293–299.

4. Fontes RA, Ogilvie CM, Miclau T. Necrotizing soft-tissue infections. *J Am Acad Orthop Surg.* 2000;8:151–158.

5. Jallali N, Withey S, Butler PE. Hyperbaric oxygen as adjuvant therapy in the management of necrotizing fasciitis. *Ann J Surg.* 2005;189:462–466.

6. Kelly EW, Magilner D. Soft tissue infections. In: Tintinalli JE, ed. *Tintinalli's Emergency Medicine: A Comprehensive Study Guide.* 7th-ed. New York, NY: McGraw-Hill; 2011:1014–1024.

7. Malangani MA. Necrotizing soft tissue infections: are we making any progress? *Surg Infect (Larchmt).* 2001;2:145–150.

8. Miller LG, Perdreau-Remington F, Rieg G, et al. Necrotizing fasciitis caused by community-associated methicillin-resistant Staphylococcus aureus in Los Angeles. *N Engl J Med.* 2005;352:1445–1453.

9. Sarani B, Strong M, Pascual J, Schwab CW. Necrotizing fasciitis: current concepts and review of the literature. *J Am Coll Surg.* 2009;208:279–288.

10. Stone DR, Gorbach SL. Necrotizing fasciitis: the changing spectrum. *Dermatol Clin.* 1997;15:213–220.

11. Trott AT, Krupp S. (). Skin and soft-tissue infections. In: Wolfson AB, ed. *Harwood-Nuss' Clinical Practice of Emergency Medicine.* 5th ed. Philadelphia, PA: Lippincott, Williams & Wilkins; 2010:875–881.

12. Tsitsilonis S, Druschel C, Wichlas F, et al. Necrotizing fasciitis: is the bacterial spectrum changing? *Langenbecks Arch Surg.* 2012:Jul26, epub ahead of print.

13. Yilmazlar T, Ozturk E, Alsoy A, Ozgue H. Necrotizing soft tissue infections: APACHE II score, dissemination, and survival. *World J Surg.* 2007;31:1858–1862.

Diabetic Foot Infections

Clare Kelleher

233

Summary Box

Disease Description: Diabetic foot infections (DFIs) are defined clinically as two or more classic findings of inflammation (eg, redness, swelling, warmth, and tenderness) or purulent drainage within an existing diabetic foot wound.

Organisms: Although many DFI are polymicrobial, the most common causative organisms are gram-positive cocci (GPC), especially *Staphylococcus* spp. *S. aureus* is the single most common organism responsible for DFI.

Treatment: For mild to moderate infections, therapy can usually be safely targeted at aerobic GPC alone.

Proven effective oral antibiotic agents include: cephalexin 500 mg PO q6 hours.

If MRSA is suspected: use clindamycin 300 mg to 450 mg PO q6 hours or vancomycin 15 mg/kg IV q12 hours.

For more severe infections, parenteral antibiotics should be initiated pending culture results.

Appropriate choices include: cefoxitin 1–2 g IV q6 to 8 hours, imipenem/cilastatin 500 mg IV q6 hours, or newer fluoroquinolones (eg, moxifloxacin 400 mg IV q24 hours or levofloxacin 500 mg IV q24 hours) plus metroniadazole 500 mg PO q8 to 12 hours or clindamycin.

If *Pseudomonas* is not suspected: consider beta-lactam/beta-lactamase inhibitors (eg, ampicillin/sulbactam 3 g IV q6 hours). If *pseudomonas* is suspected, consider piperacillin/tazobactam 3.375 g IV q12 hours.

Disease Description

Definition

DFIs are a serious and growing problem. Although diabetic foot wounds are commonplace and colonized with skin microorganisms, not all diabetic foot wounds inherently represent a DFI. DFI specifically occurs when pathogens proliferate in a wound, causing damage and eliciting a host inflammatory response.[1] Diabetic foot infections are diagnosed clinically as a diabetic foot wound with the presence of infection, which is defined as purulent drainage or two or more of either the classic findings of inflammation (ie, redness, warmth, swelling, and tenderness or pain) or additional secondary signs of infection (ie, friable or discolored granulation tissue, undermining of wound edges, and foul odor).[2]

Epidemiology

The World Health Organization estimates that close to 9% (24.5 million) of the United States population will have diabetes by the year 2025, highlighting the importance of DFI.[3] DFI can begin in any type of wound but are most often seen in neuropathic ulcerations. An estimated 15% of patients with diabetes will develop a diabetic foot ulcer (DFU) during their lifetime, which often leads to amputation (16% of patients with DFU and 36% with osteomyelitis).[4,5] DFUs have been shown to confer decreased survival compared to matched controls (72% vs 87%), and the attributable cost for a 40- to 65-year-old male with a new DFU in 2004 was $27,987 for the 2 years after diagnosis.[5] Patient factors that increase the chance of developing a DFI within an existing DFU include the presence of peripheral vascular disease, loss of protective sensation (ie, neuropathy), renal insufficiency, a history of walking barefoot, and prior foot ulcers or lower extremity amputations. Wound characteristics that increase the risk for DFI include traumatic initial wound etiology, persistence of wound or ulceration for greater than 30 days, and a positive probe-to-bone testThe PTB test is considered positive if the bone is palpable when a probe is inserted into the wound with a sensitivity of0.87 and a specificity of 0.91.

Classification of Severity

Once diagnosed clinically, DFIs should be classified by severity because this determination helps guide decisions about the need for hospitalization, imaging, and surgical consultation. According to the Infectious Disease Society of America (IDSA) 2012 guidelines, infections should be classified as mild (superficial and limited in size and depth), moderate (larger infections spreading beyond the subcutaneous tissue), or severe (accompanied by systemic signs or metabolic disturbances).[2] Mild, moderate, and severe classifications correlate to the International Working Group on the Diabetic Foot PEDIS (perfusion, extent/size, depth/tissue loss, infection and sensation) grades 2, 3, and 4, respectively. The two classification systems are outlined in Table 43.1.

Table 43.1 Classification of Diabetic Foot Infections	
IDSA Infection Severity/ IWGDF PEDIS Grade	Clinical Manifestations of Infection
Mild/Grade 1	Infection present, defined as ≥ 2 of the follow• Local swelling or induration • Erythema > 0.5–2 cm around ulcer • Local tenderness or pain • Local warmth • Purulent discharge
Moderate/Grade 2	• Erythema > 2 cm plus one sign described above OR • Infection involving the structures deeper than skin and subcutaneous tissue, such as abscess, osteomyelitis, septic arthritis, or fasciitis
Severe/Grade 3	Any foot infection with ≥ 2 of the following signs of SIRS: • Temperature > 38°C or < 36°C • Heart rate > 90 beats/minute • Respiratory rate > 20 breaths/minute • $PaCO_2$ < 32 mmHg • White blood cell count > 12,000 or < 4,000/mm³ • 10% immature (band) forms

Abbreviations: IDSA, Infectious Disease Society of America; IWGDF, International Working Group on the Diabetic Foot; PEDIS, perfusion, extent/size, depth/tissue loss, infection and sensation; SIRS, systemic inflammatory response; $PaCO_2$, partial pressure of arterial carbon dioxide.

Diagnostic Tests

Imaging

There appears to be a nearly unanimous consensus among DFI experts that all patients presenting with a new DFI should undergo imaging with plain film to evaluate for bony abnormalities, soft tissue gas, radio-opaque foreign bodies, and evidence of osteomyelitis.[2] What is often less clear is when to pursue more advanced imaging. Radiologic diagnosis of osteomyelitis is difficult for two reasons: bone changes sugges-tive of osteomyelitis may take weeks to become visible on plain film (impairing sensitivity), and diabetic neuropathy may induce rapidly progressive disorganization of joints as well as osteopenia, which can falsely suggest infection (impairing specificity).[6] When the diagnosis of osteomyelitis is in question or an abscess is suspected, magnetic resonance imaging (MRI) remains the study of choice. When MRI is contraindicated or unavailable, consideration can be given to a labeled white blood cell scan, preferably combined with a radionucleotide bone scan.[2] However, it is important to note that the IDSA defines bone culture and histology, not radiologic studies, as the gold standard for the diagnosis of osteomyelitis.

Culture

For most DFIs, definitive therapy should be guided by deep tissue culture results. For mild infections in a patient who has not recently received antibiotic therapy, cultures may be unnecessary, and empiric therapy can often be safely initiated based on local epidemiologic data.[7] For all other wounds, culture should be sent from deep tissue biopsy or curettage performed after the wound has been adequately cleaned and debrided.[2,1,7] When deep cultures are not available, cultures and Gram-stained smears of material obtained from purulent exudate may provide useful information to guide antimicrobial therapy. Although not routinely recommended, superficial swabs obtained with proper sterile technique after surgical debridement can provide remarkably reliable results. In one study, the mean number of isolates per patient at the time of initial presentation was 2.34 by superficial swabbing compared to 2.07 by deep tissue biopsy sampling.[8]

Organisms

Although many DFI are polymicrobial, the most common causative organisms are GPC, especially *Staphylococcus* spp. *S. aureus* is the single most common organism responsible for DFI. Other frequently isolated aerobes include *Enterobacteriaceae* spp., streptococci (especially groups A and B), enterococci, *Proteus* spp., *S. epidermidis, Pseudomonas aeruginosa,* and *Corynebacterium* spp. Gram-negative bacilli are most commonly seen as co-pathogens in chronically non-healing wounds and after prolonged courses of antibiotics. An ischemic or necrotic wound, especially those with a putrid smell, should raise suspicion for anaerobic copathogens such as *Peptostreptococcus, Bacteroides,* and *Clostridium* species.[1] Further com-plicating the treatment of DFIs is the increasing incidence of methicillin-resistant *S. aureus* (MRSA), which has been found in up to 30% of DFUs. Wounds infected with MRSA have longer healing times, poorer wound healing, and an increased risk of lower extremity amputation.[9,10]

Treatment

Antibiotic Therapy

Wounds without clinical evidence of soft tissue or bone infection often do not require antibiotic therapy. When infection is present, empiric antibiotic regimens must be based on the available clinical and local epidemiologic data, but definitive therapy should be based on cultures of infected tissues or clinical response.[2] For mild to moderate infections in patients who have not recent received antibiotics, therapy can usually be safely targeted at aerobic gram-positive cocci alone. A number of oral antibiotic agents have been shown to be effective in clinical trials, including cephalexin, clindamycin, and ciprofloxacin.[6] For more severe infections, broad-spectrum antibiotics are initiated pending culture results.

Proven effective oral antibiotic agents include cephalexin 500 mg PO q6 hours. If MRSA is suspected, consider clindamycin 300 mg to 450 mg PO q6 hours. For more severe infections, parenteral antibiotics should be initiated pending culture results. Appropriate choices include cefoxitin 1–2 g IV q6 to 8 hours or imipenem/cilastatin 500 mg IV q6 hours. Newer fluoroquinolones (eg, moxifloxacin 400 mg IV q24 hours or levofloxacin 500 mg IV q24 hours) plus metronidazole 500 mg po q8 to 12 hours or clindamycin can also be used.

If pseudomonas is not suspected, consider beta-lactam/beta-lactamase inhibitors (eg, ampicillin/sul-bactam 3 g IV q6 hours). If pseudomonas is suspected, consider piperacillin/tazobactam 3.375 g IV q12 hours. If MRSA is suspected consider vancomycin 15 mg/kg IV q12 hours. Consideration of MRSA coverage should be given when local prevalence is high, in patients with a prior history of MRSA infection, or when the systemic manifestations are severe.

Parenteral therapy is favored initially in some moderate and in all severe infections. IV antibiotics should be continued until culture results are available or until the patient's condition has clinically stabilized if cultures were not obtained. Duration of therapy is usually 1 to 2 weeks for mild infections, 2 to 3 weeks for moderate or severe infections, and at least 4 weeks (sometimes months) for bone infections.[2,6]

A common, difficult treatment decision for both outpatient providers and emergency physicians alike is when to hospitalize a patient with DFIs. According to the 2012 IDSA guidelines, providers should hospitalize all patients with a severe infection, patients with moderate infections and complicating features (eg, advanced age or significant peripheral vascular disease), and any patient unable to comply with outpatient regimens due to psychosocial reasons. Consideration of hospitalization should be given to any patient who is failing to improve with appropriate outpatient therapy.

Surgical Therapy
Surgical intervention plays a key role in the management of many DFIs. Urgent surgical consultation is recommended for abscess, necrotizing fasciitis, most infections accompanied by gas in the deeper tissues, and, somewhat less urgently, for wounds with substantial nonviable tissue, advancing infection despite appropriate antimicrobial therapy, or extensive bone or joint involvement.[1,2] Surgical consultation is also highly recommended in any severe or moderate DFI. Possible surgical interventions include incision and drainage, wound debridement, bone resection, tissue revascularization, and amputation.

Most deep DFIs require incision and drainage and debridement. Devitalized tissue in a wound is thought to delay wound healing and predispose to infection. Thus, current management recommendations are aimed at debridement of diabetic foot wounds in order to remove debris, eschar, and surrounding callus as well as to expose healthy tissue, decrease chronic inflammatory by-products, and shorten healing times.[11,12,13] Sharp or surgical methods, using a scalpel or tissue forceps, are generally considered most effective; but mechanical, autolytic, or larval (insects) debridement techniques are also used in certain circumstances.

Wound Off-Loading
Off-loading, or redistribution of pressure off of the wound, is a crucial and often overlooked tenet in the management of diabetic foot wounds. Off-loading promotes healing and prevents wound recurrence. Several methods have been successfully used to protect the foot from abnormal pressures, such as bed rest, non–weight bearing, total contact casts, crutches, walkers, and a myriad of orthotic devices.[2,7,13]

Vascular Assessment and Revascularization
An important consideration in the management of diabetic wounds is vascular assessment. Arterial perfusion is necessary for wound healing and antibiotic delivery. Therefore, vascular insufficiency should be suspected in all wounds that fail to heal after proper wound care and antibiotic therapy. Clinical signs suggesting lower-extremity ischemia include the absence of palpable pulses, hair loss, poor capillary refill, skin atrophy, and nail cornification.[1,7] Early consultation with a vascular surgeon is recommended in any DFI that is suspicious for ischemia, especially in any patient with critical limb ischemia. Limb revascularization success rates in patients with diabetes is comparable to those without diabetes, and these procedures can help to heal ulcerations, eliminate pain, and decrease the need for amputation at all levels.[14]

Other Key Issues

DFIs are continuing to increase in frequency and can be life-threatening. Proper care of these infections requires a multidimensional approach including imaging, appropriate antibiotic administration, wound care, surgical debridement, and properly obtaining deep wound cultures. Consideration should be given to off-loading techniques and vascular assessment.

Suggested Readings and References

1. Armstrong DG, Lipsky BA. Diabetic foot infections: stepwise medical and surgical management. Int Wound J. 2004;1:123–132.
2. Lipsky BA, Berendt AR, Cornia PB, Pile JC, Senneville E, et al. 2012 Infectious Disease Society of America Clinical practice guidelines for the diagnosis and treatment of diabetic foot infections. Clin Infect Dis. 2012;54:1679–1684.

3. King H, Aubert RD, Herman WH. Global Burden of diabetes, 1995–2025: prevalence, numerical estimates and projections. *Diabetes Care*. 1998;21:1414–1431.

4. Reiber GE, Boyko EJ, Smith DG. Lower extremity foot ulcers and amputations in diabetics. In: *Diabetes in America*. 2nd ed. Rockville, MD: National Institute of Diabetes and Digestive Health; 1995:409–428.

5. Ramsey SD, Newton K, Blough D, et al. Incidence, outcomes, and cost of foot ulcers in patients with diabetes. *Diabetes Care*. 1999;22:382–387.

6. Lipsky BA, Berendt AR. Principles and practice of antibiotic therapy of diabetic foot infections. *Diabetes Metab Res Rev*. 2000;16:S42–46.

7. Calhoun JH, Overgaard KA, Stevens CM, Mader JT. Diabetic foot ulcers and infections: current concepts. *Adv Skin Wound Care*. 2002;15:31–45.

8. Pellizzer G, Strazzabosco M, Presi S, et al. Deep tissue biopsy vs. superficial swab culture monitoring in the microbiological assessment of limb-threatening diabetic foot infections. *Diabet Med*. 2001;18:822–827.

9. Dang CN, Prasad YDM, Boulton AJM, Jude EB. Methicillin-resistant Staphylococcus aureus in the diabetic foot clinic: a worsening problem. *Diabet Med*. 2003;20:159–161.

10. Wagner A, Reike H, Angelkort B. Highly resistant pathogens in patients with diabetic foot syndrome with special reference to methicillin-resistant Staphylococcus aureus infections. *Dtsch Med Wochenschr*. 2001;126:1353–1356.

11. Lipsky BA, Baker PD, Landon GC, Fernau R. Antibiotic therapy for diabetic foot infections: comparison of two parenteral-to-oral regimens. *Clin Infect Dis*. 1997;24:643–648.

12. Steed DL, Donohoe D, Webster MW, Lindsley L. Effect of extensive debridement and treatment on the healing of diabetic foot ulcers. Diabetic Ulcer Study Group. *J Am Coll Surg*. 1996;183:61–64.

13. Armstrong DG, Lavery LA, Nixon BP, Boulton AJ. It's not what you put on, but what you take off: techniques for debriding and off-loading the diabetic foot. *Clin Infect Dis*. 2004;39:S92–99.

14. Gibbons GW, Burgess AM, Guadagnoli, LoGerfo FW, et al. Return to well-being and function after infrainguinal revascularization. *J Vasc Surg*. 1995;21:35–45.

Chapter 44

Dermatologic Manifestations of Infectious Disease

Lisa Cuttle

239

Disease Overview

According to some sources, up to 12% of patients presenting to the Emergency Department have a dermatologic complaint.[1] Following are a series of infections with pathognomonic skin findings. Many of these illnesses require rapid diagnosis and management because they are often associated with a high mortality rate.

Toxic Infectious Exfoliative Conditions

This spectrum of diseases includes staphylococcal toxic shock syndrome (TSS), streptococcal toxic shock syndrome (STSS), and staphylococcal scalded skin syndrome (SSSS). All three are mediated by bacterial toxin production and are considerations in the differential diagnosis of a febrile, hypotensive patient with a rash.

Toxic Shock Syndrome

Disease Description

TSS was first described in the 1980s in adolescent Caucasian females who were using superabsorbent tampons that were thought to serve as a reservoir for toxin-producing *Staphylococcal aureus*. Although most cases remain associated with tampon use, the prevalence of TSS due to burns, postpartum and surgical wounds, body art (eg, tattoos and piercings), sinusitis, and nasal packing is increasing. Whereas 74% of all cases of TSS were associated with menstruation and tampon use between 1979 and 1996, for example, only 59% of cases from 1987 to 1996 were related to tampon use.[2,3,4]

Patients with TSS present with sudden-onset fever and hypotension. The primary dermatologic manifestations include a generalized, blanching erythroderma, described as a "painless sunburn," followed by ulceration and bullae formation in those most severely affected patients. Mucosal surfaces may also be involved, including conjunctival and sclera hemorrhages as well as hyperemia of the vagina and oropharynx. Late skin manifestations include desquamation of the palms and soles and, later, the loss of hair and nails. Multiple organ systems can also be involved, including the following: renal (acute kidney injury), muscle (rhabdomyolysis), gastrointestinal (nausea, vomiting, and profuse, watery diarrhea), hepatic (transaminase elevation), hematologic (thrombocytopenia), and neurologic (altered mental status).

The clinical manifestations of shock, exfoliative dermatitis, and multisystem organ failure are most commonly caused by TSS toxin-1 (TSST-1), which is produced by some *S. aureus*, including both MSSA (methicillin-sensitive *Staphylococcus aureus*) and MRSA (methicillin-resistant *S. aureus*). TSST-1 is known as a super antigen because it is capable of activating large numbers of T cells simultaneously, generating massive cytokine production. Because approximately 70% to 80% of the population has antibodies to TSST-1 by late adolescence, TSS is primarily an infection that affects children, young adults, and the immunocompromised.[5] Patients with TSS often fail to develop an appropriate antibody response to TSST-1 in convalescent serum after recovery from an initial TSS infection, so they may be predisposed to relapse.

Diagnosis

The diagnosis of TSS is based purely on clinical findings. The Centers for Disease Control and Prevention defines cases as patients with fever greater than 38.9°C, hypotension, diffuse erythroderma, desquamation (unless the patient dies before desquamation occurs), and involvement of at least three organ systems. Although the vast majority of patients with TSS have *S. aureus* isolated from wound cultures or mucosal swabs, its presence is not necessary to fulfill the diagnosis. Only 5% of patients with TSS have *S. aureus* bacteremia.

Treatment

The core treatments of TSS include resuscitation with intravenous fluid, vasopressors, removal of any potential nidus of infection (eg, tampon or piercing), correction of coagulation abnormalities, and other supportive care measures. It is not certain if antibiotics alter the course of acute TSS, but they may be useful in eradicating secondary staphylococcal infection or colonization, decreasing the risk of disease recurrence.

Patients with MSSA should receive clindamycin 600 mg IV every 8 hours plus oxacillin or nafcillin 2 g IV every 4 hours. Patients with suspected MRSA should receive clindamycin 600 mg IV every 8 hours with vancomycin 30 mg/kg per day in two divided doses. Intravenous immunoglobulin 400 mg/kg as a single dose may be considered in severe cases, particularly in patients who do not respond to aggressive fluid resuscitation and vasopressors. Corticosteroids have not been shown to be useful. Patients should be screened for nasal carriage of *Staphylococcus* and treated with mupirocin if positive. Women with menstrual-associated TSS should be advised against future tampon use.

TSS mortality associated with tampons has decreased from 5.5% in 1980 to 1.8% in 1987 to 1996. The mortality in nonmenstrual cases remains unchanged at 6% from 1980 to 1996.

Streptococcal Toxic Shock Syndrome

Disease Description

STSS is defined as any Group A Streptococcal (GAS) infection (including bacteremia, pneumonia, necro-tizing fasciitis, and myonecrosis) associated with shock and multisystem organ failure.

Similar in pathophysiology to TSS, STSS is caused by toxins that act like super antigens, leading to mas-sive cytokine production. Risk factors for invasive GAS include minor trauma, soft tissue injury, recent surgery, viral infection, and the use of nonsteroidal anti-inflammatory drugs. Patients present with local-ized pain out of proportion to exam findings, typically in a limb; however, this can be noted anywhere, including intra-abdominal spaces. Dermatologic findings of STSS are often localized, beginning with dis-crete areas of erythema. These progress to vesicles and bullae, which eventually evolve into violaceous or necrotic appearing lesions. Necrotizing fasciitis or myositis may be seen in up to 70% to 80% of cases.[6] Patients often present with fever, hypotension, altered mental status, and acute renal failure. Acute respi-ratory distress syndrome develops in up to 55% of cases.

Diagnosis

The diagnosis of STTS is made confirmed by the isolation of GAS from a normally sterile site (eg, blood, cerebrospinal fluid [CSF], wound culture, or pleural or peritoneal fluid) and hypotension, along with two of the following: acute renal failure, coagulopathy, elevated transaminases, adult respiratory distress syndrome (ARDS), an erythematous rash, or soft tissue necrosis.

Treatment

Treatment includes fluid resuscitation (typically requiring up to 10–20 liters per day) and vasopressors as indicated. A low threshold for intubation is appropriate in light of the high risk of ARDS. Immediate surgical consultation is necessary and should not be delayed by imaging because many patients will need urgent debridement, fasciotomy, or amputation. Antibiotic therapy should begin with empiric clindamy-cin 900 mg IV every 8 hours in addition to a carbapenem (eg, imipenem 500 mg IV every 6 hours or meropenem 1 g IV every 8 hours) or a penicillin plus beta-lactamase inhibitor (eg. ticarcillin-clavulanate 3.1 g IV every 4 hours or piperacillin-tazobactam 4.5 g IV every 6 hours). Once the diagnosis of GAS has been confirmed by cultures, antibiotics can be narrowed to penicillin G 4 million units IV every 4 hours along with clindamycin 900 mg IV every 8 hours. Intravenous immune globulin can be considered in patients with refractory sepsis.

Staphylococcal Scalded Skin Syndrome

Disease Description

SSSS is primarily a pediatric disease caused by strains of *S. aureus* that produce exfoliative toxin. Although infants and young children are most commonly affected, risk factors for adults include renal failure (lead-ing to the inability to effectively clear toxins), malignancy, and other immunosuppressive conditions. Patients tend to be less ill than those with TSS and may present clinically with fever, malaise, and tender erythroderma, which progresses to desquamation. Nikolsky sign is present (the epidermis separates from the dermis at the basal layer with minimal horizontal tactile pressure).

Treatment

Although usually not septic appearing on presentation, SSSS patients may still need fluid resuscitation and admission. Those with extensive skin involvement should be admitted to a burn unit. Patients with smaller areas of involvement may be discharged on oral antibiotics. Antibiotics of choice include nafcillin (100 mg/kg/day IV in divided doses every 6 hours or 50 mg/kg/day PO in divided doses every 6 hours for 7 to 10 days), penicillin G procaine (300,000 units/day IM for < 30 kg or 600,000 to 1 million units/day IM for > 30 kg), amoxicillin-clavulanate (45 mg/kg/day PO in divided doses every 12 hours for 7 to 10 days), cefazolin (100 mg/kg/day IV in divided doses every 6 hours), and cephalexin (40 mg/kg/day PO in divided doses every 6 hours for 7 to 10 days). In the case of suspected MRSA, options include clindamycin (40 mg/kg/day IV or PO in divided doses every 6 hours for 7 to 10 days), sulfamethoxazole-trimethoprim (10 mg/kg/day PO in divided doses every 12 hours for 7 to 10 days), or vancomycin (10–15 mg/kg/day IV in divided doses every 12 hours, up to 1 g every 12 hours).

Meningococcemia

Disease Description

Meningococcemia is potentially fatal, and it most often affects individuals under the age of 20 years. It is extremely contagious with a short incubation period of 3 to 4 days on average. Clinically, patients present with headache, fever, neck stiffness, altered mental status, myalgias, and arthralgias. Initially, meningococcemia may be mistaken for a severe viral syndrome. The median time between the onset of symptoms and hospitalization is often less than 24 hours. Dermatologic findings include petechiae, urticaria, and hemorrhagic vesicles as well as macules that evolve into palpable purpura with grey, necrotic centers. Petechiae often begin on mucosal surfaces or at pressure points, such as the waist or sock line. Skin findings are mostly on the trunk and lower extremities. Patients may rapidly develop septic shock, disseminated intravascular coagulation (DIC), seizures, and myocardial failure. Purpura fulminans, occurring in 15% to 25% of patients with meningococcemia, is characterized by necrotic skin lesions and gangrene of subcutaneous tissue, muscle, and bone. Mortality rates are 10% to 15% despite antibiotics.[7]

In addition to basic labs, blood cultures, and CSF studies, an aspirate of the pustules or vesicles should be sent for gram stain and culture. DIC labs should also be obtained. If lumbar puncture is difficult or contraindicated because of local skin involvement or coagulopathy, empiric antibiotic treatment with ceftriaxone (1–2 g IV every 12 hours) or cefotaxime (1–2 g IV every 4–8 hours) should be started promptly. Additional gram-positive coverage with vancomycin (10 to 15 mg/kg/day IV every 12 hours, up to 1 g every 12 hours) is prudent until gram stain and culture results are available.

Disseminated Gonococcus

Disease Description

Disseminated gonococcal infection (DGI) occurs in 0.5% to 3% of patients infected with sexually transmitted *Neisseria gonorrhoeae*.[8] Risk factors for the development of DGI include recent menstruation, pregnancy or immediate postpartum state, congenital or acquired complement deficiency, and systemic lupus erythematosis. Two syndromes are readily described. In the first, patients present with tenosynovitis, dermatitis, and polyarthralgias without purulent arthritis. In the second, patients present with purulent arthritis but without skin lesions. Patients with DGI typically do not present with symptoms of acute cervicitis, urethritis, or proctitis. Skin findings consist of a limited number (typically less than 10) of painless pustular or vesicular lesions. Rarely, patients may have nodules or bullous skin changes. Tenosynovitis may involve multiple tendons, including wrists, fingers, ankles, and toes. Arthritis in DGI most commonly affects knees, wrists, and ankles. The diagnosis of DGI is made with arthrocentesis (with a mean white cell count of 50,000 cells/mm^3), blood cultures, urethral cultures, and/or cervical cultures. Patients with DGI should be treated for 7 to 10 days with ceftriaxone 1 g IV daily. All patients with *N. gonorrhea* infections should also be empirically treated for concurrent *Chlamydia trachomatis* infection with doxycycline 100 mg PO twice daily or azithromycin 1 g as single oral dose.

Ecthyma Gangrenosum

Ecthyma gangrenosum (EG) is a cutaneous manifestation sepsis due to *Pseudomonas aeruginosa*. EG is seen most frequently in immunocompromised patients, including those with diabetes. It is often seen in hospitalized patients following surgery, particularly urological procedures. Long-term indwelling catheters, intravenous lines, and tracheostomy are also risk factors. In several reported cases, patients with EG were on prolonged antibiotic therapy targeting non-pseudomonal organisms.[9] It is speculated that this may have led to elimination of normal flora, promoting pseudomonal overgrowth.

Skin lesions begin as localized areas of edema, which progress to painless nodules with central hemorrhage and necrotic ulceration. EG results from arterial and venous invasion by *Pseudomonas* with subsequent vasculitis and tissue ischemia. Although lesions may be anywhere on the body, EG predominately affects the anogenital and axillary areas. Distribution occurs with the following frequencies: gluteal or perineal region (57%), extremities (30%), trunk (6%), and face (6%).[10] Because EG is highly concerning for pseudomonal bacteremia, patients should promptly be treated with appropriate broad-spectrum parenteral antibiotics to cover *Pseudomonas*.

Rocky Mountain Spotted Fever

Rock Mountain Spotted Fever (RMSF) is the most common tick-borne disease in the United States. The etiologic agent, *Rickettsia rickettsii*, is a gram-negative obligate intracellular bacterium, most commonly transmitted by *Dermacentor variabilis* (the American dog tick). Although infection occurs throughout North and South America, it is most prevalent in the southeastern and south central states. Patients typically become symptomatic 2 to 14 days after being bitten by an infected tick with median onset of illness between days 5 and 7.

Patients present with nonspecific symptoms, such as fever, headache, myalgias, arthralgias, nausea, vomiting, and abdominal pain. The rash develops 3 to 5 days after the onset of symptoms in the majority of patients. Less than 10% of patients present without rash, which may delay the diagnosis and increase mortality due to delayed initiation of antibiotic treatment. The rash in RMSF typically starts on the ankles and wrists and spreads both centrally and to the palms and soles. It begins as a maculopapular rash, which evolves into non-blanching petechia. More severely affected patients may have altered mental status, focal neurological deficits, seizures, peripheral edema, cardiac arrhythmias, and multisystem organ failure. Mortality rates have varied from 1.1% to 4.9%.[11] Those at highest risk are the very young (ie, less than 4 years old) and the elderly. Male gender, black race, alcohol abuse, and glucose-6-phosphate dehydrogenase deficiency are additional risk factors for mortality.

The diagnosis of RMSF is primarily clinical and is based on appropriate presentation in the proper epidemiological setting. Indirect fluorescent antibody testing can be sent to confirm the diagnosis, with antibodies typically appearing 7 to 10 days after symptom onset. Convalescent antibodies can be sent 14 to 21 days after symptom onset. The minimum diagnostic titer in most labs is 1:64. Patients with RMSF should be treated with doxycycline 200 mg/day in divided doses every 12 hours in adults and children weighing more than 45 kg and with doxycycline 2.2 mg/kg per dose every 12 hours in children less than 45 kg. Pregnant women should be treated with chloramphenicol 50 mg/kg per day in four divided doses. Treatment should be continued for 3 days after the patient has defervesced, with most patients only requiring 5 to 7 days of antibiotics.

Vibrio Vulnificus

Vibrio vulnificus is a gram-negative bacterium that causes serious wound infections, sepsis, and diarrhea in patients exposed to shellfish or marine water. Those at highest risk have chronic underlying medical problems, particularly liver disease, alcohol abuse, and hemochromatosis. Wound infections occur when minor areas of skin breakdown are exposed to contaminated water, shellfish, or fish. These infections can progress into cellulitis. In high risk patients, these infections may rapidly progress to hemorrhagic bullous skin changes, myositis, and/or fasciitis. Primary septicemia can occur after eating raw shellfish, particularly oysters, and mortality rates exceed 40%.[12] The diagnosis is typically made with blood cultures. Patients should be treated with minocycline or doxycycline 100 mg by mouth twice daily plus cefotaxime 2 g IV every 8 hours or ceftriaxone 1 g IV daily.

Suggested Readings and References

1. Cydulka RK, Garber B. Dermatologic presentations. In: Marx J, Hockberger R, Walls R, eds. *Rosen's Emergency Medicine—Concepts and Clinical Practice*; 2010:1529–1556.
2. Hajjeh RA, Reingold A, Weil A, et al. Toxic shock syndrome in the United States: surveillance update, 1979–1996. *Emerg Infect Dis*. 1999;5:807–810.
3. Stockmann C, Ampofo K, Hersh AL, et al Evolving epidemiologic characteristics of invasive group A streptococcal disease in Utah, 2002–2010. *Clin Infect Dis*. 2012;55:479.
4. Jajjeh RA, Reingold A, Weil A, et al. Toxic shock syndrome in the United States: surveillance update, 1979–1996. *Emerg Infect Dis*. 1999;5:807.
5. Stevens DL, Tanner MH, Winship J, et al. Severe group A streptococcal infections associated with a toxic shock-like syndrome and scarlet fever toxin A. *N Engl J Med*. 1989;321:1.
6. Defining the group A streptococcal toxic shock syndrome. Rationale and consensus definition. The Working Group on severe Streptococcal infections. *JAMA*. 1993;269:390.
7. Heckenberg SG, de Gans J, Brouwer MC, et al. Clinical features, outcome, and meningococcal genotypye in 258 adults with meningococcal meningitis: a prospective cohort study. *Medicine (Baltimore)*. 2008;87:185.
8. O'Brien JP, Goldenberg DL, Rice PA. Disseminated gonococcal infection: a prospective analysis of 49 patients and a review of pathophysiology and immune mechanisms. *Medicine (Baltimore)*. 1983;62:395.
9. Anderson MG. Pseudomonas septicaemia and ecthyma gangrenosum. *S Afr Med J*. 1979;55:504–508.
10. Greene SL, Su WP, Muller SA. Ecthyma gangrenosum: report of clinical, histopathological and bacteriologic aspects of eight cases. *J Am Acad Dermatol*. 1984;11781–11787.
11. Centers for Disease Control and Prevention. Consequences of delayed diagnosis of Rocky Mountain spotted fever in children—West Virginia, Michigan, Tennessee, and Oklahoma, May-July 2000. *MMWR Morb Mortal Wkly Rep*. 2000;49:885.
12. Blake PA, Merson MH, Weaver RE, et al. Disease caused by marine Vibro: clinical characteristics and epidemiology. *N Engl J Med*. 1979;300:1.

Chapter 45

Mammalian and Reptile Bites

David Scordino, and Susan Peterson

Summary Box

Disease Description: Bites from animals and humans can result in significant morbidity and mortality if not managed well. Both animal and human bites can result in significant infections. Knowledge of the organisms that are associated with animal or human bites can help to direct appropriate therapy.

Organisms:
Human: *Eikenella, Staphylococcus,* and *Streptococcus*
Cat: *Pasteurella multocida* and *Bartonella henselae*
Dog: *Pasteurella, Streptococcus, Staphylococcus, Capnocytophaga canimorsus*
Rat/Squirrel/Mice: *Streptococcus moniliformis*
Livestock: *Brucella, Leptospira,* and *Francisella tularensis*
Bats/Skunk/Raccoon/Fox: *rabies virus*
Monkeys: Herpes B virus (*Cercopithecine herpesvirus 1*), *rabies virus,* and *Clostridium tetani*

Treatment:
Oral First line: amoxicillin/clavulanic acid (850 mg/125 mg or 500 mg/125 mg PO twice daily can be considered for all infectious bites unless the following are additional considerations:
Bartonella: azithromycin 10 mg/kg (max 500 mg) for day 1, and 5 mg/kg (max 250 mg) for days 2 through 5.
Herpes organisms: acyclovir 800 mg PO five times daily or valacyclovir 1 g every 8 hours for 14 days (for potential herpes simian B virus infection)
Rabies: intravenous immunoglobulin (IVIG) and rabies vaccine, supportive care

Second line: clindamycin 300 mg TID, moxifloxacin 400 mg daily, doxycycline 100 mg BID, or azithromycin 10 mg/kg (max 500 mg) for day 1 and 5 mg/kg (max 250 mg) for days 2 through 5.
For more serious infections, consider amoxicillin/clavulanic acid 1,000 mg/200 mg IV 4 to 6 times/day.

Other Specific Considerations:
Cat Scratch Disease: azithromycin 10 mg/kg (500 mg max) for the first day followed by 4 days of 5 mg/kg per day (250 mg max) [12]
Rat Bite Fever: 1.2 million units of IV penicillin per day for 5 to 7 days followed by 500 mg PO QID for 7 days. Tetracycline or streptomycin are potential alternatives for those with penicillin allergies.
Tularemia: streptomycin 10–15 mg/kg IM BID or gentamicin for 7 to 10 days.
Herpes Simian B encephalitis: acyclovir 12.5 to 15 mg/kg every 8 hours or ganciclovir 5 mg/kg every 12 hours
Tetanus: tetanus immunoglobulin, muscle relaxants (benzodiazepines), and antibiotics (penicillin, clindamycin, erythromycin, or metronidazole)
Capnocytophaga: Amoxicillin-clavulanic acid 850 mg/125 mg or 500 mg/125 mg

Other Key Issues: In general, bite wounds should not be closed unless the bite wound is in a highly vascular area such as the face.

Disease Description

Epidemiology

Reptile Bites: Venomous snake bites account for approximately 7,000 to 8,000 of animal bite cases each year in the United States, with even more from nonvenomous snakes [1]. Within the United States, native venomous snakes can be divided into two genera, *Crotalinae* and *Elapidae*. The *Crotalinae* consist of rattlesnakes, copperheads, and water moccasins/cottonmouths. These species are indigenous to different parts of the United States except Alaska, Maine, and Hawaii [2]. Although these species are diffusely distributed, the majority of cases occur in the southern and western United States during the spring and summer months [2]. The *Elapidae* genus consists of the coral snake, which is generally a more docile species, so bites are less common than with *Crotalinae* species [3]. Exotic snake bites also occur infrequently, usually in patients that work at zoos or keep exotic snakes as pets [2].

Mammalian Bites: Mammalian bites are a frequent complaint in the Emergency Department (ED), with 800,000 to 1,000,000 cases per year, accounting roughly for 1% of all ED visits; however, the majority do not seek medical attention [4, 5]. Domestic animals account for nearly 95% of animal bites presenting to the ED [4]. Deaths are infrequent from the initial attack, with 10 to 20 fatalities each year from dogs and rare deaths from other mammals in the United States [4]. Infection is common with 5% to 20% of dog bites and 28% to 80% of cat bites becoming infected, although this number is likely an overestimate because many pet owners are bitten and do not present to the hospital [4, 8, 9].

Presenting Features

Reptile Bites: The most common presentation is a young male who has attempted to catch or hold an animal and can readily admit to being bitten [1, 2, 3]. However, there are cases of individuals who are unable to provide an adequate history or who are unaware of if they were bitten or scratched. Skin evaluation in such individuals may show puncture wounds, suggesting a bite, or simple scrapes, suggesting a scratch [1, 2]. Erythema, ecchymoses, bullae, or even tissue necrosis are possible if a snake was poisonous [1, 2]. Swelling can lead to compartment syndrome or airway compromise depending on the location of the bite [1, 2].

In *Crotalinae* bites, nausea, vomiting, lethargy, confusion, coma, seizures, cardiovascular collapse, respiratory failure, or gastrointestinal or pulmonary bleeding may occur [1, 2]. However, coral snake bites may be asymptomatic initially and have no evidence of bite marks because the teeth are often very fine. These bites can later progress to numbness, weakness, lethargy, fasciculations, tremors, dysphagia, dyspnea, miotic pupils, respiratory depression, seizures, and/or paralysis [3]. Other exotic snake bites are uncommon, vary widely in presentation, and are beyond the scope of this review. The history, however, is often more straightforward in these individuals because they are often caring for these animals [2].

Other reptile bites, such as those from lizards and turtles, are often less dramatic and lack systemic symptoms, except Gila monsters, which are venomous lizards [2]. Snapping turtles can do a great deal of injury, including amputations of digits.

Mammalian Bites: The history of mammalian bites is often quite clear. The physical presentation varies based on the area that was bitten and veracity of the incident. Deep wounds to the neck or face may be associated with airway compromise and severe bleeding. Open or closed fractures are possible, particularly in children, as well as other trauma associated with fighting the animal or being attacked. Mountain lions and larger animals can do significant damage to a patient, and the patient can present with a combination of blunt and penetrating traumatic injury [5].

Diagnostic Considerations

The first consideration is the animal, the extent of injury, and the stability of the patient.

Snakes: If the patient was bitten by a snake, the type of snake involved should be identified whenever possible. A poisonous bite from a *Crotalinae* snake is unlikely if there is no evidence of tissue necrosis, severe swelling, pain out of proportion to the extent of injury, evidence of systemic illness, or the snake description is inconsistent with known poisonous morphologies [1, 2]. If the patient was bitten by a poisonous snake (or has evidence of a severe local reaction due to a bite from an unknown snake species), the patient should be assessed for stability and concomitant injury, their limb should be immobilized and elevated, and they should receive a detailed physical exam with particular focus on the wound site, marking the wound edge, and assessing tenderness every 15 to 30 minutes [1, 11]. Labs looking for disseminated intravascular coagulopathy (DIC), including a CBC, CMP, coagulation factors, D-dimer, fibrinogen, and a type and screen, should be drawn. The local poison control should be contacted [2, 11]. Keep in mind that there may be retained foreign bodies secondary to these bites, and imaging may be required.

Mammals: The force and depth of mammalian bites effects how much bacteria are inoculated and into what layers of the tissue. Deeper wounds deliver more bacteria to deeper layers of tissues, so it is more difficult to adequately clean these wounds [4, 8]. The type of animal and the rabies vaccination status of the animal are important considerations in the bite assessment. A thorough exam of the bite for evidence of contamination or infection as well as the location and type of wound is critical for wound management, follow up, and disposition. Bites to the hand and feet should be given careful consideration given the propensity of the resulting infections to enter joint capsules and/or extend into the deep tissue layers [4].

Additional considerations include the extent of the injury and the condition of vital surrounding structures such as nerves, joints, tendons, and vascular structures. Finally, medical comorbidities should be considered. Diabetes, individuals with vascular disease, immunosuppression, poor hygiene, and the very young or the very old are at higher risk of infection and complications from bites, particularly in regions with poor vascular supply, such as the feet, hands, back, and thighs [4, 5].

Typical Disease Course

Venomous Snakes: Crotalinae species "dry bite" (i.e. bite without injecting venom) approximately 25% of the time, so an isolated puncture does not always mean envenomation occurred [2, 11]. "Dry bites" are less likely in Elapids and most exotic snakes [3]. In general, a dry bite must never be assumed without 8–12 hours of observation for the development of DIC (with repeat labs) and monitoring for advancing tissue necrosis for *Crotalinae* or symptom development in *Elapidae* snakes [2, 10, 11]. If envenomation from a *Crotalinae* snake has occurred, then the course can range from local tissue swelling and necrosis to cardiac collapse and death, typically over hours to days [2, 11]. For an *Elapidae* snake, paralysis and respiratory failure can occur within hours [3]. The time course can be shorter in certain exotics.

Non-Venomous Snakes: The majority of patients have an uneventful clinical course. Basic wound care is sufficient to prevent complications, such as infection [7]. Ensure that foreign bodies are removed.

Other Reptiles (eg, lizards, turtles, alligators, etc.): The clinical course is dependent on the extent of the wound. Some bites can result in partial or complete amputations of digits or be life threatening. There is limited data about infection rates. However, there is no recommendation for empiric antibiotics [4]. Do not close deep bites primarily. You should allow for delayed or secondary closure in order to prevent infections.

Cats: Infection usually presents within one day to one week after the bite. Untreated, these can result in cellulitis, abscesses, septic joints, deep space infections, sepsis, and death [4, 5, 8].

Dogs: Local wound care maybe sufficient for minor or superficial bites. Superficial infection often presents within one day to a few weeks after the bite and most resolve with antibiotics. Untreated, these can result in cellulitis, abscesses, septic joints, deep space infections, sepsis, and death [4, 5, 8, 9].

Rodents (eg, bats, skunks, rats, etc.): Minor bite wounds are most common with an infection rate of 2–10% [5]. The wound heals with local wound care over one to two weeks with infection generally presenting a few days to one week after the bite. However, bats have a very high incidence of rabies, which can be fatal, so any patient with contact with a bat should be treated for possible rabies infection [15].

Monkeys: The incidence of monkey bites within the U.S. is low. However, proper treatment is imperative because of the risk of herpes encephalitis, rabies, and tetanus [16]. While these complications are uncommon, all have significant associated mortality. These complications can begin to develop within one week to several years (rabies) after exposure.

Large Mammals (e.g. bears, mountain lions, etc.): The course is dependent on the extent of injury, which is often extensive in these individuals. These individuals often require surgical repair of their extensive wounds [5].

Complications

Snake Bites: For non-venomous bites, few complications are generally identified. Infection is rare, so empiric antibiotics are not recommended [7]. For snake bites with envenomation, complications can range from local tissue necrosis to DIC, hemorrhage, shock, and death [1,2].

Cat scratch disease: Cat bites or scratches complicated by cat scratch disease often present with regional lymphadenitis 3 to 10 days after inoculation. Patients may present with fatigue, fever, headache, and lymphadenopathy [12].

Rabies: Rabies infection is almost universally fatal once symptoms (eg, paresthesia, numbness, itching extending from the wound site progressing to nonspecific symptoms and encephalitis) become present [13].

Rat Bite Fever: Patients present with fever, chills, arthralgias, and rash 3 to 10 days following inoculation [12]. Although typically not severe, mortality in untreated cases can be as high as 13% [12]. This entity is more common outside of the United States, so travel history should be discussed with the patient if the diagnosis is being considered.

Tularemia: Tularemia can result from rodent, rabbit, or hare bites and scratches [12]. Additionally, tick bites or the ingestion of contaminated meat can lead to infection. Patients present with sudden fever, chills, headaches, myalgias, arthralgias, and dry cough 2 to 21 days (3–6 on average) following inoculation, although further presentation varies to between six variations [18].

Herpes Simian B Encephalitis: This infection results in a potentially fatal encephalitis.

Tetanus: Tetanus is a severe bacterial infection resulting from the release of tetanospasmin, which causes muscle spasms and difficulty swallowing, followed by respiratory failure [17].

Capnocytophaga: Capnocytophaga infections are rare but often present as sepsis, and management should focus on broad-spectrum antibiotics and resuscitation. Asplenic patients, the elderly, alcoholics, and the immunocompromised are at higher risk for sepsis with *Capnocytophaga*[4].

Diagnostic Tests

The initial diagnosis is clinical, based on both history and physical exam. If the patient is seen several days later and infection is present, wound cultures should be obtained. In patients with severe systemic symptoms from snake bites, consider obtaining a DIC panel. Obtain plain films if foreign body retention is suspected or other necessary imaging for potential traumatic injuries.

Special Disorders

Cat Scratch Disease: Serologic testing available but often clinical

Rabies: Saliva polymerase chain reaction (PCR), nuchal punch biopsy, antibody testing for serum or cerebrospinal fluid (CSF)

Rat Bite Fever: Culture from blood, synovial fluid, or CSF

Tularemia: Serology or PCR

Herpes Simian B encephalitis: PCR

Tetanus: Clinical

Capnocytophaga: Blood culture

Organisms

The primary organisms associated with infections vary from animal to animal. Although the mouth is polymicrobial, only a few bacteria tend to cause pathology. These microbes are as follows:

HumanL *Eikenella, Staphylococcus,* and *Streptococcus*

Cat: *Pasteurella multocida* (75% of bites) and *Bartonella henselae*

Dog: *Pasteurella* (50% of bites), *Streptococcus, Staphylococcus, Capnocytophaga canimorsus*

Rat/squirrel/mice: *Streptococcus moniliformis*

Livestock: *Brucella, Leptospira,* and *Francisella tularensis*

Bats/skunk/raccoon/fox: *rabies virus*

Monkeys: Herpes B virus (*Cercopithecine herpesvirus 1*), *rabies virus,* and *Clostridium tetani*

Special Disorders

Cat Scratch Disease: *Bartonella henselae*

Rabies: Rabies virus

Rat Bite Fever: *Streptobacillus moniliformis* or *Spirillum minus*

Tularemia: *Francisella tularensis*

Herpes Simian B encephalitis: Herpes B virus

Tetanus: *Clostridium tetani*

Capnocytophaga: *Capnocytophaga canimorsus*

Treatment

First address the patient's airway, breathing, and circulation should they be compromised. Then, wound management should be initiated. Irrigate the wound using tap water or normal saline. No evidence supports one versus the other. Tetanus prophylaxis should be provided because the skin has been broken.

Reptile: For nonvenomous bites, basic wound care is sufficient. For venomous bites, supportive therapy and antivenom are key [2,3,6,7]. Local poison control should be contacted for all suspected or confirmed envenomations. Empiric antibiotics are not indicated, as the incidence of wound infection is small [6,7].

Mammalian: The decision to start rabies prophylaxis depends on the type of animal and the health of the animal. For dogs, cats, or ferrets that are healthy and can be observed for 10 days, prophylaxis does not need to begin unless the animal develops clinical signs of rabies during the observation period [13]. It should be noted that the Centers for Disease Control and Prevention (CDC) reports that "no one in the United States has ever contracted rabies from a dog, cat, or ferret held in quarantine for 10 days" that did not develop symptoms [14]. Rabies prophylaxis should be provided for all people who were bitten by a dog or cat that was suspected of being rabid. Rabies prophylaxis should also be provided for bat **exposure**, not just for bites or scratches [15].

Bites from raccoons, bobcats, foxes, wolves, skunks, or coyotes should also be treated with rabies prophylaxis [13]. For other animals, refer to the CDC website or local health department for further guidelines. If prophylaxis is to be provided, 20 IU/kg of rabies IVIG should be provided around the site of the wound [13]. Rabies vaccine should be provided at 0, 3, 7, and 14 days post-exposure [13]. Prior guidelines highlighted a 28-day vaccination, which has since been removed by current CDC recommendations. The health department should be notified for all cases of bites. Uncomplicated bites can be discharged with amoxicillin-clavulanic acid 875 mg or 45 mg/kg BID for 5 to 10 days [5]. For those with penicillin allergies, treatment options include clindamycin 300 mg PO TID, moxifloxacin 400 mg PO daily, doxycycline 100 mg PO BID, or azithromycin 10 mg/kg (max 500 mg) for day 1 and 5 mg/kg (max 250 mg) for days 2 through 5. Wound check should occur in 24 to 72 hours [4].

For those with complicated wounds, IV antibiotics should be provided and the appropriate surgical specialty involved. Additionally, those with bites from monkeys should be provided with prophylactic acyclovir 800 mg PO five times daily or valacyclovir 1 g every 8 hours for 14 days for potential herpes simian B virus infection [16]. Hepatitis B prophylaxis and human immunodeficiency virus prophylaxis should be considered for those with human bites obtained during a fight because blood to blood contact could have occurred.

Special Disorders

Cat Scratch Disease: Azithromycin 5mg/kg per day for 5 days [12]

Rabies: Preexposure prophylaxis

Rat Bite Fever: Penicillin 1.2 million units IV per day for 5 to 7 days followed by 500 mg PO QID for 7 days. Tetracycline or streptomycin are potential alternatives for those with penicillin allergies.

Tularemia: Streptomycin 10–15 mg/kg IM BID or gentamicin for 7 to 10 days.

Herpes Simian B encephalitis: Without central nervous system, acyclovir IV 12.5 to 15 mg/kg every 8 hours or ganciclovir 5 mg/kg every 12 hours; with neurologic symptoms, ganciclovir is recommended. [19]

Tetanus: Prevention is best with tetanus vaccination (Tdap [tetanus, diphtheria, and pertussis] preferred if not given within the last 5 years); if not vaccinated, then 3,000 to 6,000 units of IM tetanus immunoglobulin and vaccination. If clinical tetanus occurs, therapy is with tetanus immunoglobulin, muscle relaxants (benzodiazepines), and antibiotics (penicillin, clindamycin, erythromycin, or metronidazole) [17].

Other Key Issues

Wound closure is often a debated topic. Complex wounds should not be closed. Simple wounds over vascular structures, such as the face, can be considered for primary closure. For bite closures, the ethos should be, "if in doubt, don't close it."

Suggested Readings and References

1. Norris, Robert L, Bush, Sean P, Smith JC. Bites by venomous reptiles in Canada, the United States and Mexico. In: Auerbach PS. *Wilderness Medicine*. 6th ed. Philadelphia, PA: Elsevier Mosby; 2012:1011–1039.

2. Dart RC, Sullivan JB. Crotaline snake envenomation. In: Wolfson AB . . . eds. *Harwood-Nuss' Clinical Practice of Emergency Medicine*. 5th ed. Philadelphia, PA: Lippincott, Williams & Wilkins; 2010:1624–1626.

3. Dart RC, Sullivan JB. Elapid snake envenomation. In: Wolfson AB, . . . eds. *Harwood-Nuss' Clinical Practice of Emergency Medicine*. 5th ed. Philadelphia, PA: Lippincott, Williams & Wilkins; 2010:1627–1628.

4. Playe SJ. Mammalian bites and associated infections. In: Wolfson AB, . . . eds. *Harwood-Nuss' Clinical Practice of Emergency Medicine*. 5th ed. Philadelphia, PA: Lippincott, Williams & Wilkins; 2010:1648–1652.

5. Bradford JE, Freer L. Bites and injuries inflicted by wild and domestic animals. In: Auerbach PS. *Wilderness Medicine*. 6th ed. Philadelphia, PA: Elsevier Mosby; 2012:1102–1127.

6. Terry P, Mackway-Jones K. The use of antibiotics in venomous snake bite. *Emerg Med J*. 2002;1:48–49.

7. Terry P and Mackway-Jones K. Antibiotics in non-venomous snakebite. *Emerg Med J*. 2002;19:142.

8. Dendle C, Looke D. Management of mammalian bites. *Aust Fam Physician*. 2009;38: 868–874.

9. Presutti RJ. Prevention and treatment of dog bites. *Am Fam Physician*. 2001;63:1567–1573.

10. Hughes A. Observation of snakebite victims: is twelve hours still necessary? *Emerg Med (Fremantle)*. 2003;15:511–517.

11. Lavonas EJ, Ruha AM, Banner W, et al. Unified treatment algorithm for the management of crotaline snakebite in the United States: results of an evidence-informed consensus workshop. *BMC Emerg Med*. 2011;11:2.

12. Shandro JR, Jenkins JG. Wilderness-acquired zoonoses. In: Auerbach PS. *Wilderness Medicine*. 6th ed. Philadelphia, PA: Elsevier Mosby; 2012:1143–1175.

13. Wilkerson JA. Rabies. In: Auerbach PS. *Wilderness Medicine*. 6th ed. Philadelphia, PA: Elsevier Mosby; 2012:1175–1197.

14. Center for Disease Control. Rabies: Domestic Animals. Updated November 15, 2011. http://www.cdc.gov/rabies/exposure/animals/domestic.html. Accessed April 30, 2015.

15. Center for Disease Control. Rabies: bats. Updated November 15, 2011. http://www.cdc.gov/rabies/exposure/animals/bats.html. Accessed April 30, 2015.

16. Newton F. Monkey bite exposure treatment protocol. *J Spec Oper Med*. 2010;10:48–49.

17. Wu DT. Tetanus. In: Wolfson AB, . . . eds. *Harwood-Nuss' Clinical Practice of Emergency Medicine*. 5th ed. Philadelphia, PA: Lippincott, Williams & Wilkins; 2010:882–884.

18. Nguyen AB. Other tick-borne diseases. In: Wolfson AB, . . . eds. *Harwood-Nuss' Clinical Practice of Emergency Medicine*. 5th ed. Philadelphia, PA: Lippincott, Williams & Wilkins; 2010:909–910.

19. Center for Disease Control. B Virus (herpes B, monkey B virus, herpesvirus simiae, and herpesvirus B): First Aid and Treatment. Updated July 18, 2014. http://www.cdc.gov/herpesbvirus/firstaid-treatment.html#treatment Accessed April 30, 2015.

Bone and Joint Infections

Chapter 46

Septic Arthritis

Hasan E. Baydoun, Bachar Hamade, Jamil D. Bayram

Summary Box

Disease Description:
- Inflammation of a joint due to an infection
- Monoarticular more common than polyarticular

Organisms:
- *Staphylococcus aureus* is the most common
- Other organisms include *Neisseria gonorrhoeae* and gram-negative rods.

Treatment:
- IVantibiotics guided by Gram stain if positive (see following)
- Empiric IV antibiotics if Gram stain negative (see following)
- Orthopedic consultation for surgical treatment

Other Key Issues:
- Pediatric cases are often associated with bacteremia, and seeding can occur via the intra-articular physes.
- Gonococcal arthritis is a migratory arthritis associated with dermatitis and tenosynovitis.

Disease Description

Septic arthritis is an infectious inflammation of a joint.

Epidemiology

There are 20,000 reported cases of septic arthritis each year in the United States. It is most commonly seen in children and the elderly; those less than 2 years old and those greater than 65 years old comprise 30% and 45% of all cases, respectively. Monoarticular septic arthritis is more common (80%–90% of cases) than polyarticular (10%–20% of cases). S. aureus accounts for almost 50% of septic arthritis cases, and Streptococcus species account for 20%. Septic arthritis involves the large joints more often than the small joints. The knee, hip, shoulder, ankle, elbow, and wrist joints are the most common, with the knee and hip together accounting for 60% of all cases.

Method of Bacterial Joint Inoculation

Bacterial joint inoculation can result from hematogenous seeding, spread from adjacent tissue, or direct inoculation from trauma or an iatrogenic procedure.

Presenting Features

Joint pain (sensitivity 85%), swelling (sensitivity 78%), and fever (sensitivity 57%) are findings that occur in more than 50% of patients. Other features include effusion, warmth, and tenderness in the affected joint on exam. The inability to bear weight and the holding of the affected extremity in a position that maximizes intra-articular space (eg, knee extended fully or hip flexed, abducted, and externally rotated) is also seen. Patients exhibit pain with passive, non-weight-bearing motion. Pediatric patients often present with poor feeding and pseudoparalysis of the affected extremity. Sepsis occurs late in the disease course.

Diagnostic Considerations

Sexual history is important for assessing the risk of N. gonorrhoeae, and tick exposure can help determine the risk of Lyme disease. Patients should be asked about underlying joint diseases (eg, rheumatoid arthritis, osteoarthritis, gout, and others), comorbidities (eg, diabetes, cancer, and cirrhosis), and causes of immune deficiency, such as human immunodeficiency virus and corticosteroid use. In addition, patients should be asked about their vaccination histories to rule out H. influenzae and about recent joint surgery and trauma. A thorough infectious history should also be sought.

Typical Disease Course

Septic arthritis usually presents as acute, progressive pain that increases with motion and eventually leads to the inability to bear weight.

Complications

The most common complication that carries a 40% risk is damage to the articulate surface and permanent loss of the joint. Additional complications include joint contractures, leg length discrepancy, osteonecrosis, hip dislocations, deep vein thrombosis, and pulmonary embolisms. Sepsis is a potential complication, especially in immunocompromised patients.

Differential Diagnosis

The differential diagnosis for septic arthritis includes primary rheumatologic disorders (eg, vasculitis and crystalline arthritides, such as gout), reactive arthritis (eg, postinfectious diarrhea syndrome and arthritis of intrinsic bowel disease), polyarticular arthritis caused by a viral syndrome, bursitis, hemarthrosis, and cellulitis.

Diagnostic Tests

Prior to the initiation of antibiotics, joint aspiration and synovial fluid analysis is mandatory in all patients with suspected septic arthritis.

Synovial fluid analysis includes gram stain (50%–60% sensitive), culture, cell count, and crystal analysis. Septic arthritis can occur in patients with crystal arthritides, so the presence of crystals should not eliminate infection from the differential. Most septic joints have greater than 50,000 white blood cells (WBCs)/mm^3 in synovial fluids, but infection can occur in patients with lower counts, especially in cases of N. gonorrhoeae. The likelihood of septic arthritis increases with the synovial fluid WBC count. In a systematic review of the literature, counts of less than 25,000/mm^3, more than 25,000/mm^3, more than 50,000/mm^3, and more than 100,000/mm^3 gave likelihood ratios (LR) of 0.32, 2.9, 7.7, and 28, respectively. A polymorphonuclear cell count of at least 90% suggests septic arthritis with an LR of 3.4. Note that noninfectious arthritis, such as gout, may have WBC counts over 50,000/mm^3. Synovial fluid glucose is often low, and lactate is often elevated. However, neither of these is a reliable test.

Peripheral blood analysis includes WBC counts, C-reactive protein (CRP), and erythrocyte sedimentation rate (ESR). WBC counts are higher than 11,000/mm^3 in 20% to 50% of patients with septic arthritis. CRP and ESR are nonspecific markers of inflammation and can be elevated due to many other disease processes. Moreover, they are not always elevated in septic arthritis.

If positive, blood cultures can aid in diagnosis and help guide antibiotic treatment. Cultures should be drawn prior to the initiation of antibiotics. They are positive in 50% to 70% of patients with non-gonococcal arthritis. They can also be positive in the setting of negative joint cultures.

Imaging
No form of imaging can differentiate between infective and sterile effusions. In the acute setting, radiographs are typically normal but will occasionally show capsular shadows when a significant amount of swelling is present. Ultrasonography is helpful in identifying joint effusions and in performing image-guided joint aspiration. Computed tomography is a very good modality for detecting effusions and assessing the extent of bony destruction in chronic cases. Magnetic resonance imaging can measure the exact size of an effusion, demonstrate capsular engorgement and edema, and detect adjacent osteomyelitis and/or soft tissue infection.

Organisms

Microbiology
Several organisms cause septic joints, but the most common organism is *S. aureus*. Certain organisms are commonly seen among specific patient populations. *Methicillin-resistant S. aureus* (MRSA), for example, is usually the organism present in cases of septic shock. *N. gonorrhoeae* is present in 75% of septic arthritis cases in sexually active adults. *Salmonella* is typically present in sickle cell patients. In immunocompromised patients, *S. aureus* remains the most common organism; but *S. pneumoniae*, *Mycobacterium* species, and fungal species (30% of cases in immunocompromised patients) are also causes. *P. aeruginosa*, *S. aureus*, *Streptococcus* species, and Gram-negative bacilli are commonly detected in IV drug users.

Treatment

Optimal positioning of the joint to avoid future contractures is essential, and joint aspiration should be done as soon as possible.

IV antibiotics should be given only after aspiration but should not be delayed in patients with sepsis. In pediatric patients, treatment should cover *H. influenza* if documented vaccination status is unavailable. Antibiotics are typically given for 4 weeks with at least 2 weeks of IV administration. In gonococcal arthritis, the duration of IV antibiotic treatment is only 1 week.

Treatment should be guided by culture sensitivity profiles when available. The choice of empiric antibiotic therapy may rely on the Gram stain; however, Gram stain can be negative in up to 40% of cases. Antibiotics must cover *S. aureus* and *Streptococcus* species in addition to gonococci in patients who are sexually active.

First-line Recommendations
If the gram stain shows gram positive cocci characteristic of *S. aureus* or *Streptococcus* and there is no risk for MRSA, oxacillin or nafcillin should be initiated (consider clindamycin if the patient is allergic to penicillin). Vancomycin is the appropriate choice in patients at high risk for MRSA. If the gram stain reveals gram-negative cocci or rods, then third-generation cephalosporins are the appropriate choice. In cases of allergy, alternatives include aztreonam or fluoroquinolones as well as aminoglycosides if there is suspicion for *Pseudomonas*. If the Gram stain is negative and the patient is immunocompetent, ceftriaxone is an adequate empiric therapy in sexually active adults. If the risk of MRSA is high, vancomycin should be added. If the patient is immunocompromised, the appropriate therapy is vancomycin plus a third-generation cephalosporin.

Second-line Recommendations
Second-line recommendations for the treatment of *N. Gonorrhoeae* include cefixime and ciprofloxacin. For gram-negative rods, cefepime, piperacillin/tazobactam, and carbapenems are appropriate.

Bone and Joint Infections

Surgical Treatment
Orthopedic consultation is mandatory in cases of septic arthritis. Arthrotomy is warranted if osseous involvement has already occurred or if osteomyelitis is present. Arthroscopic surgery, which is less invasive, is appropriate if soft tissue involvement and abscess are absent and if the joint is readily accessible (eg, knee and shoulder). In chronic cases, open radical synovectomy is often necessary.

Nonsurgical Treatment
In cases of documented gonococcal arthritis with no suspicion for other concomitant infection, nonsurgical treatment may be considered if there is complete symptom resolution with IV antibiotics and joint aspiration. If there are contraindications to surgery, serial joint aspirations and bedside lavage with large-bore needles are recommended to decrease the bacterial count and the inflammatory mediator load in the joint.

Disposition
All patients with septic arthritis require admission.

Other Key Issues

Pediatric Population
Pyogenic seeding into the joint can occur via the following intra-articular physes: proximal humerus into the shoulder, proximal radius into the elbow, proximal femur into the hip, and distal fibula into the ankle. Immediate decompression is warranted in pediatric cases because pressure from the joint effusion may cause damage to the physeal plate, leading to osteonecrosis or growth deformities. Due to high risk of associated bacteremia in neonates, a combination of vancomycin and a third-generation cephalosporin, such as cefotaxime or ceftriaxone, is a reasonable choice for empiric coverage. In older children, oxacillin or naficillin provide adequate coverage. However, in cases of suspected MRSA, clindamycin or vancomycin should be used. For adolescents with septic arthritis, a third-generation cephalosporin suffices as adequate initial therapy.

Gonococcal Arthritis
Gonococcal arthritis is a migratory polyarticular arthritis, and patients may present with additional clinical features. Dermatitis is seen in 75% of the cases, and tenosynovitis is seen in 68% of cases. Patients may also have small, erythematous papules that progress to pustules as well as a low-grade fever. Joint aspirates usually reveal a WBC count of less than 50,000/mm^3. Cultures are usually negative and require special incubation. In cases of gonococcal arthritis, concomitant *Chlamydia* infection should be considered.

Suggested Readings and References

1. Mathews CJ, Coakley G. Septic arthritis: current diagnostic and therapeutic algorithm. *Curr Opin Rheumatol.* 2008;20:457–462.
2. Kang SN, Sanghera T, Mangwani J, Paterson JM, Ramachandran M. The management of septic arthritis in children: systematic review of the English language literature. *J Bone Joint Surg Br.* 2009;91:1127–1133.
3. Kortekangas P, Peltola O, Toivanen A, Aro HT. Synovial fluid L-lactic acid in acute arthritis of the adult knee joint. *Scand J Rheumatol.* 1995;24:98–101.
4. McCarthy JJ, Dormans JP, Kozin SH, Pizzutillo PD. Musculoskeletal infections in children: basic treatment principles and recent advancements. *Instr Course Lect.* 2005;54:515–528.
5. Rutz E, Brunner R. Septic arthritis of the hip—current concepts. *Hip Int.* 2009;19(suppl 6):S9–12.
6. Horowitz DL, Katzap E, Horowitz S, Barilla-LaBarca ML. Approach to septic arthritis. *Am Fam Physician.* 2011;84:653–660.
7. Mathews CJ, Weston VC, Jones A, Field M, Coakley G. Bacterial septic arthritis in adults. *Lancet.* 2010;375:846–855.
8. García-Arias M, Alejandro Balsa A, Martín Mola E. Septic arthritis. *Best Pract Res Clin Rheumatol.* 2011;25:407–421.
9. Nade S. Septic arthritis. *Best Pract Res Clin Rheumatol.* 2003;17:183–200.
10. Shirtliff ME, Mader JT. Acute septic arthritis. *Clin Microbiol Rev.* 2002;15:527–544.
11. Wilson ML, Winn W. Laboratory diagnosis of bone, joint, soft-tissue, and skin infections. *Clin Infect Dis.* 2008;46:453–457.

12. Margaretten ME, Kohlwes J, Moore D, Bent S. Does this adult patient have septic arthritis? *JAMA.* 2007;297:1478–1488.

13. Baker DG, Schumacher HR Jr. Acute monoarthritis. *N Engl J Med.*1993;329:1013–1020.

14. Li SF, Henderson J, Dickman E, Darzynkiewicz R. Laboratory tests in adults with monoarticular arthritis: can they rule out a septic joint? *Acad Emerg Med.* 2004;11:276–280.

15. Paakkonen M, Peltola H. Management of a child with suspected acute septic arthritis. *Arch Dis Child.* 2012;97:287–292.

Infections of the Hand

Lisa A. Steiner

Summary Box

Disease Description: Early identification and timely treatment can significantly improve the morbidity associated with infections of the hand.

Diagnostic Tests: X-ray, labs, erythrocyte sedimentation rate (ESR)/C-reactive protein (CRP), culture (wound, ± blood)

Treatment: Early antibiotics, incision and drainage, and surgical evaluation

Other Key Issues: Ensure tetanus is up to date.

Disease Description

The severity of hand infections can vary from superficial and easily treated to one involving multiple structures with the possibility of significant morbidity. Hand infections are most often caused by superficial injury or trauma to the hand. In many cases, the injury occurs days before evaluation occurs and treatment begins. Early identification and timely treatment can significantly improve the morbidity associated with infections of the hand. See Table 47.1 for a summary of diseases that affect the hand, which also includes brief description, key diagnostic information, organisms involved, and treatment recommendations.

Epidemiology

Infections of the hand are delineated by the type and location of infection, by whether they are polymicrobial versus single microbial colonization, and by the type of organism. Due to the increasing number of antibiotic-resistant hand infections, a large number are now being identified as methicillin-resistant staphylococcus aureus (MRSA) infections.

Presenting Features

Evaluation of an infection involving the hand must rely on the mechanism of injury as well as the location, progression, and severity of symptoms. Infections of the hand can present with pain, erythema, increased warmth, swelling, drainage, limitations in range of motion, fluctuance, crepitance, and systemic symptoms.

Diagnostic Considerations

In addition to determining the source and mechanism of infection, it is important to identify a number of other aspects, including tetanus immunization status, prior injury to affected area, immune status, occupation, and hand dominance.

The following factors contribute to increased severity and complications of those with hand infections: (human immunodeficiency virus) HIV/AIDS, immunosuppressive medications, diabetes mellitus, and IV drug use.

Complications

Residual effects of infections of the hand include residual joint pain/stiffness, contractures, osteomyelitis, necrotizing fasciitis, amputation, sepsis, flexor tenosynovitis, and death.

Differential Diagnosis

The differential diagnosis of hand infections includes cellulitis, paronychia, felon, bite wound, flexor tenosynovitis, herpetic whitlow, web space infection, deep space infection, open fracture, osteomyelitis.

Diagnostic Tests

X-ray should be performed to rule out foreign body (as the source of infection), fracture (if history suggests trauma), underlying gas (if there is concern for fasciitis), bone changes consistent with osteomyelitis (if infection is longstanding), and joint effusion (if concerned about septic arthritis). Ultrasound can be used to identify deep soft tissue abscess as well as fluid surrounding the tendon and/or tendon sheath in flexor tenosynovitis. Computed tomography and magnetic resonance imaging often are not necessary for diagnosis but can assist in determining the extent of the underlying infection.

Organism

The majority of hand infections are caused by S. aureus and Streptococcus pyogenes. Other sources include Neisseria, Eikenella corrodens, Pasteurella, viruses, and candida. Increasing numbers of S. aureus infections are now being identified as MRSA.

Treatment

Hand infection treatment may include the following:

- Perform appropriate evaluation of the injury/wound and referral to a hand specialist as needed.
- Incision and drainage of all infections in which an abscess has developed (in some cases by the emergency department (ED) staff, or, for more complex cases, by a surgical hand specialist).
- Rest, splinting in the position of comfort, and elevation of the affected hand are adjuncts to antibiotic treatment. Splinting is done for patient comfort, for protection, and to decrease the spread of infection.
- Frequent re-evaluation of wounds, wound marking in the case of cellulitis, and wound packing with clear instructions on when and where to return are important.

Table 47.1 Summary Information about Infectious Diseases Affecting the Hand

Disease	Disease Description	Diagnosis	Diagnostic Tests	Organism	Treatment	Medications:	Disposition
Paronychia	Infection involving the perionychium. History may include nail biting, thumb sucking, recent manicure, trauma, or an occupation in which the hands are frequently wet.	Erythema, swelling, and tenderness along the lateral nail fold. Causes include nail biting, manicure, trauma, and hangnails.	None necessary unless longstanding/untreated infection and concern for osteomyelitis. If concern for osteomyelitis: x-ray, ESR, CRP. If chronic or reoccurring: should consider culture.	S. aureus, Streptococci, Pseudomonas, Gram-negative bacilli, and Escherichia coli Chronic paronychia: consider Candida albicans.	Early infections without abscess formation: • Warm soaks followed by topical triple antibiotic ointment after each soak. Abscess formation: • Drainage of the lateral nail fold separating the paronychial fold away from the nail bed. • Oral antibiotics (in immunocompromised patients and severe infections). • Pain management. • Warm soaks. • Rest and elevation. • Splinting.	Td as needed; Amoxicillin/clavulanate 875 PO q12 h OR Cephalexin, 500 mg PO q6 h OR PCN allergy: Clindamycin, 300 mg PO q8 h; Chronic infections may benefit from topical corticosteroids.	Discharge with clear instructions for return. Patient education regarding preventing reoccurrence.
Herpetic Whitlow	Viral infection of the distal phalanx caused by Herpes simplex virus-1 (HSV-1) or Herpes simplex virus-2 (HSV-2). Lesions are painful; may be a single lesion or multiple with clear vesicular fluid.	The pulp of the finger pad will be soft unlike the tense, swollen pad of a felon.	None usually. May need to add antibiotics if overlying bacterial infection. May send culture or Tzanck smear of the vesicular lesion for confirmation.	Herpes simplex virus-1 or Herpes simplex virus-2.	No surgical treatment. • Antiviral medications for recurrent or frequent episodes. • Pain management. • Rest and elevation. • Splinting.	Acyclovir OR Famciclovir OR Valacyclovir	Discharge with clear instructions for return. Reevaluation in 48–72 hours or sooner as needed.

(continued)

Table 47.1 Continued

Disease	Disease Description	Diagnosis	Diagnostic Tests	Organism	Treatment	Medications:	Disposition
Felon	Closed-space infection of the palmer distal pulp often caused by minor cuts, punctures, and small foreign bodies.	Painful, swollen, tense distal finger pad. Swelling does not extend proximal to the DIP. Due to the likelihood of infection following septa to the periosteum, consider osteomyelitis in longstanding or refractory infections.	If history includes trauma to distal phalanx or if there is concern for foreign body: x-ray. Bedside US may help determine extent and location of abscess formation.	S. Aureus	If early: • Warm soaks and antibiotics. If late: • Drainage of the distal pad with a high lateral incision (not over midline pad). • Oral antibiotics (in immunocompromised patients and severe infections). • Pain management. • Warm soaks. • Rest and elevation. • Splinting.	Td as needed. Amoxicillin/clavulanate 875 PO q12 h OR Cephalexin, 500 mg PO q6 h OR PCN allergy: Clindamycin, 300 mg PO q8 h	Discharge with clear instructions for return. Reevaluation in 48–72 hours or sooner as needed.
Tenosynovitis	Flexor sheath infections most likely caused by penetrating trauma, less often hematogenous spread. Infection of the flexor tendon has 3 stages: • Stage 1: distension of the tendon sheath with exudative fluid • Stage 2: distension of the tendon sheath with purulent fluid • Stage 3: Septic necrosis The infection surrounding the tendon sheath impedes the gliding mechanism by creating adhesions and ultimately destroys the blood supply to the tendons and surrounding structures. Infections extending to the radial or ulnar bursa may occur.	Diagnosis can be identified using Kanavel's 4 cardinal signs: • intense pain with passive extension • flexion posture • uniform swelling • tenderness over flexor sheath	X-ray is used to identify involvement of the underlying bone and to rule out foreign body. Lab work includes CBC w/diff, BMP, ESR, CRP. Blood cultures are indicated if the patient has fever, tachycardia, tachypnea, leukocytosis, or bandemia. US evaluation in both transverse and longitudinal views may show fluid surrounding the tendon.	S. aureus Streptococcus spp. Gram- negative organisms. Atypical: fungal, Mycobacteria. Immunocompromised patients: consider mixed flora, disseminated gonorrhea, or Candida albicans.	Early identification and IV antibiotics in conjunction with elevation, splinting, and frequent re-evaluation. Late presentation or symptoms refractory to 12 hours of treatment require surgical evaluation drainage.	Td as needed; Immunocompetent individuals: Cefazolin, 1–2 g IV q6–8 h; Penicillin-allergic: Clindamycin, 600 mg IV q8 h or Erythromycin, 500–1,000 mg IV q6 h Immunocompromised individuals: Ampicillin-sulbactam 1.5–3 gm IV q6 h OR Cefoxitin 2 g IV q6–8 h; Penicillin-allergic: Clindamycin 600 mg IV q8 h PLUS Levofloxacin 500 mg IV q24 h (for adults)	Observation, admission, or surgical intervention. Ultimately patient will require physical and occupational therapy to reduce disability and return patient to fullest possible function.

Human bite wounds	Mechanism is usually direct bite or "fight bite," which is the result of striking an individual's mouth. The concern is that the usual location of a clenched fist injury occurs over the MCP. Underlying joint capsule, extensor tendon, and bone are close to the surface of the skin and can be disrupted (in up to 75% of cases).	Small puncture or laceration to the MCP joint in a majority of cases but can be anywhere on the hand in the event of a direct bite. Some may not be initially forthcoming regarding mechanism, stressing the importance of knowing if wound was caused by a tooth is vital. Overlying skin will appear as cellulitis, may be a small wound with or without discharge.	X-ray to evaluate for fracture, foreign body (teeth), gas, osteomyelitis (if untreated or late diagnosis)	Most human bite wounds are polymicrobial. • S. aureus • Streptococcus spp • Gram negative organisms • Eikenella corrodens (common in human mouth). • Viruses may also be transmitted through the human bite.	Identify underlying injuries. All human bites should receive prophylactic antibiotics. Wound will need to be evaluated for underlying structural damage and irrigated; often in operative setting. Wounds should not be closed, instead they should be dressed, splinted and elevated with wound check in 24 hours.	Td as needed; Ampicillin-sulbactam 3 g IV q6 h OR Cefoxitin 2 g IV q6–8 h; Penicillin-allergic: Clindamycin, 600 mg IV q8 h PLUS Levofloxacin 500 mg IV q24 h OR Ciprofloxacin 500 mg IV BID; If patient is immunocompromised, an IV drug user, or is failing the above treatment, consider adding Vancomycin (use proper weight- based dosing taking into account CrCl)	Due to the high infection rate and often-late presentation, observation or admission is warranted. If discharge, antibiotics and 24 hour wound check is customary.
Animal bite wounds	Animal bite wounds are common occurrences in the emergency department. Evaluate type of animal, current vaccinations of pet and recent illness or noted strange behavior. Most animal bites are from dogs, but the animal bites with the most complications are from cats. Similar to that of human bites, determine the location (will most often be a puncture).	Patient may present with a wide variety of wounds from large tear, a crush injury or a small puncture. Identifying the mechanism is important. Often the infection may be advanced due to attempted treatment at home as well as the quickly progressing infections in an immunocompromised individual.	X-ray to evaluate for fracture, foreign body (teeth), gas, osteomyelitis (if untreated or late diagnosis)	Animal bites are also polymicrobial. The most common pathogens are: • S aureus • Streptococcus • Gram-negative organisms. • Pasturella Multocida • Anaerobes are also present and should play a role in antibiotic choices.	Bite wounds should be copiously irrigated and may need to be minimally extended in order to do so. Wound should be left open to close by secondary intention. If the wound is large, delayed primary closure can be done if there is no infection present after close monitoring. Facial bite wounds require a plastic surgeon if at all possible. • Antibiotics • Close monitoring	Td as needed; Rabies vaccination as needed; Amoxicillin/davulanate 875 PO q12 h OR Doxycycline 100 mg PO q12 h OR TMP-SMX 1 double strength tab q12 h OR Moxifloxacin 400 mg PO q24 h PLUS	If early: antibiotic prophylaxis and close outpatient monitoring for immunocompetent individuals. If late or immunocompromised, IV antibiotics and close observation to antibiotic therapy.

(continued)

Table 47.1 Continued

Disease	Disease Description	Diagnosis	Diagnostic Tests	Organism	Treatment	Medications:	Disposition
						Metronidazole 500 mg PO q8 h OR Clindamycin 450 mg PO q 8 h; Cefalexin, Dicloxacillin, and Erythromycin should be avoided due to poor efficacy against *P. multocida*; Parenteral antibiotics: Piperacillin/Tazobactam 4.5 g IV q6 h OR Ampicillin-sulbactam 3 g IV q6 h OR Ceftriaxone 1 g IV q24 h PLUS Metronidazole 500 mg IV q8 h OR Ertapenem 1 g IV q24 h	
Deep space infections of the hand	Deep space infections involve the thenar, midpalmer, and the hypothenar spaces as well as the web spaces. Retained foreign body from trauma.	Areas of swelling and tenderness can help identify the location of the infection. Infection in the thenar space causes abduction of the thumb; midpalmer space infection causes swelling and tenderness on the palmar surface that is worsened with extension of the digits.	X-ray to evaluate for fracture, foreign body (teeth), gas, osteomyelitis (if untreated or late diagnosis); Ultrasound can help determine the presence or location of abscess.	• *S. aureus* • *Streptococcus* spp • Gram-negative organisms.	Early infection: • Oral antibiotics. Late infection or infection in immunocompromised • IV antibiotics. • Pain management. • Serial frequent exams. • Warm soaks. • Rest and elevation. • Splinting.	Td as needed; Parenteral Ampicillin/sulbactam 3 g IV q6 h OR Cefazolin 1 g IV q8 h OR PCN allergy: Clindamycin 600 mg IV q8 h	If early: antibiotic prophylaxis and close outpatient monitoring for immunocompetent individuals. If late or immunocompromised, IV antibiotics and close observation to antibiotic therapy

Cellulitis	Inflammation of the skin caused by bacterial seeding without the development of an abscess.	Affected skin with swelling, erythema, increased warmth. Induration without underlying fluctuance.	X-ray to evaluate for gas or osteomyelitis (if untreated or late diagnosis). Ultrasound can help determine if there is complicating abscess.	• *S. aureus* • *S. pyogenes* • Other *Streptococcus* spp • Gram-negative organisms.	Early infection: • Oral antibiotics. Late infection or infection in immunocompromised • IV antibiotics. • Pain management. • Serial frequent exams. • Warm soaks. • Rest and elevation. • Splinting.	Td as needed; Oral: Amoxicillin/clavulanate 875 PO q12 h OR Cephalexin 500 mg PO q6 h; PCN allergy: Clindamycin 300 mg PO q8 h Parenteral: Ampicillin/sulbactam 3 g IV q6 h OR Cefazolin 1 g IV q8 h; PCN allergy: Clindamycin 600 mg IV q8 h	Physical therapy and occupational therapy to ensure as close to pre-infectious function as possible.
Necrotizing soft tissue infections	Limb threatening soft tissue infection that is rapidly progressive, has early systemic signs and symptoms, and has high mortality rate. Risk factors include IV drug use, alcohol abuse, homelessness, diabetes, immunosuppression, and traumatic injuries.	Because cellulitis and necrotizing skin infections can initially present similarly, it is important to quickly identify this aggressive infection. Symptoms include significant pain, which may be out of proportion to initial exam. Initially leukocytosis and azotemia may precede hypotension and ultimately shock. Crepitus and rapid progression are keys to diagnosis.	Diagnostic tests should not delay the initiation of cultures, antibiotics, and surgical intervention, which yields definitive diagnosis and treatment. Labs should include CBC, CMP, Lactate, Cultures (blood), CRP, ESR, CK, PT, and PTT.	Currently there are two types of necrotizing soft tissue infections. Type 1 is polymicrobial: alpha- and beta-hemolytic streptococci, *S. aureus*, and anaerobes. Type 2 is most commonly caused by group A *Streptococcus*.	Early infection: • Oral antibiotics. Late infection or infection in immunocompromised • IV antibiotics. • Pain management. • Serial frequent exams. • Warm soaks. • Rest and elevation. • Splinting.	Td as needed; Vancomycin (use proper weight-based dosing taking into account CrCl) PLUS Piperacillin/Tazobactam 4.5 g IV q6 h OR Cefepime 1 g IV q8 h PLUS Clindamycin 600–900 mg IV q8 h; Severe PCN allergy: Vancomycin (use proper weight-based dosing taking into account CrCl) PLUS Ciprofloxacin 400 mg IV q8 h PLUS Clindamycin 600–900 mg IV q8 h	Physical therapy and occupational therapy to ensure as close to preinfectious function as possible

(continued)

Table 47.1 Continued

Disease	Disease Description	Diagnosis	Diagnostic Tests	Organism	Treatment	Medications:	Disposition
Septic arthritis	The majority of septic joints of the hand are the result of trauma to the hand/joint. Another cause is hematogenous spread in individuals who are at higher risk: immunocompromised, injection drug users, those with indwelling catheters, undergoing recent surgery, with rheumatoid arthritis, in the extremes of age (elderly > 80 years and neonates).	Presenting symptoms include a single joint that is exquisitely painful with motion, swelling, erythema, and increased warmth.	X-ray may identify underlying trauma or foreign body. Lab work including CBC, BMP, ESR, CRP. Synovial fluid analysis to include culture, gram stain, cell count, and crystal analysis.	Mmost common: • S. aureus • Streptococcus • Neisseria gonorrhoeae should be considered in an atraumatic septic joints. Polymicrobial septic joints are usually caused by trauma or intravenous IV drug use.	Early broad spectrum antibiotics and surgical evaluation. Depending on location, duration, and severity, washout of the joint may be necessary. Elevation, splinting in position of comfort, and pain management are all adjuncts to antibiotics and consultation.	Td as needed; Vancomycin (use proper weight- based dosing taking into account CrCl) PLUS Piperacillin/Tazobactam 4.5 g IV q6 h OR Cefepime 1 g IV q8 h PLUS Clindamycin 600–900 mg IV q8 h OR Severe PCN allergy: Vancomycin (use proper weight- based dosing taking into account CrCl) PLUS Ciprofloxacin 400 mg IV q8 h PLUS Clindamycin 600–900 mg IV q8 h	Physical therapy and occupational therapy to ensure as close to pre-infectious function as possible.

Abbreviations: BMP, basic metabolic panel; CBC, complete blood count; CMP, comprehensive metabolic panel; CK, creatine kinase; CRP, C-reactive protein; DIP, distal interphalangeal joint;ESR, erythrocyte sedimentation rate; h, hours; IV, intravenous; MCP, metacarpal phalangeal joint; PCN, penicillin; PO, oral administration; PT, prothrombin time; PTT, partial thromboplastin time; Td, tetanus vaccine; US, ultrasound.

First- and second-line antibiotic treatment recommendations for hand infections are listed in the Table 47.1. Due to the increasing frequency of antibiotic-resistant organisms, antibiotic choice is vital. Observation of a patient with a hand infection is valuable to evaluate both the progression of an infection or its response to treatment.

Disposition

Disposition varies when discussing the wide variety of hand infections. Paronychia, felon, herpetic whitlow, and some early cases of cellulitis can be treated in the ED and discharged with close follow-up. Infections caused by bite wounds, those with involvement of tendons, and deep space abscesses will require observation, admission, or the operating room depending on their severity. Disposition should always take into account a patient's comorbidities, such as diabetes, immunosuppression, injection drug use, inability to follow up for re-evaluation, and inability to fill antibiotic prescriptions after discharge.

Suggested Readings and References

1. McDonald LS, Bavaro MF, Hofmeister EP, Kroonen LT. Hand infections. *J Hand Surg*. 2011;36A:1403–1412.
2. Brook I. Paronychia: A mixed infection: microbiology and management. *J Hand Surgery Br*. 1993;18:358.
3. O'Malley M, Fowler J, Ilyas AM. Community-acquired methicillin-resistant staphylococcus aureus infections of the hand: prevalence and timeliness of treatment. *J Hand Surg*. 2009;34A:504–508.
4. Marvel BA, Budhram GR. Bedside ultrasound in the diagnosis of complex hand infections: a case series. *J Emerg Med*. 2015;48:63–68.
5. Clark DC. Common acute hand infections. *Am Fam Physician*. 2003;68:2167–2176.
6. Tosti R, Samuelsen BT, Bender S, et al. Emerging multidrug resistance of methicillin-resistant staphylococcus aureus in hand infections. *J Bone Joint Surg Am*. 2014;96:1535–1540.
7. Fleisher GR. The management of bite wounds. *N Engl J Med*. 1999;340:138–140.
8. Ray GT, Suaya JA, Baxter R. Incidence, microbiology, and patient characteristics of skin and soft-tissue infections in a U.S. population: a retrospective population-based study. *BMC Infect Dis* 2013;13:252.

Chapter 48

Prosthetic Joint Infections

David Mabey, Hasan E. Baydoun, Jamil D. Bayram

Summary Box

Disease Description: Of all prosthetic joints, 1% to 3% will become infected. Fever, joint pain, erythema, effusion, and joint loosening are common presenting features of prosthetic joint infection (PJI).

Diagnostic Tests:

- X-ray
- ESR (erythrocyte sedimentation rate)/CRP (C-reactive protein)
- CBC (complete blood count) with differential
- Imaging (see following)
- Arthrocentesis and culture*
- ^{99m}Tc (radiolabeled technetium) and ^{111}I Nuclear Scanning*
- Intraoperative frozen section and culture*

Organisms:

- Early infection: most commonly *Staphylococcus aureus* (approximately half of which is methicillin-resistant *Staphylococcus aureus* [MRSA]) or gram-negative bacilli
- Delayed infection: less virulent organisms, such as coagulase-negative Staphylococci or *Propionibacterium acnes*
- Late infection: most common are *S. Aureus, Streptococcus* spp., Gram-negative bacilli, and anaerobes

Treatment:

- Antibiotics (see "Treatment" following)
- Orthopedic consultation and admission
- Prosthesis exchange vs retention with early surgical washout and debridement

Other Key Issues: Those with PJI generally require admission for appropriate management.

*In general, these diagnostic modalities should be pursued by the orthopedic surgeons who will be managing the patient's definitive care. Primary and acute care providers should avoid performing or requesting these studies in patients with a suspected prosthetic joint infection without first consulting the definitive care team and instead should refer these patients for admission.

Disease Description

PJI represents a devastating complication of joint replacement surgery, often requiring prolonged hospitalization, additional surgical procedures, and long-term antibiotics. The estimated average cost of care for an infected prosthetic joint is $96,000. Fortunately, there have been many advances that decrease the risk of infection, such as the use of perioperative antimicrobial prophylaxis and intraoperative laminar airflow, which reduces the risk of surgical infection.

Epidemiology

Overall, 1% to 3% of all prosthetic joints will become infected. In patients with primary joint replacement, the infection rate in the first 2 years is usually < 1% in hip and shoulder prostheses, < 2% in knee prostheses, and < 9% in elbow prostheses. In some studies, the risk of infection in those with joint replacement revision is 10 times higher than the risk of the primary joint replacement; incidences of joint revision infection ranges from 5% to 45%. Among revision joint replacements, the rate of infection in revision prostheses is four times higher in those who underwent revision for infectious versus aseptic complications of the primary prosthesis.

Presenting Features

Presenting signs and symptoms of PJI are related to the subtype of infection: early, delayed, or late.

Early infections are the most common subtype, accounting for up to 90% of PJI. By definition, early infections manifest within 3 months of joint replacement. Patients present with the classic findings of fever, acute-onset joint pain and erythema, joint effusion and warmth, and swelling at the implant site. Cellulitis and the formation of a sinus tract with purulent discharge may occur.

Delayed infections occur 3 to 24 months following surgery. Symptoms are indolent and often non-specific (ie, persistent moderate pain). This may explain why delayed prosthetic infections are often overlooked as the cause of chronic joint pain. Although patients usually have an elevated ESR and CRP, leukocytosis may be absent, and patients may remain afebrile.

Late infections occur more than 2 years after surgery and are often due to hematogenous spread from dermatologic, respiratory, dental, or urinary tract infections. Patients usually complain of sudden, local joint pain and systemic symptoms. Depending on the causative microorganism, patients with late infections may present with a more indolent course like those with delayed infection.

Diagnostic Considerations

Patient characteristics that increase the risk of developing PJI include diabetes mellitus, rheumatoid arthritis, psoriasis, malignancy, corticosteroid use, obesity, recurrent urinary tract infection, and an immunocompromised state. Important features of the medical history include comorbidities, history of immunodeficiency, trauma to the joint, the surgical timeline (particularly surgery duration), whether the joint in question contains a primarily placed or a revision prosthesis, and if the indication for the joint replacement procedure was infectious or aseptic.

Complications

Complications for PJI are related to the destruction of local tissue, as well as joint loosening and failure. In addition, there is a risk of systemic spread and sepsis.

Differential Diagnosis

Other conditions that may confound the diagnosis of PJI include aseptic joint loosening, cellulitis, and bone fracture.

Diagnostic Tests

Although there are no definitive criteria for diagnosing PJI, the gold standard is culture and histopathology taken from at least three intraoperative biopsy sites, which should include any grossly abnormal sites, the interface between the bone and the prosthesis, and the interface between the anchoring cement and bone. Intraoperative frozen section has a positive predictive (PPV) value of 100% and a negative predictive value (NPV) of 73%. Thus, it can be used to rule in PJI but not to rule it out. These interventions should be handled by the operating surgeon or the orthopedic team admitting the patient. The main diagnostic tests for PJI that are utilized by acute and primary care providers are listed below and ultimately can lead to admission for definitive surgical diagnosis.

Imaging

Plain radiographs are most useful in identifying the presence of an infection if studied serially after implantation. Even if previous radiographs are not available, however, radiography is still widely accepted as a first-line imaging modality. This is because radiographs, despite not providing a definitive diagnosis in most cases, are able to detect or rule out numerous noninfectious sources of joint pain and joint failure. Evidence of infection that can be identified on plain radiographs includes prosthetic migration, periosteal reaction, osteopenia, osteolysis, and transcortical sinus tracts at the bone-cement or bone-prosthesis interface. However, aseptic migration of the implant (especially if uncemented) and aseptic periprosthetic osteolysis can also occur, which limits the ability of radiographs to definitively diagnose infection.

Computed tomography provides better contrast between normal and abnormal tissue when compared to plain radiography, but artifacts caused by metal implants limit its use.

Magnetic resonance imaging (MRI) can be performed in patients with non-ferromagnetic implants (eg, titanium or tantalum) that are safe for MRI with minimal artifact and good tissue resolution for the detection of soft tissue pathology.

Radionuclide scans have become the imaging modalities of choice for diagnosing PJI. One study of ^{99m}Tc and ^{111}I bone scanning revealed a PPV of 30% and a NPV of 88% while another study of ^{99m}Tc and ^{111}I-labeled leukocyte scan revealed a PPV of 54% and a NPV of 95%. In general, the high NPV of both the bone scan and the labeled leukocyte scan make them useful in ruling out PJI; however, these tests cannot reliably diagnose infection due to their poor PPV.

Laboratory Evaluation

Leukocytosis and bandemia are not accurate enough to predict the presence or absence of infection.

ESR and *CRP* are inflammatory markers that are much more accurate than leukocytosis, but they have variable characteristics. An ESR of greater than 30 mm/hour has a sensitivity of 61% to 96% and a specificity of 79% to 100%. CRP of greater than 10 mg/L has a better sensitivity of 91% to 96% and specificity of 88% to 92%. In general, the high sensitivity and specificity of CRP and ESR make them valuable tools for establishing or ruling out PJI.

In one prospective study of 202 hip replacements, for example, the probability of PJI when both ESR and CRP were within normal limits was 0 percent, and the probability of PJI with positive ESR and positive CRP was 83%. However, CRP and ESR can both be elevated postoperatively as well as in various other inflammatory conditions, such as rheumatologic disease. CRP levels typically return to normal within 3 weeks after surgery, whereas ESR levels can remain elevated as long as 1 year postoperatively. Thus, CRP proves more useful for diagnosing PJI in a recent postoperative patient. Additionally, CRP levels show less variability among patients, so a single CRP level provides more reliable diagnostic information than a single ESR level, which typically needs to be followed serially within a given patient to establish a trend. In general, serial levels of both CRP and ESR are superior to isolated values.

Joint Fluid Analysis: In general, joint fluid sampling should only be performed by the orthopedic team. Cell count, differential, and culture can be very useful. Depending on the cutoff values chosen to define an abnormal result, sensitivity and specificity for PJI range from 56% to 75% and 95% to 100%, respectively. One study of 168 synovial fluid specimens found that a leukocyte count of greater than a cutoff of 1,760 cells/µL yielded a sensitivity and specificity of 90% and 99%, respectively. In that same study, a neutrophil percentage of greater than 73% was also suggestive of PJI, with a sensitivity and specificity of 93% and 95%, respectively. Joint fluid cultures have a sensitivity and specificity of 90% and 97%, respectively, and they provide the additional benefit of microbial speciation and antibiotic sensitivities. However, prior antimicrobial treatment decreases the sensitivity of cultures.

In suspected cases of PJI during the first few weeks postoperatively, joint fluid analysis can help clarify whether increases in ESR and CRP are due to PJI or a normal physiologic response to surgery. Of note, cultures of sinus tracts should not be performed due to the risk of contamination from the surrounding skin flora. Unless specifically trained in joint fluid aspiration, acute and primary care providers should consult the appropriate service (eg, orthopedics or rheumatology) to perform this diagnostic procedure (see Figure 48.1).

Organisms

Microbiology

Organisms causing prosthetic joint infections often grow in biofilms, which make them difficult to treat. Biofilms create a physical barrier both to antibiotics and to the host immune response. Additionally, many of the organisms inside the biofilm are in a sessile state, so they are less susceptible to antibiotics. Biofilms serve as a nidus of chronic infection, so treatment for chronic PJI must eradicate the biofilm. This typically requires surgery. Sequestra, which are islands of bone that are devitalized by infection, also represent a protected nidus of infection because the lack of circulation within sequestra prevents the adequate delivery of immune cells and antibiotics to fight infection.

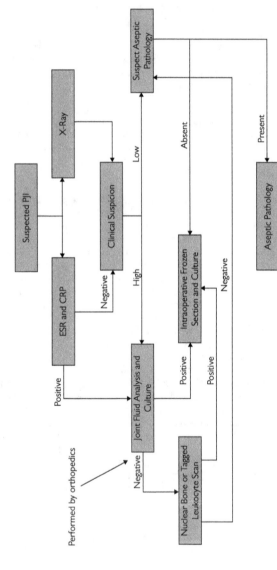

Figure 48.1 Suggested Approach to a suspected prosthetic joint infection.

S. aureus, about half of which is methicillin resistant, is the most common cause of PJI, accounting for over 50% of cases. Other Gram-positive and Gram-negative bacilli account for 20% to 25% of infections. Anaerobes, including P. acnes, account for another 10%. In addition, P. acnes is the most common cause of infected total shoulder arthroplasties. Between 10% and 30% of PJI are polymicrobial. These polymicrobial infections are associated with poorer outcomes, as are S. aureus infections.

To a degree, the type of infection correlates to the organisms involved. Early infections are commonly caused by the more virulent microorganisms, such as S. aureus and Gram-negative bacilli, whereas delayed PJI is often caused by less virulent agents, such as coagulase-negative Staphylococci and P. acnes. Late PJI is often due to hematogenous spread from skin, respiratory, dental, and urinary tract infections. The most frequently isolated bacterium is S. aureus, followed by Streptococcus, Gram-negative bacilli, and anaerobes.

Treatment

Orthopedic surgeons should be consulted as early as possible because effective treatment requires both surgical intervention and antibiotic administration. Surgical treatment options include one or two-stage prosthesis exchange, debridement with retention of the prosthesis, resection arthroplasty, arthrodesis, or amputation.

Antibiotic therapy should be continued for 3 months following surgical debridement, and therapy should be guided by intraoperative cultures and decided on in consultation with the infectious disease service. Intravenous treatment should be administered for the first 2 to 6 weeks, followed by oral therapy. Oral therapy is continued to give a total of 3 months of antibiotic therapy in hip replacements and 6 months in knee replacements.

Intravenous antibiotic therapy decreases the sensitivity of both arthrocentesis and cultures, limiting the ability to narrow antibiotic coverage. For this reason, empiric antibiotics should be reserved for septic patients. In these patients, broad spectrum antibiotics, usually a combination of rifampin plus vancomycin and cefepime (or piperacillin/tazobactam) is a reasonable choice. In stable patients, intravenous therapy should be guided by Gram stain and culture. When combined with rifampin 450 mg IV q12 hours, acceptable initial treatments for stable patients include the following regimens:

Negative or unavailable gram stain: vancomycin 15 mg/kg IV q12 hours plus ceftriaxone 1 g IV q24 hours
Gram-positive cocci: vancomycin 15 mg/kg IV q12 hours
Gram-negative rods: ceftriaxone 1 g IV q12 hours, cefepime 2 g IV q8 hours, or piperacillin-tazobactam 3.375 to 4.5 g IV q6 to 8 hours
Patients with penicillin allergy: aztreonam 1 to 2 g IV q8 hours

As for oral antibiotics, rifampin (450 mg PO q12 hours) is commonly used in PJI because of its increased bone and biofilm penetration. However, it must always be combined with another drug, such as a quinolone (levofloxacin 750 mg PO q24 hours or ciprofloxacin 750 mg PO q12 hours), to prevent resistance. Because of increasing resistance to quinolones, co-trimoxazole, minocycline, and fusidic acid have also been used in combination with rifampin with good results. Linezolid and daptomycin are also active against gram-positive bacteria, including MRSA.

Other Key Issues

Disposition
Consult the orthopedic service for any patient in whom PJI is suspected. These patients generally require admission to an orthopedic inpatient service.

Pediatric Considerations
PJI is rare in pediatrics because prosthetic joint replacement in this age group is uncommon. When infections do occur, infectious disease consultation is even more important than in adults.

Suggested Readings and References

1. Osom DR, Berendt AR, Lew D, et al. Diagnosis and management of prosthetic joint infection: clinical practice guidelines by the Infectious Diseases Society of America. Clin Infect Dis. December 6, 2012. doi:10.1093/cid/cis803.
2. Widmer AF. New developments in diagnosis and treatment of infection in orthopedic implants. Clin Infect Dis. 2001;33(suppl 2):S94–106.

3. Peel TN, Cheng AC, Buising KL, Choong PF. Microbiological etiology, epidemiology, and clinical profile of prosthetic joint infections: are current antibiotic prophylaxis guidelines effective? *Antimicrob Agents Chemother.* 2012;56:2386–2391.

4. Edward JR, Peterson KD, Mu Y, et al. National Healthcare Safety Network (NHSN) report: data summary for 2006 through 2008, issued December 2009. *Am J Infect Control.* 2009;37:783–805.

5. Shuman EK, Urquhart A, Malani PN. Management and prevention of prosthetic joint infection. *Infect Dis Clin North Am.* 2012;26:29–39.

6. Aslam S, Darouche RO. Prosthetic joint infections. *Curr Infect Dis Rep.* 2012;14:551–557.

7. Del Pozo JL, Patel R. Clinical practice: infection associated with prosthetic joints. *N Engl J Med.* 2009;361:787–794.

8. Westberg M, Grogaard B, Sorrason F. Early prosthetic joint infections treated with debridement and implant retention. *Acta Orthop.* 2012;83:227–232.

9. Costerton JW, Stewart PS, Greenberg EP. Bacterial biofilms: a common cause of persistent infections. *Science.* 1999;284:1318–1322.

10. Maduka-Ezeh AN, Greenwood-Quaintance KE, Karau MJ, et al. Antimicrobial susceptibility and biofilm formation of *Staphylococcus epidermidis* small colony variants associated with prosthetic joint infection. *Diagn Microbiol Infect Dis.* August 14, 2012. doi:10.1016/j.

11. Zimmerli W, Widmer AF, Blatter M, et al. Role of rifampin for treatment of orthopedic implant-related staphylococcal infections: a randomized controlled trial. Foreign-Body Infections (FBI) Study Group. *JAMA.* 1998;279:1537–1541.

12. Schäfer P, Fink B, Sandow D, Margull A, Berger I, Frommelt L. Prolonged bacterial culture to identify late periprosthetic joint infection: a promising strategy. *Clin Infect Dis.* 2008;47:1403–1409.

13. García-Arias M, Balsa A, Mola EM. Septic arthritis. *Best Pract Res Clin Rheumatol.* 2011;25:407–421.

14. Kaandorp CJ, Dinant HJ, van de Laar MA, et al. Incidence and sources of native and prosthetic joint infection: a community based prospective survey. *Ann Rheum Dis.* 1997;56:470–475.

15. Koeppe J, Johnson S, Morroni J, Siracusa-Rick C, Armon C. Suppressive antibiotic therapy for retained infected prosthetic joints: case series and review of the literature. *Infect Dis Clin Pract.* 2008;16:224–229.

16. Trampuz A, Zimmerli W. Prosthetic joint infections: update in diagnosis and treatment. *Swiss Med Wkly.* 2005;135:243–251.

17. Suarez J, Griffin W, Springer B, Fehring T, Mason JB, Odum S. Why do revision knee arthroplasties fail? *J Arthroplasty.* 2008;23(6): 99–103.

18. Mortazavi J, Schwartzenberger J, Austin MS, Purtill JJ, Parvizi J. Revision total knee arthroplasty infection: incidence and predictors. *Clin Orthop Relat Res.* 2010;468: 2052–2059.

19. Bori G, Soriano A, Garcia S, Mallofre C, Riba J, Mensa J. Usefulness of histological analysis for predicting the presence of microorganisms at the time of reimplantation after hip resection arthroplasty for the treatment of infection. *J Bone Joint Surg Am.* 2007;89:1232–1237.

20. Parvizi J, Ghanem E, Menashe S, Barrack RL, Bauer, TW. Periprosthetic infection: what are the diagnostic challenges? *J Bone Joint Surg.* 2006 88(suppl 4):138–147.

21. Larson S, Thelander U, Friberg S. C-reactive protein (CRP) levels after elective orthopedic surgery. *Clin Orthop Relat Res.* 1992;275:237–242.

22. Greidanus NV, Masri BA, Garbuz DS, et al. Use of erythrocyte sedimentation rate and C-reactive protein level to diagnose infection before revision total knee arthroplasty: a prospective evaluation. *J Bone Joint Surg.* 2007;89:1409–1416.

23. Spangehl MJ, Masri BA, O'Connell JX, Duncan CP. Prospective analysis of preoperative and intraoperative investigations for the diagnosis of infection at the sites of two hundred and two revision total hip arthroplasties. *J Bone Joint Surg Am.* 1999;81:672–683.

24. Bauer TW, Parvizi J, Kobayashi N, and Krebs V. Diagnosis of periprosthetic infection. *Am J Bone Joint Surg.* 2006;88: 869–882.

Osteomyelitis

Lisa A. Steiner

Summary Box

Disease Description: Osteomyelitis is an infectious process that affects any part of the bone, including the periosteum, the cortex, or the marrow. Depending on the time course of the infection, it can be an acute, subacute, or chronic process. Osteomyelitis is often characterized by its source: contiguous or hematogenous spread of bacterial infection or the consequence of vascular insufficiency.

Diagnostic Tests: X-ray, complete blood count (CBC), erythrocyte sedimentation rate (ESR), C-reactive protein (CRP) ± magnetic resonance imaging (MRI) and computed tomography (CT)

Organisms: Most commonly *Staphylococcus aureus*; also, *Streptococcus* species, gram-negative bacilli, *Pseudomonas aeruginosa*, and *Staphylococcus epidermidis*

Treatment: Broad spectrum empiric antibiotic treatment should begin immediately if the patient is unstable or if there are no immediate plans to obtain bone biopsy.

Consider oxacillin 1 to 2 g IV q6 hours; if methicillin-resistant *S. aureus* (MRSA) is suspected, consider vancomycin 25 mg/kg (initial dose), then 15 mg/kg IV q12 hours* and cefepime 2 g IV q8 hours. If chronic osteomyelitis is suspected, consider vancomycin as well as piperacillin-tazobactam 3.375 to 4.5 g IV q6 hours.

Other key issues: Consult appropriate services (eg, orthopedics and infectious diseases) for long-term management and biopsy.

*Adjust for creatinine clearance CrCl.

Disease Description

Osteomyelitis is an infectious process affecting one or more portions of bone, including the periosteum, the cortex, or the marrow. The infection often results in bone destruction, as the inflammatory process increases intramedullary pressure, which can cause necrosis of the periosteum, the cortex, or marrow. Osteomyelitis is often the result of contiguous spread or hematogenous spread of infection. A third category of osteomyelitis originates from vascular insufficiency, usually occurring in patients with diabetes mellitus and some degree of neuropathy who develop a soft tissue foot infection that extends to the bone.

In addition, osteomyelitis can be described as an acute, subacute, or chronic process depending on the time course of the infection. Although the time course classification can sometimes be arbitrary, the distinction can be important, as acute osteomyelitis can be successfully treated with appropriate antibiotics. In contrast, chronic osteomyelitis can be associated with significant bone necrosis, sometimes requiring months to years of treatment with antibiotics as well as surgical debridement.

Epidemiology

Contiguous infections occur most often and onset begins when an organism is introduced directly to the bone. Examples include trauma, open fractures, bone surgery, and joint replacements. Trauma and open fractures usually result in polymicrobial infection, whereas surgery or joint replacements often result in monomicrobial infections.

Hematogenous osteomyelitis occurs when the organism is spread from another location; this is more common in children but does occur in adults, especially the elderly or those who have risk factors, such as central venous catheters, dialysis, urinary tract infections, or intravenous drug use.

Osteomyelitis related to vascular insufficiency most frequently occurs in patients with diabetes mellitus and sickle cell disease.

Several of the following conditions can increase the risk of developing osteomyelitis: diabetes mellitus, malignancy, sickle cell disease, acquired immunodeficiency disorder, intravenous drug use, steroid use, alcoholism, malnutrition, tobacco use, osteoarthritis, lymphedema, venous stasis, open fractures, and orthopedic surgeries.

Osteomyelitis can involve any bone, but it most often occurs in lower extremities.

Presenting Features

Presenting features vary based upon the location of the infection, the host state, and the severity of the infection. Acute osteomyelitis presents gradually, beginning with dull pain and then progressing to tenderness. There is often warmth of the overlying skin, fatigue, malaise, swelling, fever, and rigors. When the site of infection is located near or involves a joint, the presentation can be similar to that of a septic joint. Some of the previously noted signs may be masked when infection is located in the hips, pelvis, or vertebrae.

Subacute infections may present only with pain and without systemic symptoms.

Chronic osteomyelitis can present with pain, erythema, and swelling. In patients with a sinus tract and associated draining or discharge, chronic osteomyelitis must be considered.

Immobility of an affected area may be a presenting feature in any form of osteomyelitis.

Complications

Untreated, undertreated, and undiagnosed osteomyelitis can have significant ramifications. Associated tissues and joints can become involved, pathologic fractures can occur, and infections can spread to the blood, resulting in sepsis. Individuals with osteomyelitis of a long bone have a greater chance of developing deep vein thrombosis. Those with vertebral involvement can have associated neurologic involvement.

Diagnostic Tests

Laboratory evaluation

Lab work for suspected osteomyelitis includes CBC, ESR, and CRP. Testing should be initiated during the patient's presentation and repeated throughout treatment as ESR and CRP are helpful for following the infection over time. If there is a concern for joint involvement, gram stain, culture, cell count, and crystal analysis should be obtained.

It is best to obtain blood cultures in stable patients before antibiotics are administered. Wound cultures should not be obtained from the surface of the skin but, instead, should be reserved for intraoperative wound exploration, drainage, and biopsy. Consultants may be able to obtain a bone culture to help identify the offending organisms and their sensitivities in individuals who do not have positive blood cultures.

Imaging

Standard x-rays may initially be negative during an early presentation. In some cases, plain films of the affected areas can help to identify soft tissue swelling, joint effusions, periosteal reaction/elevation, or cortical or medullary lucencies. More sensitive studies include CT and MRI, as these can detect earlier evidence of bone destruction as well as cortex and marrow changes. CT and MRI can also help to identify the extent of a sinus tract and help to better characterize overlying abscesses. In patients with vertebral osteomyelitis, MRI should be considered. If the patient has hardware that precludes the use of CT or MRI, the next study of choice is a bone scan.

Organism

Microbiology

It is vital to identify the organism(s) as well as antibiotic susceptibility to ensure effective and complete treatment. The most commonly seen pathogens are S. aureus, Streptococcus species, gram-negative bacilli, P. aeruginosa (often seen in IV drug users), and S. epidermidis (seen in postsurgical and diabetic foot infections). For individuals with sickle cell anemia, S. aureus and Salmonella should be considered. S. aureus is the most common causative agent of osteomyelitis. Recently, MRSA has become a concern and should be considered as a potential agent. Both S. aureus and S. epidermidis can form biofilms, which resist antibiotic penetration.

Treatment

Empiric antibiotic treatment should begin immediately if the patient is unstable or if there is no immediate plan to obtain a bone biopsy. Antibiotic choice is based on location, type of inciting injury, and patients' comorbidities. Initial antibiotic therapies are listed in Table 49.1 and should cover both gram-positive and gram-negative organisms. Once an organism has been identified, antibiotic choice and dosing should be adjusted accordingly and should be continued for 4 to 8 weeks. The patient's tetanus immunization status should be verified.

Disposition

Consultation with orthopedic service (or spine service for vertebral osteomyelitis) should be considered. Vascular service consultation should occur if there is a concern for osteomyelitis of the foot in a patient with diabetes mellitus. These patients often require admission to the hospital for follow up

Table 49.1 Initial Antibiotic Therapy for Osteomyelitis		
Organism	First Line	Second Line
MSSA	Oxacillin 1–2 g IV q6 h	Cefazolin 1 g IV q8 h
MRSA	Vancomycin 25 mg/kg (initial dose), then 15 mg/kg IV q12 h* And Cefepime 2 g IV q8 h	Oxacillin 2 g IV q4 h Or Nafcillin 2 g IV q4 h And Ceftazidime 2 g IV q8 h
Chronic or severe osteomyelitis	Vancomycin 25 mg/kg (initial dose) then 15 mg/kg IV q12 h* And Piperacillin-tazobactam 3.375–4.5 g IV q6 h Or Ampicillin/sulbactam 3 g IV q6 h Or Ciprofloxacin 400 mg IV q8 h	Vancomycin 25 mg/kg (initial dose) then 15 mg/kg IV q12 h* And Cefepime 2g IV q8 h Or Piperacillin-tazobactam 3.375–4.5 g IV q6 h

Abbreviations: MSSA, methicillin-sensitive *Staphylococcus aureus*; MRSA, methicillin-resistant *Staphylococcus aureus*; CrCl, creatinine clearance; IV, intravenous; h, hours.
*Adjust for CrCl.

of culture and sensitivity, parenteral antibiotics, serial exams, and possible operative debridement and biopsy.

Suggested Readings and References

1. Gentry L. Management of osteomyelitis. *Int J of Antimicrob Agents.* 1997;9:37–42.

2. Lew DP, Waldvogel FA. Osteomyelitis. *Lancet.* 2004;369–379.

3. Roesgen M, Hierholzer G, Hax PM. Post-traumatic osteomyelitis: pathophysiology and management. *Arch Orthop Trauma Surg.* 1989;108(1):1–9.

4. Lew DP, Waldvogel FA. Osteomyelitis. *N Engl J Med.* 1997;336:999.

5. Pineda C, Vargas A, Rodriguez AV. Imaging of osteomyelitis: current concepts. *Infect Dis Clin North Am.* 2006;20:789–825.

6. Sammak B, Abd El Bagi M, Al Shahed M, et al. Osteomyelitis: a review of currently used imaging techniques. *Eur Radiol.* 1999;9:894–900.

7. Wheat J. Diagnostic strategies in osteomyelitis. *Am J Med.* 1985;78:218–224.

8. Black J, Hunt TL, Godley PJ, Matthew E. Oral antimicrobial therapy for adults with osteomyelitis or septic arthritis. *J Infect Dis.* 1987;155:968.

9. Spellberg B, Lipsky BA. Systemic antibiotic therapy for chronic osteomyelitis in adults. *Clin Infect Dis.* 2012;54:393.

10. Lew DP, Waldvogel FA Osteomyelitis. *Lancet.* 2004;364(9431):369–379.

Vector-Borne Infections

Chapter 50

Lyme Disease

Zach Smith

Summary Box

Disease Description: Lyme disease is a tick-borne illness caused by *Borrelia burgdorferi*. It causes a range of symptoms over days to months, including rash, constitutional symptoms, arthritis, and neurologic or cardiac abnormalities.

Organism: *B. burgdorferi* is a spirochete that is transmitted by the deer tick *Ixodes scapularis* in the United States.

Treatment:

Oral first line: Doxycycline 100 mg TID for 14 to 21 days for adults, 1 to 2 mg/kg BID for children over 8 years

   Pregnant/lactating women: Amoxicillin 500 mg TID for 14 to 21 days

   Children under age 8: Amoxicillin 50 mg/kg/day divided TID

Oral second line: Cefuroxime axetil 500 mg TID for 14 to 21 days, 30 mg/kg per day divided BID for children

Parenteral: Ceftriaxone 2 g daily for 14 to 28 days for adults, 75 to 100 mg/kg/day for children; or Penicillin G 18 to 24 million units/day divided every 4 hours for adults, 200,000 to 400,000 units/kg/day divided every 4 hours for children.

Other Key Issues: *B. burgdorferi* is not thought to be transmitted via transfusion. It can, however, be transmitted in pregnancy through the placenta to the fetus if mothers are not treated effectively. *Ixodes scapularis* can transmit *Theileria microti*, which is the vector of babesiosis, and *Anaplasma phagocytophilum*, which leads to human granulocytic anaplasmosis (HGA).

Epidemiology

Transmitted by *I. scapularis* ("deer tick"), Lyme Disease (LD) is caused by the spirochete *B. burgdorferi* and is the most common vector-borne zoonotic infection in the United States. In 2011, there were over 24,000 confirmed cases. The two major geographic foci are the Northeast and upper Midwest, with a significant number of cases also occurring in the mid-Atlantic region. LD has been reported in all 48 continental states, Alaska, and even worldwide. Most cases occur in the warmer months, both because outdoor activity is highest and nymphal tick activity is at its peak.

Presenting Features

LD presents in three stages: primary, early disseminated, and tertiary disseminated. Notably, each stage is highly variable in onset and presentation, and symptoms may manifest across multiple stages.

The primary stage begins as a localized infection at the site of the tick bite. Most commonly, the nymphal form of the tick attaches to the skin and inoculates *B. burgdorferi* during feeding. Symptoms begin 7 to 10 days later. The most common presenting symptom is erythema migrans (EM), which is seen in up to 80% of patients. EM skin lesions occur at the site of the tick bite and appear as an expanding, red macule that spreads in a centrifugal pattern over days to weeks. Lesions are frequently seen at the belt line or in the axillary, inguinal, or popliteal region. Lesions are not painful, but they may burn or itch and are often warm to the touch. EM may reach a diameter of 20 cm and often demonstrates a bull's eye appearance. Although the Centers for Disease Control and Prevention surveillance criteria require a diameter of at least 5 cm, smaller EM lesions may be found. If treated with antibiotics, EM fades within days. Untreated lesions typically persist for 28 days. However, the range is broad, so lesions may persist for months.

Constitutional symptoms are common in LD; because they are nonspecific, however, early LD may go undiagnosed. This is particularly common if EM is not identified or if the patient does not recall a tick bite (only 25% of patients report bite). In a review of 79 patients with culture-confirmed EM, the following symptoms were reported: fatigue (54%), anorexia (26%), headache (42%), neck stiffness (35%), myalgias (44%), arthralgias (44%), regional lymphadenopathy (23%), and fever (16%).[1] Less common symptoms include sore throat, abdominal pain, nausea, and vomiting. Headache with photophobia and neck stiffness may occur. However, meningeal findings are absent, and cerebrospinal fluid (CSF) studies are normal.

In the primary stage, laboratory studies are typically normal, but patients may have an elevated sedimentation rate, elevated creatinine phosphokinase, anemia, thrombocytopenia, and leukopenia or leukocytosis.

The secondary stage, also called early disseminated infection, has a variable onset, ranging from days to weeks after the tick bite. Cutaneous manifestations are common in this stage and are characterized by multiple annular lesions that are smaller than those found in the early stage; these usually spare the palms, soles, and mucous membranes. Neurologic symptoms may be present in 15% of patients. Among these, a fluctuating meningoencephalitis is the most common finding, but other neurologic manifestations include cranial neuropathy (most commonly unilateral or bilateral Bell's palsy), peripheral neuropathy, and radiculopathy. As in the early stage of LD, headache, nausea, vomiting, and lethargy are common; meningeal signs are typically absent. In contrast to the primary stage, CSF studies may show a lymphocytic pleocytosis and elevated protein.

Cardiac involvement occurs in up to 8% of patients. It presents as myopericarditis with varying degrees of atrioventricular block, which may require temporary pacemaker placement. Symptoms preceding diagnosis include palpitations, chest pain, lightheadedness, or shortness of breath. Rarely, ocular abnormalities occur in early disseminated infection, including conjunctivitis, optic neuritis, keratitis, uveitis, and even blindness.

Tertiary disseminated or late stage infection occurs months to years after the initial tick bite and is characterized primarily by joint complaints. It typically involves arthritis of the larger joints (with a predilection for the knee) and can be either monoarticular or asymmetric polyarticular in distribution. Prior data suggest 60% of untreated patients with Lyme disease may develop monoarticular or oligoarticular arthritis. Of this population, 10% may have a persistent monoarthritis affecting the knee.[2] Exacerbations become less frequent over years, and chronic arthritis is less common now because Lyme disease is more commonly identified and treated at an earlier stage.

Neurologic symptoms in tertiary disease are widely variable and often difficult to diagnose due to their similarity to other chronic neurologic diseases. Subtle symptoms include changes in mood, memory, cognition, and sleep. Together, these have been labeled "Lyme encephalopathy." A chronic axonal poly-neuropathy may also be present with radicular pain and distal parasthesias. These patients will uniformly have abnormal CSF studies.

"Post Lyme disease syndrome" describes nonspecific symptoms, such as fatigue, headache, and body aches, that 10% to 20% of patients experience after appropriate treatment with antibiotics for Lyme disease. The Infectious Disease Society of America recommends the following criteria for defining this syndrome: 1. Prior history of Lyme disease treatment with an acceptable regimen with initial symptom resolution 2. Onset of subjective symptoms (fatigue, musculoskeletal pain, and/or cognitive distur-bances) within 6 months of treatment and lasting more than 6 months. These patients have normal labs and CSF studies. There is no current evidence that these symptoms are related to active infection, and further antibiotic treatment is not indicated.[3]

Diagnostic Tests

Diagnosis of early LD with EM is made on clinical grounds alone, and patients with consistent skin find-ings who live in an endemic area should be treated without serological testing.

For patients being evaluated for early disseminated or late disease, the recommended initial laboratory test is the enzyme-linked immunosorbent assay (ELISA). ELISA tests for immunoglobulin (Ig) G (IgG) and IgM response to antigens of whole Borrelial organisms. It has a sensitivity of 89% and specificity of 72%, which yields many false positives. Positive or equivocal ELISA tests may be confirmed with the more specific Western blot. Patients with a positive ELISA but a negative Western blot do not have Lyme disease and do not require treatment. Conversely, patients with late disease uniformly have a positive Western blot.

The limitations of ELISA are due to the variability in host antibody response to B. burgdorferi and the high rates of false-negative and false-positive results. Typically, IgM antibody titers peak 6 weeks after illness onset and return to normal within 10 to 12 weeks after the onset of symptoms. Alternatively, the IgM response may persist for months or years despite treatment; because IgM antibodies can persist, serologic testing for IgM is not a reliable indicator of recent inoculation. IgG antibodies peak around 12 months and are present in late disease, but they may be detected as early as 2 months after the tick bite or seen in patients who have been effectively treated.

It is recommended to send serological testing on patients who live in or have recently traveled to endemic areas, who have risk factors for a tick bite, and who have symptoms of early disseminated or late LD. Follow up serology after appropriate treatment is not recommended. False-positive ELISA results are possible when serology cross reacts with other similar antigens, such as other Borrelial diseases (relapsing fever), spirochete infection (syphilis), other active infections (infective endocarditis, Epstein-Barr virus, malaria), and autoimmune disease. Up to 5% of the population may have a false-positive ELISA test.

Culture of B. burgdorferi from blood, tissue, or body fluids is not helpful. Polymerase chain reaction (PCR) is more useful in identifying B. burgdorferi DNA, but PCR only has a 20% sensitivity in CSF testing, causing a high rate of false negatives. A Lyme urine antigen test exists but is not recommended due its unreliability.

Organisms

I. scapularis has a life cycle of 2 years, and it exists in four stages: egg, larva, nymph, and adult male or female. After the egg hatches, each stage requires a blood meal to survive. When the tick attaches to its host, it inserts a feeding tube, which has barbs and secretes saliva with cement-like properties and anesthetic capabilities. The tick will feeds for several days until it detaches, falls off, and begins the next stage of its life cycle. If a tick feeds on an organism infected with LD, it may become infected itself and subsequently infect future hosts.

The white-footed mouse is the reservoir for B. burgdorferi and is the most common blood meal for the larval stage of I. scapularis. The nymphal tick is the most active life form in the late spring and summer, and it is the most common form to infect humans, who are more likely to be active outside during this time. Due to its small size, the nymphal tick is often not identified, and therefore is able to remain attached for the time necessary to transmit infection. The white-tailed deer is a common blood meal for adult ticks, and migra-tion of deer into suburban areas increases the spread of infected ticks among areas where humans live.

Treatment

If a tick is found attached to human skin and removed within the first 72 hours, the likelihood of infection with *B. burgdorferi* is low. In endemic areas, patients suspected of having a tick attached for at least 36 hours with signs of engorgement should receive a single dose of 200 mg doxycycline, which is effective in preventing LD (pediatric dose is 4 mg/kg). When LD is diagnosed, treatment varies depending on the stage and severity of symptoms. One must keep in mind that patients with early stages of LD are often seronegative, so the decision to treat is clinical. A history of a tick bite plus EM is a clear indication for antibiotics. Although treatment is not urgent, early antibiotics may reduce the severity and duration of symptoms.

In the primary or secondary stages, oral doxycycline 100 mg BID for 14 to 21 days is recommended for adults, and 1 to 2 mg/kg BID is recommended for children over age 8. In pregnant or lactating women, amoxicillin 500 mg TID for 14 to 21 days can be used. In children under 8 years, amoxicillin 50 mg/kg/day divided TID (maximum dose of 500 mg/dose) is appropriate. Cefuroxime axetil is also effective at a dose of 500 mg BID for 14 to 21 days in adults and 30 mg/kg/day divided BID for children. Macrolides are less effective, but they can be used if the patient is intolerant or allergic to doxycycline and penicillin.

In Lyme meningitis, ceftriaxone 2 g IV daily for 14 to 28 days in adults and 75 to 100 mg/kg/day for children should be used. Alternative medications include doxycycline, penicillin G, or cefotaxime. For patients with isolated facial nerve palsy (Bell's palsy) and no signs of meningitis, oral doxycycline is adequate. If patients with facial nerve palsy have headache or neck stiffness, strongly consider elective lumbar puncture, and use IV ceftriaxone for patients with abnormal findings.

For mild cardiac disease (asymptomatic patients with PR interval of < 300 ms), the same regimen used for primary and secondary LD can be used. For severe cardiac disease (second- or third-degree heart block, first-degree block with PR > 300 ms, or symptomatic patients), ceftriaxone at the same dosing as for meningitis can be used. Ceftriaxone or penicillin G may also be used as a parenteral option for arthritis found in late disease.

Typically, patients have resolution of symptoms within 20 days, although nonspecific subjective symptoms of fatigue, muscle pain, and headache may persist for weeks to months.

Other Key Issues

A vaccine is not available at this time. There is no transmission of LD through people, food, or water. There are no known cases of contraction through blood transfusion; however, *B. Burgdorferi* has been identified as living in stored donated blood. If acquired during pregnancy, LD can be transmitted through the placenta to the fetus. If mothers are treated effectively, no known harm to the fetus has been identified.

Finally, *I. scapularis* can transmit other parasitic infections, including *T. microti*, which is the vector of babesiosis, and *A. phagocytophilum*, which leads to human granulocytic anaplasmosis (HGA). Babesiosis is seen in 2% to 40% of patients with Lyme disease and HGA in 2% to 12% of patients, complicating the diagnosis and treatment.[4]

Suggested Readings and References

1. Nadelman RB, Nowakowski J, Forseter G, et al. The clinical spectrum of early Lyme borreliosis in patients with culture-confirmed erythema migrans. *Am J Med*. 1996;100:502.

2. Steere AC, Schoe RT, Taylor E. The clinical evolution of Lyme arthritis. *Ann Intern Med*. 1987;107:725

3. Halperin JJ. Prolonged Lyme disease treatment: enough is enough. *Neurology*. 2008;70:986.

4. Wormser GP. Clinical practice early Lyme disease. *N Engl J Med*. 1996;354:2794.

Chapter 51

Ehrlichia, Anaplasma, and Rickettsia

Susan Tuddenham

Summary Box

Disease Description: *Ehrlichia* and *Anaplasma* are tick-borne infections that present with an abrupt, febrile, and flu-like illness along with headache, nausea, vomiting, and abdominal pain. These diseases show significant similarity, often with elevated liver function tests (LFTs), leukopenia, and thrombocytopenia. Rash is less common in *Anaplasma* infections but accompanies approximately 30% of *Erlichia* infections. Severe infections and complications are more common with Human Monocytic Ehrlichiosis (HME, caused by *E. chaffeensis*) than Human Granulocytic Anaplasmosis (HGA, caused by *A. phagocytophilum*) or Human Ewingii Ehrlichiosis (HEE, caused by *E. ewingii*). Rickettsial diseases generally present with a febrile illness accompanied by headache and rash. Patients may have elevated LFTs, thrombocytopenia, leukocytosis, and, occasionally, leukopenia. In particular, Rocky Mountain spotted fever (RMSF) and typhus can lead to very serious disease, including shock, multiorgan failure, pulmonary edema, acute respiratory distress syndrome (ARDS), myocarditis, and encephalitis with delirium and coma.

Organisms:
> *Ehrlichia* and *Anaplasma*: *E. chaffeensis*, *E. ewingii*, *E. muris* (not seen in the United States), *Ehrlichia* Wisconsin HM543746 (recently identified and currently unnamed), and *Anaplasma phagocytophilum*.
> *Rickettsial* species: *R. rickettsii* (RMSF), *R. australis* (Australian tick typhus), and *R. parkerii*. The typhus bacteria proper group includes *R. prowazekii* (epidemic typhus) and *R. typhi* (murine/endemic typhus). The scrub typhus group (no longer classified within the *Rickettsia* genus) includes *Orientia tsutsugamushi* (not seen in the United States).

Treatment:
> **Oral first line:** Doxycycline
> **Second line:** *Rickettsia*: Tetracycline, ciprofloxacin, and chloramphenicol
> *Anaplasma* and *Ehrlichia*: Rifampin
> **Parenteral:** Doxycycline

Other Key Issues: Diagnostic tests for all of these organisms are imperfect. If disease is suspected, empiric treatment should be started without delay because some patients may progress rapidly to fulminant disease. Note that the lack of a rapid response to doxycycline in a patient with suspected HGA should prompt consideration of coinfection with *Babesia* (which is not cured by doxycycline) and/or reconsideration of the diagnosis of HGA.[1] Coinfection with HGA and Lyme disease can be treated with doxycycline.[2]

Disease Description

Epidemiology

Ehrlichia and Anaplasma

E. chaffeensis occurs across the south-central, southeastern, and mid-Atlantic states, as does *E. ewingii*.[2] Cases of *E. chaffeensis* are most commonly reported in Missouri, Oklahoma, Tennessee, Arkansas, and Maryland.[3]

A. *Phagocytophilum* is found in the Northeastern, mid-Atlantic, upper Midwest, and Pacific Northwest states, including California. It is also found in Europe and in parts of Asia, including China, Russia, and Korea. *E. muris* is found in Eastern Europe, Japan, and is very similar to a new *Ehrlichia* species found recently in Wisconsin and Minnesota.

Rickettsia

R. rickettsia (ie, RMSF) is seen in South and Central America, the desert regions of the Southwestern United States, the northern Pacific coast, the upper Midwest, New England, Southern and southeastern United States, and southern Canada.[4]

R. parkerii is seen in the eastern and southern United States, particularly along the coast.[5]

R. typhii is seen in the Southwestern United States, particularly along the border with Mexico, as well as in Hawaii.[6]

R. prowazekii is very rare in the United States but has occurred in some rural and suburban areas of the eastern United States. A case has also been reported in California.[7]

Presenting Features

HME, HEE, and HGA

Ehrlichia and *Anaplasma* infections present similarly with abrupt, febrile, and flu-like illness often accompanied by elevated LFTs, leukopenia, and thrombocytopenia. Most of the *Ehrlichia* cases reported to the Centers for Disease Control and Prevention have onset of illness during the summer months, so any patient presenting with the preceding constellation of symptoms and laboratory abnormalities in a region with endemic ticks should be evaluated for *Ehrlichia* and *Anaplasma*. Note that only 68% of patients with Ehrlichiosis report a specific history of tick bite within 14 days of illness onset, so the absence of this history does not rule out infection.[3] A meta-analysis comparing patients with HME and HGA found common symptoms, signs, and laboratory findings, which are roughly summarized and found in Table 51.1.

Rickettsia

Rickettsial disease can present similarly to *Ehrlichia* and *Anaplasma* infections with a febrile illness and headache as well as elevated transaminases, thrombocytopenia, leukopenia, or leukocytosis.[3] The classic

Table 51.1 Percentages of Patients with Symptoms and Lab Findings Associated with HME and HGE

Symptom, Sign or Lab Finding	HME*	HGA*
Fever	+++++	+++++
Myalgia	+++	++++
Malaise	+++++	+++++
Headache	++++	++++
Vomiting	++	++
Diarrhea	++	+
Nausea	++++	++
Cough	++	+
Rash	++	+
Stiff neck	+	++
Confusion	+	+
Leukopenia	++++	+++
Thrombocytopenia	++++	++++
Elevated AST or ALT	+++++	++++

Abbreviations: HME, Human Monocytic Ehrlichiosis; HGA, Human Granulocytic Anaplasmosis; AST, aspartate aminotransferase; ALT, alanine transaminase.
*Percentages: 0–20 +, 21–40 ++, 41–60 +++, 61–80, ++++, 81–100 +++++.

286

clinical triad for RMSF includes fever, headache, and rash. This triad is present in less than 5% of patients in the first 3 days of illness but is seen in 60% to 70% by the second week of illness. The rash of rickettsial disease is characteristically centripetal (ie, beginning in the extremities and progressing toward the trunk) and develops in most patients between the 3rd and 5th days of illness. Detection of a skin rash may be difficult in dark-skinned individuals, and rash is completely absent in 10% of RMSF cases. Rickettsial diseases other than RMSF are often associated with a "tache noir," or dark eschar at the inoculum site.[5]

The source of these skin findings is rickettsial infection of endothelial cells, causing vasculitis, which can lead to potentially life-threatening damage to the brain, lungs, and other vital organs in addition to rash. In particular, RMSF as well as typhus can lead to very serious disease, including shock, multiorgan failure, pulmonary edema, ARDS, myocarditis, and encephalitis with delirium and coma. RMSF itself can present with widespread endothelial and microangiopathic thrombosis.[4] Because of the potential for a rapidly lethal illness in those affected by RMSF, therapy should not be delayed while awaiting diagnostic tests.

Hyponatremia is the most common biochemical disturbance in RMSF, occurring in up to half of all cases. Elevated creatinine, blood urea nitrogen, and creatinine kinase can be seen as well.

Diagnostic Considerations/ Diagnostic Tests

HME, HEE, and HGA

Diagnosis can be challenging, and empiric treatment should not be delayed while confirmatory testing is pending. Wright-stained peripheral blood smears may show morulae (intracytoplasmic inclusions) in monocytes (HME) or neutrophils (HGA and HEE). Note that the absence of morulae does not rule out disease, as morulae are present at presentation in less than 10% of cases of HME and only 25% to 75% of reported cases of HGA. Also, treatment with doxycycline decreases the sensitivity of blood smear for both infections.[2]

Polymerase chain reaction (PCR) tests exist but are not available everywhere. The sensitivity of PCR is reported to be about 60% to 85% for HME and 67% to 90% for HGA. PCR can also be done for HEE. Note that doxycycline treatment decreases PCR sensitivity. Culture of E. chaffeensis and Anaplasma is possible, but the cell culture techniques that are required are not generally available in most clinical laboratories.[2]

Serologic diagnosis with detection of a fourfold change in antibody titer during the convalescent phase of illness is the most sensitive way to confirm the diagnosis of HME or HGA, although like rickettsial infections, this is of limited utility during the acute presentation. Therefore, a negative serologic test early in the infection cannot be used to exclude the diagnosis. It is important to note that serologic testing is complicated by the fact that there is a background of high seroprevalence rates in asymptomatic individuals in some geographic regions, that IgG antibodies can persist for months or years after infection, and that a number of other diseases can be associated with false-positive serologic tests.[2]

Rickettsia

Because of the potential for a rapidly lethal illness in those affected by Rickettsia in general and RMSF in particular, therapy should not be delayed while awaiting diagnostic tests. Confirming a clinical diagnosis of rickettsial disease through laboratory tests can be challenging. Diagnosis of rickettsial infection is not possible from blood smears, as it may be confused with Ehrlichia or Anaplasma infection. The Weil-Felix test lacks adequate sensitivity and specificity and is no longer recommended. Serologic diagnosis is the gold standard for the diagnosis of rickettsial diseases, and indirect fluorescent antibody testing is commonly used. Unfortunately, as with Ehrlichia and Anaplasma, this is not generally useful in acute illness. Sensitivity is poor in the first 10 to 12 days of symptoms, although it increases to 94% if a convalescent serum sample is obtained from days 14 through 21. Therefore, it can be useful in confirming a diagnosis of rickettsial disease later in the clinical course.[4] A fourfold increase in titer in paired samples, or a convalescent titer greater than 1:64, is considered diagnostic.[8] Cross reactivity between the different rickettsial diseases is very common, so it is difficult to distinguish between them based on antibodies alone.[4]

There are other options for testing. Direct immunofluorescence or immunoperoxidase tests specific to R. rickettsii can be done on skin biopsies of the rash or from formaldehyde-fixed tissues. This has an approximate sensitivity and specificity of 70% and 100%, respectively. Blood cultures for Rickettsia species are sensitive and specific. However, neither of these tests is generally available outside of specialized centers.[4]

Typical Disease Course/Complications

Infections with Ehrlichia and Anaplasma may be mild and self-limited but may also present with more serious complications. Approximately 40% of patients with HME and 33% to 50% of patients with HGA require hospitalization. Immunocompromised patients are at higher risk for severe complications. HME infections are frequently more severe than HGA infections (17% of identified patients with HME suffer a life-threatening complication versus 7% of patients with HGA). A fulminant syndrome similar to septic shock can develop, as can respiratory distress, pneumonia, and ARDS; again, this is more common in HME than HGA. Meningoencephalitis or meningitis is seen more commonly in HME, but peripheral neuropathies are more common in HGA and may persist for months. Fatalities occur in around 3% of reported HME infections and 0.7% of HGA. HEE appears to have far fewer complications than those from HME and HGA.[2]

Rickettsial infections, particularly those from RMSF, can be life threatening. The mortality rate for RMSF is thought to be approximately 20% for those who are untreated and 5% among those treated, although the accuracy of these numbers may be affected by unreported disease. The rash in RMSF is related to small vessel vasculitis, and may rarely be complicated by frank skin hemorrhage, larger areas of skin necrosis, or even gangrene. Digital infarction can rarely occur. Pulmonary vasculitis, edema, and ARDS can occur. Neurologic symptoms, including focal neurologic deficits, meningismus, confusion, or meningoencephalitis can occur. Renal impairment, sometimes requiring dialysis, is common in severe RMSF and is usually due to a combination of acute tubular necrosis from hypotension, intravascular thrombosis, and interstitial vascular inflammation. Multiorgan failure, including respiratory and cardiac failure, can occur with severe RMSF.[4]

Organisms

Microbiology/ Life Cycle

Both *Ehrlichia* and *Anaplasma* are transmitted by ticks. *E. chaffeensis* is transmitted by *Amblyomma americanum* (the Lone Star Tick) and possibly by other tick vectors, such as *Dermatocenter variabilis*. The white-tailed deer is the major host of lone star ticks and is a natural reservoir for *E. chaffeensis*. *E. ewingii* is also transmitted by *A. americanum*, although infection has principally been reported in dogs.[3] *Ehrlichia* Wisconsin HM543746 is likely transmitted by the *Ixodes scapularis* (ie, deer tick).[9] *Anaplasma* is also transmitted by *I. scapularis* as well as *I. pacificus*, the same vectors that transmit *Borrelia burgdorferi* (ie, Lyme disease). *Babesia* species can also be transmitted by *I. scapularis* and is seen as a coinfection with *B. burgdorferi* and *Anaplasma*. Deer, elk, and wild rodents are thought to be the primary reservoirs.[3] When transmitted to humans via a tick bite, *E. chaffeensis* has a predilection for monocytes, whereas *A. phagocytophilum* and *E. ewingii* usually infect granulocytes. The causative agents multiply in cytoplasmic membrane-bound vacuoles as microcolonies called morulae.[3]

R. rickettsii: In the eastern, central, and Pacific coastal United States, *D. variabilis* (ie, American dog tick) is the primary vector of *R. rickettsii*. In the western United States, *Dermacentor andersoni* (ie, Rocky Mountain wood tick) is an important vector. *Rhipicephalus sanguineus* (ie, Brown dog tick) has been implicated in Arizona and is an important vector in Mexico. *Amblyomma cajennense* (ie, cayenne tic) is an important vector in Central and South America and has also been implicated in Texas.[3]

R. typhi (ie, endemic/murine typhus) is transmitted by fleas. Outbreaks are usually limited to southern Texas, Southern California, and Hawaii. It is transmitted by the *Xenopsylla cheopis* (ie, rat flea) and *Ctenocephalides felis* (ie, cat flea).[6]

R. prowazekii (ie, epidemic typhus) is the classically spread by *Pediculus humanus corporis* (ie, body louse). In the United States, it appears that the reservoir may be flying squirrels.[7]

Treatment

Ehrlichia and Anaplasma

Doxycycline 100 mg PO or IV every 12 hours for symptomatic adult patients is the preferred first-line treatment for both Ehrlichiosis and Anaplasmosis. Tetracycline is an alternative, although it is more poorly tolerated and must be dosed every 6 hours. Pregnant patients have been successfully treated in the past with rifampin, but such patients should be carefully monitored for treatment response. Antibiotic therapy should be continued for 3 to 5 days after fever subsides.[2] The minimum total course is usually 5 to 7 days, although severe or complicated disease may require longer courses of up to 14 days. Patients with HGA may be treated with doxycycline for 10 to 14 days to cover possible coinfection with *B. burgdorferi*.[3] Lack of a rapid response to doxycycline in a patient with suspected HGA should prompt consideration of coinfection with *Babesia* and/or reconsideration of the diagnosis of HGA.

Rickettsia

Doxycycline is also the preferred agent for Rickettsial infections, and the dosage is the same as for *Ehrlichia* and *Anaplasma* infections. Tetracycline is an alternative. Chloramphenicol can be used to treat RMSF in pregnant women or patients with serious hypersensitivity reactions to tetracyclines. However, data on the efficacy of chloramphenicol in humans is limited, and data from in vitro and animal models suggests that it is significantly less effective than doxycycline in patients with RMSF. Treatment times for rickettsial diseases are similar to those for *Ehrlichia* and *Anaplasma*. Treatment should be continued for at least 3 days after the patient defervesces.[4]

Suggested Readings and References

1. Wormser GP, Dattwyler RJ, Shapiro ED, et al. The clinical assessment, treatment, and prevention of lyme disease, human granulocytic anaplasmosis, and babesiosis: clinical practice guidelines by the Infectious Diseases Society of America. *Clin Infect Dis.* 2006;43(9):1089–1134.

2. Dumler JS, Madigan JE, Pusterla N, Bakken JS. Ehrlichioses in humans: epidemiology, clinical presentation, diagnosis, and treatment. *Clin Infect Dis.* 2007;45(suppl 1):S45–51.

3. Chapman AS, Bakken JS, Folk SM, et al. Diagnosis and management of tickborne rickettsial diseases: Rocky Mountain spotted fever, ehrlichioses, and anaplasmosis—United States: a practical guide for physicians and other health-care and public health professionals. *MMWR Recomm Rep.* 2006;55(RR-4):1–27.

4. Chen LF, Sexton DJ. What's new in Rocky Mountain spotted fever? *Infect Dis Clin North Am.* 2008;22(3):415–432, vii–viii.

5. Paddock CD, Finley RW, Wright CS, et al. Rickettsia parkeri rickettsiosis and its clinical distinction from Rocky Mountain spotted fever. *Clin Infect Dis.* 2008;47(9):1188–1196.

6. Outbreak of Rickettsia typhi infection—Austin, Texas, 2008. *MMWR Morb Mortal Wkly Rep.* 2009;58(45):1267–1270.

7. Epidemic typhus associated with flying squirrels—United States. *MMWR Morb Mortal Wkly Rep.* 1982;31(41):561–562.

8. Dantas-Torres F. Rocky Mountain spotted fever. *Lancet Infect Dis.* 2007;7(11):724–732.

9. Pritt BS, Sloan LM, Johnson DK, et al. Emergence of a new pathogenic Ehrlichia species, Wisconsin and Minnesota, 2009. *N Engl J Med* 365:422–429.

Malaria and Dengue Fever

Dana Mueller

Summary Box

Malaria

Disease Description: Vector-borne parasitic illness characterized by acute fever, headache, chills, and vomiting.

Uncomplicated: symptomatic malaria without evidence of vital organ dysfunction

Complicated: symptomatic malaria with severe anemia, metabolic acidosis, and respiratory distress; or cerebral malaria

Organisms: *P. falciparum, P. vivax, P. ovale, P. malariae*

Treatment: Artemisinin-based combination therapy (ACT) is almost always indicated, as are antipyretics and supportive treatment.

First line: Artemisinin-based therapy (4 mg/kg per day) for 3 days with long-acting second agent for 7 days (7 days of coverage total)

Second line: Quinine + clindamycin for 7 days

Parenteral: Artesunate is available in intramuscular and rectal forms. Quinine and artemether are also available in intramuscular preparations.

Other Key Issues: Country-specific recommendations for prophylaxis can be found in the Centers for Disease Control and Prevention (CDC)'s annual Health Information for International Travel (also known as the "Yellow Book") Protection against mosquito bites, such as protective clothing, usage of bed nets, and insect repellent is important to consider along with prophylactic medications.

Disease Description

Epidemiology

World Malaria Report estimates that in 2012, there were 207 million cases of malaria with an estimated 627,000 deaths worldwide. Mortality rates have dropped significantly since the year 2000. Most deaths occur among children living in Africa. Parasites are spread to people through the bites of infected *Anopheles* mosquitoes. Adults in endemic areas are likely to have an uncomplicated course due to malaria tolerance developed through exposure to malarial antigens before the maturation of their immune system. In contrast, if nontolerant travelers acquire an infection abroad, they are at high risk of progressing to fatal, severe malaria, often at parasite loads that would produce only mild symptoms in endemic citizens.

Presenting Features

Malaria presents as an acute febrile illness. Initial symptoms are nonspecific: fever, headache, chills, and vomiting. *P. falciparum* can progress rapidly to severe illness, so history and clinical suspicion are essential for diagnosis.

Diagnostic Considerations

Diagnosis requires clinical suspicion. Confirmation requires an appropriate history and parasites in the blood. Cerebral malaria rarely presents with signs of meningeal irritation.

Typical Disease Course

In the nontolerant, symptoms generally appear 7 to 15 days after the infective bite. If untreated, the cycle of fevers, chills, and sweats may recur repeatedly. Cerebral malaria presents secondary to severe *P. falciparum* infection with neurologic manifestations (most often coma with Glasgow Coma Score <11). Other complications include respiratory distress and severe anemia.

Diagnostic Tests

The World Health Organization (WHO) recommends that all cases of suspected malaria be confirmed with parasite-based diagnostic testing before initiating treatment. Parasitological diagnosis can result in 15 minutes or less, and the modality of diagnosis depends on availability. Confirmatory diagnosis is based on microscopic (thick or thin smear) or rapid diagnostic testing.

Organisms

Plasmodium are protozoan parasites. *P. falciparum, P. vivax, P. ovale,* and *P. malariae* are the only *Plasmodium* species that are infectious to humans. *P. falciparum* and *P. vivax* are the most common forms. *P. falciparum* is also the most deadly. Infected mosquitos spread sporozoites into the host blood stream, which then invade host hepatocytes. Intra-hepatocyte maturation of schizonts (which can take up to 2 years) results in the release of thousands of merozoites, which can infect host red blood cells. Within the erythrocyte, the merozoite develops into a gametocyte, which can then be transmitted to the appropriate vector mosquito, or into an erythrocytic schizont, which can release merozoites that are capable of infecting other red blood cells (see Figure 52.1).

Treatment

Treatment should be initiated after diagnosis is confirmed. In the absence or delay of parasitological diagnosis beyond 2 hours of presentation, treat empirically if severe malaria is suspected. Medications must attack the causes of clinical malaria while also eliminating the parasite's inactive forms. They must be active against schizontocides, gametocytocides, and merozoitocides. Thus, the current first-line recommendation is for schizontocidal ACT combined with a longer-acting, second-line medication that will eliminate the gametocyte and merozoite forms. There is no difference in efficacy between the different formulations of ACT, although fixed-dose combination pills are preferred. When patients are unable to tolerate oral medications, there are parenteral preparations. Artesumate is available in intramuscular and rectal forms. Quinine and artemether are also available in intramuscular preparations. However, a standard oral course should be initiated when gastrointestinal symptoms resolve.

Other Key Issues

During the first trimester of pregnancy, treatment regimens should consist of quinine and clindamycin. Person-to-person transmission can occur via sharing of blood products or during pregnancy. Vertical

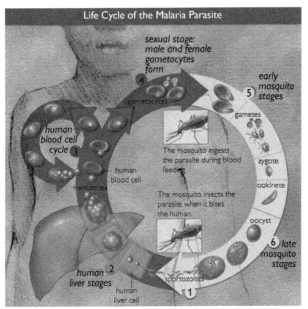

Figure 52.1 The "Life Cycle of the Malaria Parasite," differentiating between the parasite's development inside the mosquito vector and development inside the human host, specifically inside the liver hepatocytes and red blood cells circulating in the blood. Image by National Institute of Allergy and Infectious Diseases from CDC.gov. Public Health Image Library (PHIL). https://www.niaid.nih.gov/topics/Malaria/Pages/lifecycle.aspx

transmission appears to be most common in semi-immune populations. It is possible to contract malaria even while on prophylactic medications because resistance is widespread. Preventing transmission is very important, as are malaria prophylaxis medications. Country-specific recommendations for prophylaxis can be found in the CDC's annual Health Information for International Travel (also known as the "Yellow Book") Protection against mosquito bites—such as protective clothing, usage of bed nets, and insect repellent—is important to consider along with prophylactic medications.

Suggested Readings and References

1. Baron S, ed. *Medical Microbiology*. 4th ed. Galveston, TX: University of Texas Medical Branch at Galveston; 1996.
2. Bisoffi Z, Gobbi F, Angheben A, Van den Ende J. (2009). Role of rapid diagnostic tests in managing malaria. *PLoS Med*. 6(4):e1000063.
3. Malaria. About malaria. Biology. Centers for Disease Control and prevention website. http://www.cdc.gov/malaria/about/biology/index.html. 2010.
4. Enyati A, J. Hemingway. Malaria management: Past, present, and future. *Annu Rev Entomol*. 2010;55:569–591.
5. World Health Organization Malaria [Fact sheet]. http://www.who.int/mediacentre/factsheets/fs094/en/index.html. 2012.

Summary Box

Dengue Fever

Disease Description: Vector-borne viral infection that causes a flu-like illness with occasionally lethal complications.

Organisms: Four serotypes of the *Flavivirus dengue virus* may cause dengue fever (DEN-1, DEN-2, DEN-3, and DEN-4).

Treatment: There is no specific treatment for dengue fever. All treatment is supportive and may range from oral rehydration to intravenous fluid administration and vasopressor support. Aspirin and nonsteroidal anti-inflammatory drugs (NSAIDs) for the management of fever and arthralgias are contraindicated in this population.

Disease Description

Epidemiology

Dengue fever is primarily seen in tropical and sub-tropical regions, particularly in urban and semi-urban areas. The vector for dengue fever, the *Aedes* mosquito, breeds mostly in manmade containers. The incidence of dengue fever has increased thirtyfold in the last 50 years, likely due to increased urbanization, population growth, international travel, and global warming. The WHO currently estimates that there may be up to 100 million *dengue virus* infections annually and that 40%of the world population may be at risk of infection. Severe dengue fever is becoming more prominent, with endemic status now reached in more than 100 countries. Most patients with dengue fever recover without residual problems, and mortality is low with appropriate treatment. Still, there are an estimated 500,000 cases of severe dengue fever that require hospitalization each year. Many of these cases occur in children. By some estimates, up to 5% of those affected die, even with appropriate treatment. Without treatment, mortality is estimated at 20% to 25%.

Presenting Features

The hallmark of a *dengue virus* infection is a high fever (at least 40°C) accompanied by at least two of the following symptoms: severe headache, retro-orbital pain, myalgias, arthralgias, nausea, vomiting, swollen glands, or rash.

Diagnostic Considerations

See Table 52.1.

Disease Course

An incubation period of 4 to 10 days following an infected *Aedes* mosquito bite is typical. Symptoms usually last for 2 to 7 days. In most cases, infection is self-limited. After resolution, the patient will have lifelong immunity against the infecting serotype. The patient will remain susceptible to the other three infecting serotypes, however. In some cases, severe dengue develops as a complication 3 to 7 days after the onset of symptoms. Severe dengue is characterized by severe bleeding, hypotension, and respiratory distress due to plasma leakage and fluid accumulation. End organ damage is not uncommon. The initial 24 to 48 hours after the development of complications can be deadly. In individuals who have already been infected with one serotype, a second infection seems to result in an increased risk of developing severe dengue (formerly dengue hemorrhagic fever) and dengue shock syndrome (DSS). This increased risk is thought to be due to antibody-dependent enhancement.

Table 52.1 Suggested Dengue Classification and Levels of Severity[a]

CRITERIA FOR DENGUE + WARNING SIGNS		CRITERIA FOR SEVERE DENGUE
Probable dengue	**Warning signs***	**Severe Plasma leakage leading to:**
Lives in / travel do Dengue endemic area, Fever and 2 of the following criteria:	• Abdominal pain or tendermess	• Shock (DSS)
• Nausea and vomiting	• Persistent vomiting	• Fluid occumulation with respiratory distress
• Rash	• Clinical fluid accumulation	
• Aches and pains	• Mucosal bleed	**Severe bleeding**
• Tourniquet test positive	• Lethargy, restlessness	as evaluated by clinician
• Leukopenia	• Liver enlargement >2 cm	
• Any warning sign	• Laboratory: Increase in HCT concurrent with rapid decrease in platelet count	**Severe organ involvement**
		• Liver: AST or ALT >= 1000
Laboratory-confirmed dengue		• CNS: Impaired consciousness
(Impartant when no sign of plasma leakage)		• Heart and other organs

Abbreviations: HCT, Hematocrit; AST, aspartate aminotransferase; ALT, alanine transaminase.

[a]Adapted from Image from WHO Dengue guidelines.

*(requiring strict observation and medical intervention)

Table 52.2 Antibody, NS1, and Viral Levels in Dengue Infection Over Time		
Levels	Primary Dengue Infection Days Post Onset of symptoms	Secondary Dengue Infection Days Post Onset of symptoms
Virus	0–6, peaks at approximately 3d	0–6, peaks at approximately 3d
NS1	0–45, peaks early	0–30, peaks early
IGM	5–90, peaks at approximately 45 d	5–45, peaks at approximately 30 d
IGG	45 days to years, Rises over years	0–years, Peaks over years

(Adapted from CDC—Laboratory Guidance—Dengue)

³d, day

Diagnostic Tests

Due to the rapid onset of severe disease and the lack of available laboratory equipment, diagnosis is usually clinical. Although there have been recent advances in serum testing, studies show that the use of the WHO criteria in Table 52.2 is almost as sensitive as the NS1 (nonstructural protein 1) PCR (polymerase chain reaction) test, which detects a secreted glycoprotein in patient samples prior to antibody development. The NS1 test is less sensitive in hyperendemic areas and in secondary infection. Antibodies to *dengue virus* develop around 5 days after infection and can be found circulating at detectable levels after that point. The year 2012 marked the release of a PCR test that can be run on the same equipment as that used to diagnose influenza, which may make rapid PCR diagnosis more accessible.

Other laboratory features include leukopenia, lymphocytosis, and atypia. The development of Severe Dengue or DSS is marked by laboratory markers of bleeding diathesis and end-organ dysfunction. See Table 52.3.

Organisms

Dengue virus is a single-stranded RNA virus of the Flaviviridae family. There are four serotypes known to cause the clinical presentation of dengue fever, appropriately named DEN-1 through DEN-4. The *Dengue virus* is transmitted to the human host via the bite of an infected *Aedes* mosquito, at which point it enters the Langerhans cells of the skin and travels to the lymph nodes, where its replication results in the clinical symptoms of infection. Mature virus particles are released via exocytosis, which then can infect other leukocytes prior to destruction via T-cell mediated destruction and phagocytosis.

Treatment

There are no specific treatments for dengue fever. All treatment is supportive and may range from oral rehydration to intravenous fluid administration and vasopressor support. During initial presentation, frequent vitals and lab checks are indicated, as the onset of severe dengue and DSS may be very rapid. Aspirin and NSAIDs for management of fever and arthralgias are contraindicated in this population due to the increased risk of bleeding, but other antipyretics are accepted.

Other Key Issues to Consider

Person-to-person transmission can occur via sharing of blood products or during pregnancy, although vertical transmission is rare.

Table 52.3 Laboratory Markers of Severe Dengue	
High Values	Low Values
Packed cell volume	Platelets (< 100)
Prothrombin time	Fibrinogen
Partial Thromboplastin time	Factor 8
Thrombin time	Factor 12
Transaminases	

Suggested Readings and References

1. Laboratory guidance and diagnostic testing—Dengue homepage. Centers for Disease Control and prevention website. http://www.cdc.gov/dengue/clinicallab/laboratory.html. Accessed October 3, 2012.

2. New CDC test for dengue approved [Press release]. Centers for Disease Control and prevention website. http://www.cdc.gov/media/releases/2012/p0620_dengue_test.html. 2012.

3. Chaterji S. et al. Evaluation of the NS1 rapid test and the WHO dengue classification schemes for use as bedside diagnosis of acute dengue fever in adults. *Am J Trop Med Hyg.* 2011;84(2):224–228.

4. Teixeira M, M Baretto. Diagnosis and management of dengue. *Br Med J.* 2009;339:1189–1193.

5. World Health Organization. Dengue: guidelines for diagnosis, management, treatment and control. 2009.

6. Dengue and severe dengue [Fact sheet]. World Health Organization website. http://www.who.int/mediacentre/factsheets/fs117/en/. 2012.

West Nile Virus

Matthew Finn

Disease Description: West Nile virus (WNV) is a single-stranded RNA virus of the flavivirus family that is transmitted via a mosquito vector, typically causing fever and capable of causing meningoencephalitis. WNV is a leading cause of domestically acquired arboviral disease. It is most commonly seen in late August and early September.

Organisms: WNV is part of the Japanese encephalitis serocomplex that contain a similar viral hemagglutinin. Other members of this class include: Japanese encephalitis, St. Louis encephalitis, Murray Valley fever, and Kunjin virus.

Treatment: Currently there are no clinically proven treatments. Therapy is supportive.

Other Key Issues: WNV is a nationally notifiable disease. Cases should be reported to local health departments. Prevention remains the key to controlling this disease. Reducing the breeding grounds of the *Culex* mosquito and using insect repellant to prevent bites (diethyltoluamide or DEET, less than 50%) are two important strategies.

Disease Description

WNV is a single-stranded RNA virus of the flavivirus family and part of the Japanese encephalitis sero-complex. WNV is usually asymptomatic but is known to cause sudden onset fevers, malaise, and weakness. Although mortality is low, it can lead to debilitating neuroinvasive disease in some patients.[1]

Epidemiology

The first case of WNV was identified in the West Nile region of Uganda in 1936. Subsequent outbreaks of the virus mainly occurred in Europe, Africa, and the Middle East. The first cases in the United States were reported in New York in 1999, with 62 reported cases and 12% mortality. Over the past decade, WNV has become the most common cause of domestically acquired arboviral (group of viruses that are transmitted by arthropod vectors) disease in the United States.[2] In 2011, there were 712 cases of WNV infection in the United States, of which 72% were classified as neuroinvasive with 6% mortality.[3] In 2012, a significant outbreak occurred, with over 4,000 cases in the contiguous United States. Approximately 40% of these cases occurred in Dallas, Texas, and the surrounding area. As of 2012, every state in the contiguous United States, except Maine, had a documented case.[5]

The rate of WNV infections is seasonally dependent. The peak incidence of WNV tends to occur in late August and early September. In the more temperate Southern and Western states, the virus can cause infections year round.[1]

Presenting Features

Approximately 75% to 80% of infected patients will never develop symptoms.[5] Of the 20% who do develop symptoms, the most common presenting features are fever, myalgias, and malaise of sudden onset (see Table 53.1).

The presentation of neuroinvasive WNV can be variable, and its prevalence varies broadly from year to year. In 2012, over 50% of cases in the United States were classified as being neuroinvasive. The most common manifestations of neuroinvasive disease include meningitis, encephalitis, or more rarely poliomyelitis. Flaccid quadriplegia was seen in approximately 10% of cases in the 1999 New York outbreak.[10] Facial weakness, cranial nerve palsies, dysarthria, dysphagia, seizures, cerebellar dysfunction, and chorioretinitis have also been described.[1,8] According to the June 20, 2014, Morbidity and Mortality Report by the Centers for Disease Control and Prevention, in 2013 there were nearly 2,500 cases of WNV. Fifty one percent were described as neuroinvasive cases, coming from 47 states. (See Figure 53.1.) The median age of patients was 55 years, with 58% being male. Five percent died, and the median age of patients who died was 78 years.[19]

Diagnostic Considerations

A high degree of clinical suspicion is warranted in older adults with fever and meningeal symptoms, especially when presenting in the late summer and early fall. One should also consider WNV in otherwise unexplained cases of meningitis or encephalitis. It is important to note that transmission can occur year round in more temperate climates.

Risk factors for developing neuroinvasive disease include age greater than 50, immunocompromised status, and the presence of diabetes.[10] History of transplantation has been shown to increase the risk of neuroinvasive disease fortyfold. Malignancies, particularly of hematologic origin, have also been associated with development of neurologic pathology.[16] Other reported risk factors include alcohol abuse, renal disease, and hypertension.

Typical Disease Course

The clinical course of WNV is variable. The incubation time is reported to be from 2 to 14 days. With the onset of symptoms, development of a high fever is characteristically rapid. Symptoms typically last from

Table 53.1 WNV Most Common Presenting Symptoms	
Symptom	Prevalence %
Fever	90
Weakness	56
Headache	47
Altered mental status	46
Stiff neck	19
Rash (erythematous, maculopapular)	19

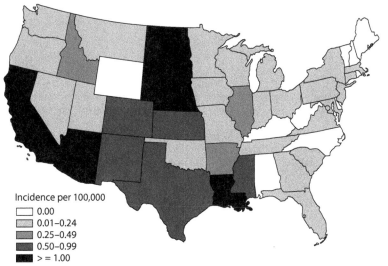

Figure 53.1 West Nile virus neuroinvasive disease incidence reported to ArboNET by state, United States, 2014.
West Nile virus neuroinvasive disease incidence maps present data reported by state and local health departments to CDC's ArboNET surveillance system. This map shows the incidence of human neuroinvasive disease (e.g., meningitis, encephalitis, or acute flaccid paralysis) by state for 2014 with shading ranging from 0.01-0.24, 0.25-0.49, 0.50-0.99, and greater than 1.00 per 100,000 population.
Neuroinvasive disease cases have been reported to ArboNET from the following states for 2014: Arizona, Arkansas, California, Colorado, Connecticut, District of Columbia, Florida, Georgia, Idaho, Illinois, Indiana, Iowa, Kansas, Louisiana, Maryland, Massachusetts, Michigan, Minnesota, Mississippi, Missouri, Montana, Nebraska, Nevada, New Jersey, New Mexico, New York, North Carolina, North Dakota, Ohio, Oklahoma, Oregon, Pennsylvania, South Carolina, South Dakota, Tennessee, Texas, Utah, Virginia, Washington, and Wisconsin.

Reprinted with permission from Centers for Disease Control and Prevention. http://www.cdc.gov/westnile/resources/pdfs/data/wnv-neuro-incidence-by-state-map_2014_06052015.pdf.

3 to 8 days; however, in some cases, the disease can persist up to 2 months or longer. Seizures, unlike similar arbovirus disease, are not typically an early manifestation of the disease but can occur several days into the disease course. Status epilepticus is also a possible complication.[14,16]

Patients who develop neuroinvasive disease commonly experience significant long-term disability. In a 1-year follow up study to the 1999 New York epidemic, 67% of patients had significant fatigue, 50% had memory loss, and 49% had gait difficulties.[17]

Diagnostic Tests

Initial testing should consist of cerebrospinal fluid (CSF) fluid analysis and WNV immunoglobulin M (IgM) enzyme-linked immunosorbent assay (ELISA) of serum and/or CSF. Serum blood counts typically show a normal or elevated WBC. Hyponatremia can be seen on serum chemistry. CSF fluid testing characteristically demonstrates a pleocytosis with a lymphocytic predominance. Protein levels are elevated, and glucose levels are typically within reference limits.

The sensitivity of IgM ELISA testing ranges from 90% to 95% in serum or CSF. IgM antibodies develop very rapidly with the onset of viremia. One study showed a median time from viral RNA detection to the development of IgM of approximately 4 days.[1,11]

Patients can have false-positive WNV IgM ELISA testing if they have recently received the yellow fever or Japanese encephalitis vaccines. If there is concern for a false positive, further evaluation with plaque reduction neutralization testing (PRNT) can be performed. PRNT is the primary means used to distinguish among the viruses of the Japanese encephalitis serocomplex and is the most specific test for WNV.

Other testing modalities include viral RNA PCR amplification and viral culture/histology. PCR is highly specific; however, it has low sensitivity due to low levels of viremia in the human host (WNV PCR sensitivity is approximately 55% in CSF and 10% in serum). Viral culture also has poor sensitivity. Histology on postmortem pathologic examination typically demonstrates a mononuclear infiltrate with microglial nodularity throughout the grey and white matter. In autopsy studies of patients with neuroinvasive disease, the most extensive invasion was localized to the brain stem, particularly to the medulla.[1,10]

Magnetic resonance imaging is frequently abnormal in patients with neuroinvasive meningitis.[15] Abnormal signals are most characteristically seen in the deep gray matter and brain stem but have also been observed in the white matter and the spinal cord. Computed tomography scans are not helpful in detecting pathologic changes of WNV.

Organism

WNV transmission typically occurs via the Culex mosquito vector. Birds are considered to be the primary amplifying hosts. Birds infected with the virus usually do not die from the infection and are capable transmitting WNV to other mosquitoes. Humans, horses, and several other vertebrates are incidental (dead-end) hosts. Incidental hosts are not capable of transmitting the virus to other mosquitoes, as levels of viremia are typically low. To date, there are no known cases of human to human or animal to animal transmission.[4]In the incidental host, the virus is taken up by epithelial Langerhans cells where the virus replicates. The Langerhans cells then migrate to regional lymph nodes where the virus further replicates and enters the blood stream to infiltrate multiple organ systems.[14]

Other modes of transmission have been documented, including blood and fresh frozen plasma transfusions, organ transplantation, and occupational transmission from percutaneous or conjunctival exposures. The possibility of transplacental and breast milk transfer of the virus is still under investigation but is thought to be possible.[4,12]

Treatment

There are currently no proven treatments available. Care is considered primarily supportive, including intravenous fluids, respiratory support when needed, and prevention of secondary infections.[4,5] Interferon, ribavirin, and intravenous immunoglobulin have been studied as potential therapies; however, no randomized trials exist that prove efficacy.[7]

Other Key Issues

WNV is a nationally notifiable disease; as such, clinicians and laboratories are required to report WNV disease cases to local health departments.

The health care community has increasingly focused on prevention. There are two primary routes to improve prevention. The first is to decrease the number of mosquito vectors. Communities have attempted to improve drainage with a goal of reducing the number of mosquito breeding grounds. Additionally, spraying (typically with organophosphates or pyrethroid aerial sprays) has been demonstrated to diminish the frequency transmission.

The second method is to decrease the number of mosquito bites. This can be done by avoiding the outdoors and minimizing exposed skin when outdoors. Additionally, insect repellants, particularly DEETS (diethyltoluamide), have been shown to be effective and safe when used in adults in concentrations of less than 50%.[1]

Suggested Readings and References

1. Petersen LR, Marfin AA. West Nile virus: a primer for the clinician. Ann Intern Med. 2002;137(3):173.
2. Reimann CA, Hayes EB, DiGuiseppi C, et al. Epidemiology of neuroinvasive arboviral disease in the United States, 1999–2007. Am J Trop Med Hyg. 2008;79:974–979.
3. West Nile virus disease and other arboviral diseases—United States, 2011. MMWR Morb Mortal Wkly Rep. 2012;61(27):510–514.
4. West Nile Virus: Epidemiologic information for clinicians. Centers for Disease Control and Prevention website. http://www.cdc.gov/ncidod/dvbid/westnile/clinicians/pdf/wnv-epidemiology-clinguidance.pdf, Accessed September 29, 2004.
5. Petersen LR, Fischer M. Unpredictable and difficult to control—the adolescence of West Nile virus. N Engl J Med. 2012;367(14):1281–1284.
6. Sejvar JJ, et al. Neurologic manifestations and outcome of West Nile virus infection. JAMA. 2003; 290(4):511–515.
7. Morrey JD et al. Effect of interferon-alpha and interferon-inducers on West Nile virus in mouse and hamster animal models. Antivir Chem Chemother. 2004;15(2): 101–109.
8. Avis LE, et al. West Nile virus neuroinvasive disease. Neurology. 2006;60(3):286–300.
9. Petersen LR, Roehrig JT. Emerg Infect Dis. 2001;7(4):611–614.
10. Nash D, Mostashari F, Fine A, et al. The outbreak of West Nile virus infection in the New York City area in 1999. N Engl J Med. 2001;344:1807–1814.

11. Busch MP, et al. Virus and antibody dynamics in acute West Nile virus infection. *J Infect Dis*. 2008;198(7):984–993.

12. Pealer LN, et al. Transmission of West Nile virus through blood transfusion in the United States in 2002. West Nile Virus Transmission Investigation Team. *N Engl J Med*. 2003;349(13):1236–1245.

13. Petersen LR. Epstein Problem solved? West Nile virus and transfusion safety. *N Engl J Med*. 2005;353(5):516.

14. Gea-Banacloche J, et al. West Nile virus: pathogenesis and therapeutic options. *Ann Intern Med*. 2004;140(7):545–553.

15. Petropoulou KA, Gordon SM, Prayson RA, Ruggierri PM. West Nile virus meningoencephalitis: MR imaging findings. *Am J Neuroradiol*. 2005;26(8):1986.

16. Watson JT, et al. Clinical characteristics and functional outcomes of West Nile Fever. *Ann Intern Med*. 2004;141(5):360–365.

17. West Nile virus surveillance and control: an update for healthcare providers in New York City. City Health Information. New York Department of Health. 2001;20.

18. Weiss D, et al. Clinical findings of West Nile virus infection in hospitalized patients, New York and New Jersey, 2000. *Emerg Infect Dis*. 2000;7(4):645–658.

19. Lindsey NP, Lehman JA, Staples JE, Fischer M. West Nile Virus and other arboviral diseases—United States, 2013. *MMWR Morb Mortal Wkly Rep*. 2014;63(24):521–526.

Infection in Special Populations

Chapter 54

Infection in the Cancer Patient

Sri Raghavan

Epidemiology

Cancer patients are a specialized subset of patients with increased susceptibility to a variety of both common and atypical infections. With the steady increase in outpatient chemotherapy regimens, these patients are presenting more often to the emergency department when acutely ill as opposed to being monitored throughout treatment in an inpatient setting. In addition to being relatively immunocompromised from their underlying disease, chemotherapy regimens lead to neutropenia, deficits in cellular and humoral immunity, and disruption of mucosal barriers that predispose oncology patients to severe and rapidly progressive presentations with high morbidity and mortality rates.

Some estimates suggest that patients with cancer are 10 times more likely to develop sepsis than patients without cancer. Cancer patients have a 30% higher rate of death from sepsis, and sepsis accounts for nearly 10% of all deaths related to cancer.[1,2,3,4] As such, it is important the emergency physician to be able to rapidly recognize and manage infections and infectious complications in this population. Although there are different subsets of oncologic patients who are predisposed to specific types of infections (ie, those with hematologic malignancies, bone marrow transplant patients, and solid tumor patients), outlined below are several key principles for managing these patients and their most common presentations to the emergency department.

Neutropenic Fever

Diagnosis and Course

One of the most common presentations of oncologic patients undergoing active or recent chemotherapy is neutropenic fever. Neutropenia is defined as an absolute neutrophil count (ANC) below 500 cells/mm^3 or an ANC expected to drop below 500 cells/mm^3 within 48 hours. Neutropenic fever includes neutropenia and either one oral temperature above 38.3°C (101°F) or two measurements separated by at least 1 hour above 38°C (100.4°F). Some patients may be functionally neutropenic even if their ANC appears normal if they have recently received chemotherapy or if their underlying hematologic malignancy compromises the function of their immune cells. Given their immunocompromised state, these patients can rapidly develop sepsis and have high mortality rates.[1,3,4] On presentation, patients should be risk-stratified, with low-risk patients constituting only those with a short anticipated duration of neutropenia (less than 7 days) and few comorbidities.[5] In general, all neutropenic patients require early initiation of antibiotics and prompt inpatient admission (Table 54.1).

The source of neutropenic fever is often unclear, as these patients' immune response is blunted. Consequently, careful history and physical examination are needed to identify any possible source of infection. Most patients require early computed tomography (CT) imaging, as a pneumonia is often revealed by CT on a high number of patients with normal chest x-rays.[6,7] At some centers, routine chest and sinus CTs are obtained on all patients with new onset neutropenic fever to evaluate for sinopulmonary disease, with additional abdominal/pelvic imaging if warranted.

Where possible, intravenous contrast should be avoided because most oncology patients, in particular those with hematologic malignancies, receive numerous other nephrotoxic agents (including chemotherapy and frequent antibiotics). In addition, these patients should undergo broad laboratory and microbiological evaluation, including cultures from blood (both peripherally and from each lumen of

Table 54.1 Common Bacterial Pathogens in Neutropenic Patients[a]

Gram-Positive Organisms	Gram-Negative Organisms
Coagulase-negative staphylococci	Escherichia coli
Staphylococcus aureus (including MRSA)	Klebsiella species
Enterococcus species (including VRE)	Pseudomonas aeruginosa
Viridans group streptococci	Enterobacter species
Streptococcus pneumoniae	Citrobacter species
Streptococcus pyogenes	Acinetobacter species
Corynebacterium species	Stenotrophomonas maltophilia

Abbreviations: MRSA, methicillin-resistant Staphylococcus aureus: VRE, vancomycin-resistant enterococci.

[a]Adapted with permission from Freifeld AG et al. Clin Infect Dis. 2011;52:e56–e93.

in-dwelling catheters), sputum, urine, stool, and cerebrospinal fluid as indicated. After initial diagnostic workup, principles of early goal-directed therapy are generally followed with broad antibiotic coverage, aggressive fluid resuscitation, and blood products if needed.

Bacterial Organisms and Treatment

A wide host of organisms can cause neutropenic fever. Consequently, initial therapy is typically very broad (Table 54.1). The primary sites of infection leading to bacteremia include the lung, gastrointestinal (GI) tract, and sites of indwelling hardware.[5,8] In patients who have recently received chemotherapeutic agents that induce intestinal mucosal injury, gram-negative bacteria have translocated from the gut with *Escherichia coli, Pseudomonas* species, and *Klebsiella* species most commonly implicated.[5,8] As such, these patients are generally initiated on broad gram-negative coverage with piperacillin/tazobactam, cefepime, or a carbapenem.

Anaerobes are rarely involved in neutropenic fever, but can include *Bacteroides* species, *Clostridium* species, or *Fusobacterium*; additional coverage for anaerobes can be added if clinical suspicion is high.[5,8,9] In patients with indwelling central venous catheters, oral mucosal breakdown, skin infections, or pneumonia, infection with gram-positive organisms should be considered; it is important to consider initiating therapy with parenteral vancomycin or other gram-positive agents.[5,9,10] The most common gram-positive organisms include *Staphylococcus aureus*, coagulase-negative *Staphylococcus* species, *Enterococcus* species, and *Corynebacterium* species. *Stenotrophomonas maltophilia* most commonly involves the sinuses but can manifest as bacteremia and is treated with high-dose trimethoprim-sulfamethoxazole.

Fungal organisms and treatment

In addition to the bacterial infections discussed previously, oncology patients are highly susceptible to fungal infections, with high mortality in these cases.[8] Most patients with neutropenia are on prophylactic antifungal agents, so generally they are not started empirically on broader antifungal coverage unless there is clinical suspicion for a fungal etiology or if fevers persist despite broad antibiotic coverage for more than 4 days.[5,11,12] *Candida* species, including *albicans, glabrata, tropicalis,* and *parapsilosis,* are the most common infectious fungal agents.[5,8] *Aspergillus* species, most commonly *Aspergillus fumigatus*, are often colonizers of the lung and sinuses and can progress to pneumonia or invasive aspergillus in the setting of neutropenia or immunocompromise secondary to chemotherapy.

Patients present less frequently with cryptococcal infection or *Pneumocystis jiroveci* pneumonia. CT typically demonstrates pulmonary macronodules (≥ 1 cm) with a halo sign that represents edema or blood around the nodule.[5,7] Studies have not clearly identified optimal empiric coverage for fungal species, but guidelines recommend parenteral administration and switching to a different class of antifungal if previously on antifungal coverage.[5] Micafungin, voriconazole, or amphotericin B are commonly used depending on the degree of concern and other associated comorbidities.

Sinus infection by aspergillus or mucormycosis represents an oncologic emergency as these organisms can erode through the sinuses and invade the cranium. Due to the angio-invasive nature of these fungal species, the potential for acute hemorrhage or thrombosis and tissue necrosis is high. As such, neutropenic patients who present with headache or sinus symptoms should undergo urgent sinus and head CT scans followed by magnetic resonance imaging if needed. If these studies are concerning for fungal sinus infection, it is imperative that these patients be covered early and broadly with antifungals. Only amphotericin B and posaconazole have activity against mucormycosis, and, in general, amphotericin B is the first-line treatment in suspected cases.[12] Patients with invasive fungal disease will likely need to be transferred to a tertiary care center where appropriate evaluation can be undertaken by otolaryngology, neurosurgery, ophthalmology, and infectious disease specialists, as these patients may need urgent, coordinated surgical debridement. After the fungal organisms are speciated from tissue biopsy samples, antifungal coverage can be narrowed.

Viral Organisms and Treatment

As with fungal prophylaxis, most neutropenic patients are also on viral prophylaxis, decreasing the need for empiric viral treatment on presentation to the emergency department. Patients with respiratory symptoms and cough should undergo testing for respiratory viruses.[5] However, given the side effects of parenteral antivirals and their propensity to further suppress the bone marrow and prolong neutropenia, these agents should generally only be initiated if clinical suspicion is high for a viral source. Herpes simplex virus and cytomegalovirus are most commonly seen in the hematologic malignancy and bone marrow transplant populations, at times with viremia but more commonly with pneumonitis.[8] Respiratory syncytial virus, varicella zoster virus, influenza, parainfluenza, and *metapneumovirus* are also common viral illnesses in the oncologic population, as in the general population.

Neutropenic patients with suspected exposure to influenza or symptoms of influenza-like illness should be initiated empirically on neuraminidase inhibitors pending the results of respiratory virus testing.[5]

Neutropenic Enterocolitis and Typhlitis

In addition to neutropenic fever, oncologic patients can present to the emergency department with a variety of other infectious processes. Patients with hematologic malignancies, particularly those undergoing chemotherapy or bone marrow transplant, can present with neutropenic enterocolitis or typhlitis (inflammation of the cecum with high risk for bacterial translocation and possible perforation). Oncologic patients presenting to the emergency department with abdominal pain (particularly in the right lower quadrant) and diarrhea should be evaluated with an abdominal CT scan. If the CT demonstrates bowel inflammation, empiric coverage against gram-negative organisms should be started as discussed previously.

Given the wide spectrum of antibiotic exposure of most of these patients, it is also important to evaluate for *Clostridium difficile* infection as a possible etiology for diarrhea and abdominal pain. If there are peritoneal signs concerning for perforation, prompt surgical evaluation is required as these patients may need partial bowel resection despite their immunocompromised state. Many solid tumor patients, particularly those with hepatobiliary malignancies, can present in the acute setting with biliary obstruction or cholangitis. These are generally managed in the same manner as non-oncologic patients with similar conditions: early diagnostic evaluation, initiation of antimicrobials, and possible intervention to drain fluid collections or relieve obstruction.

Catheter-Associated Blood Stream Infection

Many oncologic patients have indwelling catheters or mediports and, thus, are at risk for developing catheter-associated blood stream infections. In addition to skin and mucosal colonizers, such as *S. aureus*, coagulase-negative *Staphylococcus*, and *Candida* species, catheters can become colonized by gram-negative organisms that have translocated from the GI tract to the bloodstream or by mycobacteria.[5,9,10] On presentation, blood cultures through the catheter and from peripheral blood should be drawn simultaneously prior to initiating antibiotics, as several studies have demonstrated that there is a high likelihood of catheter infection if the catheter culture returns positive before the peripheral culture.[5,10] The infected line should be removed urgently, and empiric coverage should be initiated if there is high suspicion for catheter-associated infection with *S. aureus, Pseudomonas*, fungi, or mycobacteria. Empiric treatment is also warranted if the patient has evidence of septic thrombosis, endocarditis, port pocket infection, sepsis, or persistent bacteremia despite antibiotic treatment for over 72 hours.[5,8] If the only organism documented is coagulase-negative *Staphylococcus*, the catheter can be retained with appropriate systemic antibiotics.[5]

In summary, oncologic patients represent a specialized patient population with a variety of acute presentations related to their immunocompromised status. Effective management of these patients hinges on rapid diagnostic evaluation with imaging and cultures followed by early initiation of antimicrobial therapy. Early therapeutic intervention started in the emergency department upon presentation can help decrease morbidity and mortality in this growing patient population.

Suggested Readings and References

1. Danai PA, Moss M, Mannino DM, et al. The epidemiology of sepsis in patients with malignancy. *Chest.* 2006;129:1432–1440.
2. Safdar A, Armstrong D. Infectious morbidity in critically ill patients with cancer. *Crit Care Clin.* 2001;17:531–570, vii–viii.
3. Angus DC, Linde-Zwirble WT, Lidicker J, et al. Epidemiology of severe sepsis in the United States: analysis of incidence, outcome, and associated costs of care. *Crit Care Med.* 2001;29:1303–1310.
4. Williams MD, Braun LA, Cooper LM, et al. Hospitalized cancer patients with severe sepsis: analysis of incidence, mortality, and associated costs of care. *Crit Care.* 2004;8:R291–298.
5. Freifeld AG, Bow EJ, Sepkowitz KA, et al. Clinical practice guideline for the use of antimicrobial agents in neutropenic patients with cancer: 2010 update by the infectious diseases society of America. *Clin Infect Dis.* 2011;52(4):e56–93.

6. Heussel CP, Kauczor HU, Heussel GE, et al. Pneumonia in febrile neutropenic patients and in bone marrow and blood stem-cell transplant recipients: use of high-resolution computed tomography. *J Clin Oncol.* 1999;17:796–805.

7. Marom EM and Kontoyiannis DP. Imaging studies for diagnosing invasive fungal pneumonia in immunocompromised patients. *Curr Opin Infect Dis.* 2011;24:309–314.

8. Thirumala R, Ramaswamy M, Chawla S. Diagnosis and management of infectious complications in critically ill patients with cancer. *Crit Care Clin.* 2006;26:56–91.

9. Wisplinghoff H, Seifert H, Wenzel RP, et al. Current trends in the epidemiology of nosocomial bloodstream infections in patients with hematological malignancies and solid neoplasms in hospitals in the United States. *Clin Infect Dis.* 2003;36:1103–1110.

10. Raad I, Hachem R, Hanna H, et al. Sources and outcome of bloodstream infections in cancer patients: the role of central venous catheters. *Eur J Clin Microbiol Infect Dis.* 2007;26:549–556.

11. Wingard JR. Empirical antifungal therapy in treating febrile neutropenic patients. *Clin Infect Dis.* 2004;39:S38–S43.

12. Kontoyiannis DP. Invasive mycoses: strategies for effective management. *Am J Med.* 2012;125:S25–S38.

Chapter 55

Infections in the HIV Patient

Michelle Henggeller

Worldwide, there are approximately 35 million people living with human immunodeficiency virus (HIV) (27). At the end of 2011 in the United States, this figure was measured at over 1.2 million people infected with HIV, with up to 14% of this population unaware of their diagnosis (13). The incidence of new HIV infections has been relatively constant in the United States at approximately 50,000 new cases estimated per year (9). The group that retains the highest risks for transmission of HIV is men who have sex with other men. The disease also continues to be more prevalent in the African American population (9).

The virus that causes HIV leads to deficiencies in cell mediated immunity by both inactivating and depleting CD4 T lymphocytes as well as affecting B lymphocytes, monocytes, and polymorphonuclear cells (26). The disease processes that are the primary basis of morbidity and mortality in HIV are a reflection of this impaired immunity. The CD4 count can be used as an initial estimation of the measurement of cell-mediated immunological activity. A CD4 count of 200 cells/microL has been used as the threshold for delineation between HIV infection and AIDS in the absence of AIDS defining illnesses (31).

With the advent and widespread implementation of effective antiretroviral therapy (ART), there has been an overall decline in opportunistic infections, disease transmission, and death from HIV(31). However, it has been estimated that less than one-third of HIV infected individuals in the United States are adequately virally suppressed (31). This number represents a combination of undiagnosed HIV infection, poor medication compliance, and financial and social barriers to care; it results in a large number of patients with HIV presenting for care with significant disease processes despite the development of ART (31).

Infection with CD4 Count >200

In general, the etiologies of infection in patients with HIV with CD4 counts above 200 cells/microL are reflective of those found in the general population (6,7). Several conditions, however, occur with increased frequency and severity in patients with CD4 counts above 200 cells/microL (6,7). These include fungal infections, such as thrush and vaginal candidiasis, and bacterial infections, such as bacillary angiomatosis, *Staphylococcus aureus* (as well as methicillin-resistant *Staphylococcus aureus* [MRSA]), *Streptococcus pneumoniae*, and Syphilis. Similarly, viral infections are more frequent due to both the patient's underlying HIV as well as shared risk factors (eg, IV drug use) that can lead to co-infection with HIV and other virsuses. These include Hepatitis B, Hepatitis C, Herpes Simplex Virus, Varicella Zoster Virus, and Human Papillomavirus (6,7).

Infection with CD4 Count < 200

The hallmark of the acquired immunodeficiency syndrome (AIDS) patient (an HIV patient with a CD4 count below 200) is the development of opportunistic infections. Although the use of ART has decreased the incidence of these infections, they continue to be a major case of morbidity and mortality in the patient with HIV and remain important for inclusion in the differential diagnosis during medical evaluation (31). The major opportunistic infections are presented in the following by major system involved.

Cough or Shortness of Breath

Pneumocystis pneumonia (PCP)
PCP, the most frequently identified opportunistic respiratory infection in HIV, is caused by the ubiquitous airborne fungus *Pneumocystis jirovecii* (32).

Clinical Manifestations
PCP is characterized by fever, cough, progressive dyspnea, and chest discomfort. The resting exam is frequently normal, although diffuse rhonchi or rales may be auscultated. Hypoxia frequently occurs with PCP infection, and a widened A-a gradient is seen in up to 90% of patients (35). An elevated lactate dehydrogenase (LDH), although nonspecific, is common in PCP infection (31). Chest radiographs are normal in up to one quarter patients presenting with PCP, although classically, the radiograph will show bilateral diffuse interstitial infiltrates in a butterfly pattern (31,35). Upper lobe alveolar infiltrates and pneumothoraces may also be seen. In patients with a normal chest radiograph, a high resolution computed tomography (CT) that demonstrates patchy or nodular ground-glass attenuation is highly suggestive of PCP (35).

Diagnosis
Definitive diagnosis of PCP requires direct visualization of the trophic or cystic forms of the *P. jirovecii* organism obtained through induced sputum or preferably tissue or bronchoalveolar lavage (35).

Treatment
Patients with mild to moderate disease (room air $PaO_2 > 70$ or A-a gradient < 35 mm Hg) can be treated with 21 days of the following oral regimens:
- Trimethoprim-sulfamethoxazole (TMP-SMX) at a dose of TMP 320 mg plus SMX 1600 mg (two double-strength tablets) PO every 8 hours
- Trimethoprim can be given at a dose of 5 mg/kg PO every 8 hours with dapsone 100 mg

PO daily; prior to therapy, G6PD (glucose-6-phosphate dehydrogenase) deficiency testing should be performed as dapsone can lead to hemolysis in these patients.
- Clindamycin 450 mg PO every 6 hours plus primaquine base 15 mg PO per day; G6PD deficiency testing should be performed prior to therapy as primaquine can lead to hemolysis in these patients.
- Atovaquone suspension 750 mg PO every 12 hours

Patients requiring intravenous antibiotics for severe illness (room air $PaO_2 < 70$ or A-a gradient > 35 mm Hg) or for mild to moderate disease not tolerating oral medications, the following regimens are recommended:
- TMP-SMX 15 to 20 mg/kg IV of the TMP component to be administered in divided doses every 6 to 8 hours.
- Pentamidine 4 mg/kg IV daily (although significant adverse events including hypotension, hypoglycemia, and renal failure can occur in up to 70% of patients).
- Clindamycin 600 mg IV every 8 hours with primaquine base 30 mg PO daily. (Adapted from Sax, 2012 and Panel on Opportunistic Infections in HIV-Infected Adults and Adolescents)

Corticosteroids should be started in all patients meeting criteria for severe illness.
- Prednisone 40 mg every 12 hours for 5 days, followed by
- Prednisone 40 mg daily for 5 days, followed by
- Prednisone 20 mg daily for 11 days.

IV methylprednisolone should be substituted for patients not tolerating PO therapy.
(Adapted from Sax, 2012)

Mycobacterium Tuberculosis Infection
Tuberculosis (TB) is caused from inhaling an aerosolized droplet containing *Mycobacterium Tuberculosis* bacilli spread from an infected person. The pulmonary system is the primary focal point for infection, although in the HIV population, extra pulmonary disease occurs with increasing frequency as the immune system declines (28). Active TB can occur in the HIV population with primary infection or with reactivation of latent infection (31). TB continues to be a leading cause of death in the worldwide HIV population while also posing the threat of transmission to the public and health care workers (17).

Clinical Manifestations
Pulmonary symptoms of TB vary with the degree of immunosuppression in patients with HIV. Patients with early HIV present with symptoms of fever, cough, night sweats, fatigue, and weight loss (28). The chest radiograph in these patients is likely to show a classical TB presentation with apical cavitary lesions and upper lobe fibronodular infiltrates (31). Patients with declining immunocompetence have variable presentations that can range from an acute fulminant multiorgan disease to a subacute disease with fever, weight loss, malaise, and dysfunction of various organ systems (8).

Extrapulmonary and disseminated TB are more common in this group with findings of lymphadenopathy, pleural effusions, pericarditis, meningitis, liver disease, and bone and joint involvement (8,28). Chest radiographs in patients with TB and advanced HIV more frequently show lower lobe, middle lobe, miliary, or interstitial infiltrates without classic cavitary lesions. Chest radiographs can also demonstrate nonspecific or normal findings in this population (28,31). CT can be helpful because pulmonary lesions are more visible than on plain radiograph, and the characteristic appearance of hypodense rim-enhancing lymph nodes with contrast studies makes the diagnosis more likely (28).

Diagnosis
Definitive diagnosis of TB is made with acid fast smear and culture of *M. tuberculosis* from sputum or other body fluid. Aspirates from lymph nodes, pleural fluid, pericardial fluid, ascites, or cerebrospinal fluid (CSF) along with blood and urine cultures can be diagnostic in appropriate patients (28,31). Fluorescence microscopy and Nucleic Acid Amplification can also be used for diagnosis of active TB when available (28). All cultures should be tested for drug susceptibility and resistance.

Treatment

The initial recommended treatment for tuberculosis includes 2 months of combined therapy with all of the following:

- Isoniazid (isonicotinylhydrazine [INH]) 15 mg/kg (maximum 900 mg) PO once, twice, or three times weekly
- Pyrazinamide 15 to 30 mg/kg PO (maximum 2000 mg) once daily or 50 mg/kg (maximum 2000 mg) PO twice weekly
- Ethambutol 15 to 20 mg/kg PO (maximum 1000 mg) PO once daily or 50 mg/kg (maximum 2500 mg) PO twice weekly
- Rifampin 10 mg/kg (maximum 600 mg) PO daily, twice weekly, or three times weekly; or rifabutin

Patients with suspected multidrug-resistant TB are recommended to start the preceding treatment with the addition of capreomycin and moxifloxacin or levofloxacin. Pyridoxine should also be prescribed in all HIV patients taking INH to diminish risks of peripheral neuropathy.

(Adapted from Maartens, 2014)

Aspergillosis

Aspergillosis infections occur from inhalation of spores from the ubiquitous fungus, *Aspergillus*, in an immunocompromised individual (3). The inhaled spores germinate and invade lung tissue and local vascular structures, causing an invasive, disseminated disease process (3).

Clinical Manifestations

The majority of HIV infected patients with disseminated aspergillosis present with pulmonary involvemen, which can include tracheobronchitis or a necrotizing pneumonia (3,31). The most common symptoms of aspergillosis infection are cough, dyspnea, and fever. Patients also report chest pain, hemoptysis, malaise, and weight loss (3). With primary involvement of the tracheobronchial tree, patients may present with cough, dyspnea, and wheezing due to direct fungal invasion of the tracheobronchial mucosa and cartilage. Invasion can result in thick mucus plugs of *Aspergillus* and necrotic debris in the airways (3). Although less commonly seen, disseminated infection can involve the central nervous system (CNS), heart, kidneys, bone, or sinuses (3,31).

Diagnosis

Radiographic findings in pulmonary aspergillosis include predominantly upper lobe cavitary lesions; focal alveolar infiltrates; pleural-based lesions; and diffuse nodular, reticulonodular, or interstitial bilateral infiltrates (3). Chest CT scan may show a pulmonary nodule surrounded by a low attenuation halo or a cavitary lesion (31). Currently, fungal culture with histopathology is the mainstay of diagnosis of infection with *Aspergillus* (5). Respiratory secretions sent for culture on specific fungal media are optimal for isolating *Aspergillus* species (5). The challenge of differentiating colonization from infection with a positive culture is aided by histopathologic findings of *Aspergillus* hyphae invading into tissue structures (5).

Treatment

Prompt treatment while remaining cognizant of possible drug–drug interactions is indicated in suspected or definitively diagnosed invasive aspergillosis, as the mortality in HIV-infected patients is nearly 75% (5). Recommendations include the following:

- Voriconazole 6 mg/kg IV every 12 hours for 1 day, followed by 4 mg/kg IV every 12 hours in patients with proven or probable aspergillosis. Alternatively, the oral formulation of 200 mg every 12 hours can be used.
- Amphotericin B lipid complex 5 mg/kg daily or Liposomal amphotericin B 3 to 5 mg/kg daily is recommended when the diagnosis is unclear and pending further diagnostic data.

(Adapted from Baddley, 2014b)

Coccidioidomycosis

Coccidioides immitis and *Coccidioides posadasii* are soil residing fungi endemic to the southwestern desert areas of the United States and South and Central America (15). Inhalation of the spores of these species of fungus leads to coccidiodomycosis in susceptible populations (31).

Clinical Manifestations

Coccidioidomycosis customarily presents with cough, fever, and a focal pneumonia in immunocompetent patients or in HIV patients with CD4 counts greater than 250 cells/mm^3 (16,31). The infiltrate is commonly associated with night sweats, fatigue, and lymphadenopathy in the hilar and mediastinal region as well as a peripheral eosinophilia on white blood cell differential (16). In more immunocompromised patients, a diffuse pulmonary disease is most frequently seen with accompanying fevers, dyspnea, and night sweats (16). Disseminated coccidioidomycosis is also common in advanced HIV infection with presentations of meningitis, cutaneous disease, lymph node infection, and liver involvement (16,31).

Diagnosis

Patients with diffuse coccidioidomycosis pulmonary infection frequently present with a nonspecific bilateral reticulonodular infiltrate on chest radiograph. Definitive diagnosis is made through histopathological tissue examination or with positive culture of the organism from clinical specimens (16,31). Serological tests for coccidioidal immunoglobulins are less frequently positive in patients with HIV than their immunocompetent counterparts (16).

Treatment

Recommended treatment for immune compromised patients with focal pneumonia includes:

- Fluconazole 400 mg daily for at least 6 months

Recommended combination two-drug treatment for patients with diffuse pulmonary or disseminated disease includes:

- Amphotericin B deoxycholate 0.7 to 1.0 mg/kg per day for patients with normal renal function or a lipid formulation of amphotericin B 4-6 mg/kg per day in patients with renal insufficiency.
- Fluconazole 400 mg daily for patients with diffuse pulmonary disease; or itraconazole, 200 mg three times daily for patients with extrathoracic dissemination.

(Adapted from Galgiani and Ampel, 2014)

Change in Mental Status

Toxoplasmosis gondii Encephalitis

Toxoplasmosis encephalitis (TE), the most common CNS infection in susceptible HIV patients, is caused by the protozoan *Toxoplasmosis gondii* (18). This protozoa is ingested in the oocyte stage from contaminated soil, cat feces, undercooked meat, or raw shellfish. Once ingested by humans, the parasites can become latent in cyst form in nucleated cells (18). Reactivation of the cyst in the CNS is the most common etiology of the disease (31).

Clinical Manifestations

Patients presenting with TE generally present with complaints of headache, confusion, and fever (18). They may also present with focal neurological deficits, seizures, or psychiatric complaints (18,31). Progression of the disease can cause mental status changes that progress from confusion and flat affect to stupor and coma (18,31). Less commonly, toxoplasmosis can present with chorioretinitis, pneumonia, focally infection in other organ systems, or as a disseminated disease (18).

Brain CT and magnetic resonance imaging (MRI) are both used in the evaluation for TE. However, MRI is more sensitive for visualizing the multiple ring-enhancing lesions with edema that characterize the disease, making it the study of choice (18). Serum testing for anti-Toxoplasma IgG antibodies is nearly uniformly positive in patients with TE; however, this is not diagnostic, although a negative test makes TE less likely (18).

Diagnosis

Using CSF obtained from spinal tap in appropriate patients, *T. gondii* can be detected with polymerase chain reaction (PCR). Although specificity with PCR is high (96%–100%), the sensitivity has been reported as low as 50% (31). Definitive diagnosis of TE requires brain biopsy for positive staining of *T. gondii* in brain tissue (18). However, as brain biopsy is invasive with significant morbidity and mortality, a presumptive diagnosis of TE can be made in patients with a CD4 count < 100 cells/microL who have not been on appropriate prophylaxis for Toxoplasmosis and who meet the following three criteria:

- Clinical syndrome consistent with TE infection
- Positive serum *T. gondii* antibodies
- Classic multiple ring-enhancing lesions on brain imaging

(Adapted from Heller, 2014)

Treatment

Patients with presumed TE should be started on appropriate ART along with antimicrobial therapy for *T. gondii*, to be continued for 6 weeks (31). The preferred regimen is as follows:

- Sulfadiazine 1000 mg every 6 hours for patients ≤ 60 kg or 1500 mg every 6 hours for patients > 60 kg PLUS
- Pyrimethamine 200 mg loading dose, then 50 mg daily for patient ≤ 60 kg or 75 mg daily for patients > 60 kg PLUS

- Leucovorin 10 mg daily (to prevent pyrimethamine-induced hematologic toxicity)
  Alternative regimens include:
- Clindamycin 600 mg IV or PO every 6 hours PLUS
- Pyrimethamine 200 mg loading dose, then 50 mg daily for patient ≤ 60 kg or 75 mg daily for patients > 60 kg plus
- Leucovorin 10 mg daily
- Trimethoprim-sulfate in doses of 5 mg/kg of trimethoprim and 25 mg/kg of sulfamethoxazole twice daily was effective and well tolerated in a small trial.
  (Adapted from Heller, 2014).

Cryptococcus Meningoencephalitis

The fungal species *Cryptococcus neoformans* is the primary agent in the estimated one million cases of cryptococcal meningitis worldwide (31). Although the pathogen initially invades the respiratory system to cause pulmonary infections, the presentation in the immunosuppressed HIV patient is primarily with a meningoencephalitis (10).

Clinical Manifestations

Patients typically report gradual onset of fever, headache, and malaise over 1 to 2 weeks (10). Only one-fourth to one-third of patients present with the more classic triad of meningismus, photophobia, or vomiting (10). Global changes in mental status and lethargy with personality changes, memory loss, and visual or hearing loss are also seen along with cough, dyspnea, and molluscum-appearing skin lesions (10,31).

Diagnosis

In cryptococcal meningoencephalitis, neuroimaging may be suggestive of increased intracranial pressure or hydrocephalus (10). Mass lesions are rarely seen in HIV patients with *C. neoformans* central infection (10). CSF obtained from lumbar puncture is required to perform cryptococcal cultures, India ink staining, and cryptococcal antigen testing (10). In patients unable to undergo lumbar puncture, serum antigen testing has sensitivity comparable to that of CSF. Similarly, blood, urine, and sputum should be sent, as *C. neoformans* is frequently cultured from these media as well (10).

Treatment

Recommended treatment for cryptococcal meningoencephalitis includes antifungal therapy for an induction phase of at least 2 weeks, followed by consolidation therapy for at least 8 weeks.
  Induction Therapy:
- Amphotericin B deoxycholate 0.7 mg/kg IV daily PLUS
- Flucytosine 100 mg/kg PO daily in four divided doses
  Consolidation Therapy:
- Fluconazole 400 mg PO daily
  (Adapted from Cox and Perfect, 2014b)

Progressive Multifocal Leukoencephalopathy/JC Virus Infection

The John Cunningham (JC) Virus is a common childhood virus that remains dormant in kidneys and lymphoid organs in most adults (21,22). This virus can reactivate in the setting of immunosuppression, causing lytic infections of myelin-producing oligodendrocytes (21,22). This results in the demyelinating CNS disorder, Progressive Multifocal Leukoencephalopathy (PML) (21).

Clinical Manifestations

PML usually has an insidious onset with a varied presentation that depends on the area of the CNS involved (31). The patient may portray focal white matter symptoms such as monoparesis or hemiparesis, ataxia, hemianopia, or diplopia (21,22). Cortical manifestations are also seen from lesions in white matter that affect cortical function and from direct JC viral infection found in cortical neurons (21,22). These patients may present with aphasia, symptoms of cortical blindness, or general altered mental status (22). Seizures are also seen in nearly 20% of patients (31).

Diagnosis

Diagnosis of PML is made with a combination of the clinical picture, neuroimaging, CSF analysis, and, occasionally, brain biopsy to establish a diagnosis (31). Head CT imaging typically shows PML lesions as confluent or patchy hypodense white matter regions (22). MRI helps to delineate distinct lesions in the white matter in areas that correspond to the clinical findings and appear hyperintense on T2-weighted and fluid-attenuated inversion recovery sequences and hypointense on T1-weighted sequences (31). Definitive diagnosis can be established with the positive finding of JC virus DNA on analysis of CSF using PCR. The gold standard of brain biopsy with histological examination of suspect lesions is reserved for those patients with negative CSF findings in the absence of an alternative diagnosis (21,22).

Treatment

PML continues to be a progressive and frequently fatal disease in patients with advanced HIV (21,22). Optimizing the patient's immune system with appropriate ART treatment gives the best chance for survival (21,22). However, even with ART therapy, patients with HIV who develop PML have a 1-year survival rate of about 50%. There is no specific current therapy for the JC virus infection or PML (21,22).

Abdominal Pain and Diarrhea

Cryptosporidium Infection

The *Cryptosporidium* protozoan parasite is one of the most common causes of diarrhea in HIV immunosuppressed patients in developing countries (31). In the United States it is the causative agent in less than one in one thousand person-years of patients with AIDS (31). The infecting oocytes can be spread from infected feces through direct contact from animals or people or by contamination of recreational or public water supplies. (31)

Clinical Manifestations

Cryptosporidium infection is characterized by watery diarrhea, which can be severe and is associated with nausea, vomiting, and crampy lower abdominal pain (23). It can also be accompanied by fever and usually results in malabsorption states (23). Less commonly, the biliary tract can be involved, with ascending cholangitis and pancreatitis seen (31).

Diagnosis

Laboratory findings may include elevated alkaline phosphatase, and the gallbladder may be observed to be thickened and enlarged with dilated hepatic ducts on ultrasound or CT (23). Visualizing the oocytes from stool or tissue samples under microscopy with immunofluorescence or acid fast staining makes the definitive diagnosis of *Cryptosporidium* (31). Alternatively, enzyme immunoassays and PCR are equally or more sensitive, respectively (23).

Treatment

The mainstay of treatment for *Cryptosporidium* is to improve immunocompetence with ART along with supportive care, fluid and electrolyte replacement, and antidiarrheal medication (25). Nitazoxanide 1000 mg PO twice daily for 2 to 8 weeks has been recommended in patients with severe disease; however, a recent meta-analysis has shown it to be of little benefit in reducing parasitemia or improving symptoms in immunocompromised patients (25).

Microsporidiosis

Microsporidia are ubiquitous protists known to cause primarily a diarrheal disease in the immunosuppressed population, although recently seen more frequently in non-HIV infected people, including travelers, children, contact wearers, and the elderly. (31)

Clinical Manifestations

Infections with Microsporidia are usually associated with watery diarrhea, crampy abdominal pain, weight loss, nausea, and vomiting with resulting malabsorption (24). These infections rarely produce fever, and symptoms are related to the specific infecting species (31). Other disease processes caused by the variable species of Microsporidia can range from encephalitis and keratoconjunctivitis to infection of the sinuses, lung, liver, and disseminated disease (24,31).

Diagnosis

The diagnosis is made when the spores are seen under direct microscopy in the absence of significant blood or leukocytes in stool, body fluid, or tissue samples (24). Laboratories should be notified to specifically to stain for microsporidia, as routine ova and parasite evaluation does not generally detect these spores (24). Alternatively, tissue cultures, indirect immunofluorescence, and serological assays can also be used to diagnose Microsporidia infection (24).

Treatment

Rehydration, electrolyte repletion, antidiarrheal medication, and ensuring the patient is on appropriate ART assists the patient in eradicating the Microsporidia spores.

- Albendazole 400 mg orally twice daily is recommended for treatment of intestinal Microsporidiosis

No effective treatment currently is available for infection secondary to the *E. bieneusi* species of Microsporidia diarrhea.

(Adapted from Leder and Weller, 2014b)

Fever or Nonspecific Symptoms

Disseminated *Mycobacterium avium* Complex Disease

Mycobacterium avium Complex (MAC) includes infections caused by either mycobacterium species *M. avium* or *M. intracellulare* (12). Infection is thought to occur through ingestion or inhalation of the ubiquitous mycobacterium (12).

Clinical Manifestations

MAC disease can present as a multiorgan disseminated infection or a localized manifestation (31). Disseminated disease presents with nonspecific symptoms, including fever, weight loss, cough, diarrhea, night sweats, and abdominal pain (12). Localized disease frequently presents with focal lymph node inflammation found on exam or imaging study with or without fever (12,31). Focal MAC infection can also include pneumonitis, pericarditis, skin ulcers or abscesses, or CNS infection (31).

Diagnosis

Culture of mycobacterium from blood, lymph node, bone marrow, or other body fluid is diagnostic for MAC disease (31). DNA probes are used to differentiate *M. avium* and *M. intracellulare* from *M. tuberculosis* (12,31).

Treatment

Two or more antimicrobial drugs are recommended for initial therapy for MAC disease to decrease drug resistance.

Preferred first antibiotics:

- Clarithromycin 500 mg PO every 12 hours OR
- Azithromycin 600 mg PO once daily in patients who cannot tolerate clarithromycin

Preferred second antibiotic:

- Ethambutol 15 mg/kg PO once daily

If the patient is not on a protease inhibitor, the efficacy of Clarithromycin and Ethambutol may be increased with the addition of:

- Rifabutin 450 mg PO daily

If the patient is severely immunosuppressed or has high bacterial loads, the addition of amikacin, streptomycin, or one of the fluoroquinolones could be considered.

(Adapted from Currier, 2014 and Panel on Opportunistic Infections in HIV-Infected Adults and Adolescents)

Histoplasmosis

The fungus *Histoplasma capsulatum* exists in the soil throughout the world, although it is more prevalent in the Mississippi and Ohio River Valley areas in the United States (29). Infection is more likely in patients who travel to endemic areas or participate in activities that aerosolize bird or bat guano like caving or bird handling (2,29). Disease occurs through inhalation of the *H. capsulatum* spores (2).

Clinical Manifestations

Although frequently an isolated pulmonary infection in the immunocompetent patient, histoplasmosis is more likely to present as a progressive disseminated disease in the patient with advanced HIV (2). Primary symptoms in disseminated histoplasmosis can be nonspecific and include fever, weight loss, fatigue, night sweats, and nausea (2). Cough, dyspnea, and chest pain are present in approximately half of reported cases (31). CNS symptoms including seizures and altered sensorium along with gastrointestinal and cutaneous symptoms can also occur (31). Up to 10% of patients can present with multiorgan failure and shock.

Diagnosis

Pancytopenia, elevated aminotransferases, and elevated LDH are commonly seen in patients with disseminated disease (2). Radiographic findings on chest x-ray commonly include diffuse interstitial infiltrates or reticulonodular infiltrates, although pleural effusions, granulomas, adenopathy, cavitary disease, or a normal exam can be seen (2). In patients with disseminated disease, *Histoplasma* antigen detection is the most sensitive and specific diagnostic test (4). Culture of sputum, blood, or tissues along with direct microscopy is frequently used in resource-limited areas, although culture durations of 4 to 6 weeks and lower sensitivities of direct microscopy make this a less desired alternative (4).

Treatment

Patients with moderately severe to severe disseminated histoplasmosis should receive the following:

- Liposomal amphotericin B 3 mg/kg IV daily for 2 weeks or clinical improvement

Patients with less severe disease and patients completing IV amphotericin B should be started on the following oral regimen:

- Itraconazole 200 mg PO 3 times daily for 3 days, then
- Itraconazole 200 mg PO twice daily for up to 12 months

(Adapted from Panel on Opportunistic Infections in HIV-Infected Adults and Adolescents)

Bartonellosis

Bartonellosis encompasses infections caused by over thirty *Bartonella* species of the gram-negative intracellular bacteria that have been identified worldwide (1). However, less than half of these species have been isolated from humans, and only two, *Bartonella henselae* and *Bartonella quintana*, cause significant clinical disease in immunocompromised patients with HIV (1,34,35). *B. henselae* is transmitted by contact, usually a scratch, from a cat carrying *Bartonella*-infected flea feces in its claws (34). The cat is the reservoir, and the fleas become infected when they feed from the cat. Humans are thought to be the reservoir for *B. quintana*, and the disease is transmitted by bites from body lice and, as such, is more predominant in the homeless population (34). Infection with *Bartonella* causes a range of disease processes, including cat scratch disease, retinitis, trench fever, relapsing bacteremia, endocarditis, bacillary angiomatosis (BA) and bacillary peliosis hepatis (31). However, BA and bacillary peliosis hepatis only occur in immunocompromised patients (31).

Clinical Manifestations

Patients with BA can present with generalized constitutional symptoms, such as fever, chills, headache, malaise, and anorexia (34). Although BA vascular lesions have been found in most organ systems, the cutaneous manifestations occur most frequently (34). These lesions tend to originate as small red to purple papules, but may vary greatly with papular, nodular, pedunculated, or verrucous appearances (34). Along with skin lesions, patients may present with smooth purple plaques and papules in oral mucosa, tender subcutaneous nodular lesions, painful bony lesions, and involvement of lymph nodes, gastrointestinal tract, respiratory tract, and CNS (34). Patients with bacillary peliosis hepatis can present with fever and abdominal pain with evidence of hepatomegaly with or without splenomegaly (34). Laboratory values can show elevated alkaline phosphatase with thrombocytopenia or pancytopenia (34). CT of the abdomen and pelvis usually shows organomegaly with scattered hypodense lesions (34). Unexplained fever in a patient with HIV should also prompt consideration of *Bartonella* infection, as cases of bacteremia and endocarditis have also been reported in this population (31,34).

Diagnosis

Diagnosis of Bartonellosis is made through histopathological examination of tissue biopsy with modified silver staining (31,33). Although culture and isolation of the organism makes a definitive diagnosis, *Bartonella* is an extremely fastidious bacterium that makes this difficult to accomplish (31,33). Serological testing can be supportive if positive; however, studies suggest that some patients with advanced HIV would not produce the antibodies to *Bartonella* necessary to effect a positive test (31).

Treatment

Recommendations for patients with BA, peliosis hepatitis, and osteomyelitis are the following:

- Doxycycline 100 mg PO twice daily or erythromycin 500 mg PO every 6 hours

Oral therapy is recommended for BA and IV therapy for patients with peliosis hepatitis or osteomyelitis. Recommendations for patients with *Bartonella* CNS disease include the following:

- Doxycycline 100 mg PO or IV twice daily
- Rifampin 300 mg PO or IV twice daily has been advocated by some experts, although there is not significant data to support this use in HIV-infected patients.

Recommendations for patients with *Bartonella* bacteremia are the following:

- Doxycycline 100 mg PO or IV twice daily PLUS
- Gentamicin 1 mg/kg IV every 8 hours for the first 14 days

The addition of rifampin 300 mg IV to IV doxycycline listed previously should be considered for any unstable patient with life-threatening infection.

(Adapted from Spach, 2014a)

Cytomegalovirus Retinitis

Cytomegalovirus (CMV) is a double-stranded DNA virus whose initial infection is followed by a latent phase, similar to other viruses in the herpes family (31). Studies have shown about 40% to 80% of adults in the United States to be seropositive for CMV, with a higher percentage seen in African American and Mexican American populations (14). The majority of disease in immunocompromised patients is from reactivation of the latent virus with advanced immunosuppression, although reinfection with novel strains has also been demonstrated (19,31).

Clinical Manifestations

Although other systems can be affected by CMV end organ disease, the most common presentation of CMV infection in HIV positive patients is retinitis (19,31). Two-thirds of patients with CMV retinitis will present with unilateral symptoms, although without appropriate treatment, bilateral eye involvement will frequently occur (19,31). As CMV causes a full thickness necrotizing retinitis, symptoms will depend upon the severity of infection, the location on the retina, and the presence of retinal detachment. Patients may report blurred vision, blind spots, floaters, photopsia, and central or peripheral visual field deficits (19,31).

CMV colitis can occur in 5% to 10% of patients with AIDS and presents with abdominal pain, diarrhea, weight loss, and malaise (31). Similarly, a small subset of patients may present with odynophagia, nausea, and chest discomfort with CMV esophagitis or, even less commonly, with fever, cough, and dyspnea associated with CMV pneumonitis (31).

CMV involvement in the nervous system produces a spectrum of disease processes. CMV encephalitis results in confusion, lethargy, and fever (31). CMV ventriculoencephalitis produces focal neurological signs, including cranial nerve palsies and nystagmus with a potentially rapid decline to death (31). CMV polyradiculomyelopathy can present with slow progression over weeks and can result in loss of bowl and bladder control as well as lower extremity flaccid paraplegia (31).

Diagnosis

CMV retinitis is usually a clinical diagnosis on indirect ophthalmoscopy with the findings of yellow-white, fluffy, or granular retinal lesions located near retinal vessels with associated hemorrhage (19,31). Cultures, PCR, and antigen assays for CMV have poor sensitivity and specificity for determining end organ disease (19). CMV esophagitis and colitis are diagnosed based on the findings of ulcerations on endoscopic visualization and characteristic histopathologic findings of intranuclear inclusion bodies on biopsy specimens (31). CMV is usually thought to be an incidental finding when found in the evaluation of pneumonitis in immunosuppressed patients (31). Diagnosis is usually made in the context of pulmonary interstitial infiltrates on chest radiograph, appropriate clinical picture, multiple CMV inclusion bodies on cytopathology or histopathological examination, and the absence of an alternative diagnosis (31). CMV neurological disease is diagnosed from CSF or brain tissue biopsy, usually via PCR (31).

Treatment

Recommended therapy for CMV retinitis is valganciclovir 900 mg PO twice daily for 14 to 21 days. An initial intravitreal injection of ganciclovir 2 gm/infection or foscarnet 2.4 mg/injection can also be given for more rapid control of infection. Less research is available for the appropriate therapy for CMV esophagitis, colitis, pneumonitis, or CNS disease. The current recommendation to use IV ganciclovir or IV foscarnet in this population, with some experts recommending dual therapy with both gancicliovir and foscarnet in rapidly progressive CMV neurological disease.

(Adapted from Jacobson, 2014b and Panel on Opportunistic Infections in HIV-Infected Adults and Adolescents.)

Suggested Readings and References

1. Angelakis E, Raoult D. Pathogenicity and treatment of Bartonella infections. *Int J Antimicrobial Agents.* 2014;44(1):16–25. doi: 10.1016/j.ijantimicag.2014.04.006.

2. Baddley J. Epidemiology and clinical manifestations of histoplasmosis in HIV-infected patients. UpToDate website. 2013. Updated Month day, year. Accessed Month day, year.

3. Baddley J. Epidemiology and clinical manifestations of pulmonary aspergillosis and invasive disease in HIV-infected patients. UpToDate website. 2013.

4. Baddley J. Diagnosis and treatment of histoplasmosis in HIV-infected patients. UpToDate website. 2014.

5. Baddley J. Diagnosis and treatment of invasive Pulmonary Aspergillosis in HIV-infected patients. UpToDate website. 2014.

6. Bartlett J. Overview of primary prevention of opportunistic infections in HIV-infected patients. UpToDate website. 2015.

7. Bartlett J. The natural history and clinical features of HIV infection in adults and adolescents. UpToDate website. 2015.

8. Burnardo J. Clinical manifestations, diagnosis, and treatment of extrapulmonary and miliary tuberculosis. UpToDate website. 2015.

9. HIV/AIDS. HIV in the United States: *at a glance*. Centers for Disease Control and Prevention website. http://www.cdc.gov/hiv/statistics/basics/ataglance.html Accessed March 5, 2015.

10. Cox G, Perfect J. Epidemiology, clinical manifestation, and diagnosis of cryptococcus neoformans meningoencephalitis in HIV-infected patients. UpToDate website. 2014.

11. Cox G, Perfect J. Treatment of cryptococcus neoformans meningoencephalitis in HIV-infected patients UpToDate website. 2014.

12. Currier J. Mycobacterium avium complex (MAC) infections in HIV-infected patients. UpToDate website. 2014.

13. Diagnoses of HIV Infection in the United States and Dependent Areas, 2013. HIV Surveillance Report. 25. Centers for Disease Control and Prevention website. http://www.cdc.gov/hiv/pdf/library/reports/surveillance/cdc-hiv-surveillance-report-vol-25.pdf. Accessed March 14, 2015.

14. Friel T. Pathogenesis, clinical manifestations, and diagnosis of AIDS-related cytomegalovirus retinitis. UpToDate website. 2014.

15. Galgiani J. Coccidioidal meningitis. UpToDate website.

16. Galgiani J, Ampel N. Coccidioidomycosis in compromised hosts. UpToDate website. 2014.

17. Havlir D, Getahun H, Sanne I, Nunn P. Opportunities and challenges for HIV care in overlapping HIV and TB epidemics. *JAMA*. 2008;300(4). doi: 10.1001/jama.300.4.423.

18. Heller H. Toxoplasmosis in HIV-infected patients. UpToDate website. 2014.

19. Jacobson M. Pathogenesis, clinical manifestations, and diagnosis of AIDS-related cytomegalovirus retinitis. UpToDate website. 2014.

20. Jacobson M. Treatment of AIDS-related cytomegalovirus retinitis. UpToDate website. 2014.

21. Koralnik I. Progressive multifocal leukoencephalopathy: treatment and prognosis. UpToDate website. 2015.

22. Koralnik I. Progressive multifocal leukoencephalopathy: epidemiology, clinical manifestations, and diagnosis. UpToDate website. 2015.

23. Leder K, Weller P. Epidemiology, clinical manifestations, and diagnosis of cryptosporidiosis. UpToDate website. 2014.

24. Leder K, Weller P. Microsporidiosis. UpToDate website. 2014.

25. Leder K, Weller P. Treatment and prevention of cryptosporidiosis. UpToDate website. 2014.

26. Lee C-C, Hsieh C-C, Chan T-Y, Chen P-L, Chi C-H, Ko W-C. Community-onset febrile illness in HIV-infected adults: variable pathogens in terms of CD4 counts and transmission routes. *Am J Emerg Med.* 2015;33(1):80–87. doi: 10.1016/j.ajem.2014.10.013.

27. Lucas S, Nelson AM. () "HIV and the spectrum of human disease," *J Pathol.* 2014;235(2):229–241. doi: 10.1002/path.4449.

28. Maartens G. Epidemiology, clinical manifestations, and diagnosis of tuberculosis in HIV-infected patients. UpToDate website. 2014.

29. McLeod DSA, Mortimer RH, Perry-Keene DA, et al. Histoplasmosis in Australia. *Medicine.* 2011;90(1):61–68. doi: 10.1097/md.0b013e318206e499.

30. HIV/AIDS. Opportunistic infections. Centers for Disease Control and Prevention website. 2015. http://www.cdc.gov/hiv/basics/livingwithhiv/opportunisticinfections.html. Accessed March 5, 2015.

31. Panel on Opportunistic Infections in HIV-Infected Adults and Adolescents. Guidelines for the prevention and treatment of opportunistic infections in HIV-infected adults and adolescents: recommendations from the Centers for Disease Control and Prevention, the National Institutes of Health, and the HIV Medicine Association of the Infectious Diseases Society of America. http://aidsinfo.nih.gov/contentfiles/lvguidelines/adult_oi.pdf. Accessed March 5, 2015.

32. Sax P. Treatment of pneumocystis infection in HIV-infected patients. UpToDate website. 2012.

33. Spach D. Diagnosis, treatment, and prevention of Bartonella infections in HIV-infected patients. UpToDate website. 2014.

34. Spach D. Epidemiology and clinical manifestations of Bartonella infections in HIV-infected patients. UpToDate website. 2014.

35. Tietjen P, Sax P. Clinical presentation and diagnosis of Pneumocystis pulmonary infection in HIV-infected patients. UpToDate website. 2013.

Chapter 56

Infections in the Transplant Patient

Alexander Billioux

Summary Box

Disease Description:
There are three phases of infectious risk in solid organ transplant patients:

- Early (< 1 month): Typical postoperative infections, such as urinary tract infection (UTI), central line-associated blood stream infection, hospital-acquired pneumonia/ventilator-associated pneumonia/health care-associated pneumonia, and surgical site infection
- Intermediate (1–6 months): Opportunistic infections due to immunosuppression, such as *Cytomegalovirus* (CMV), *Pneumocystis jirovecii*, *Cryptococcus* species, other fungal infections, and *Nocardia* species
- Late (> 6 months): Common community infections and pathogens, such as bacterial pneumonia, viral pneumonia, and UTIs; also seen are recurrent CMV, *P. jirovecii*, and *Cryptococcus* in patients with more intense immunosuppression

Organisms and Treatment:

- Early: Empiric coverage for hospital-acquired and drug-resistant bacteria, such as methicillin-resistant *Staphylococcus aureus* (MRSA), *Pseudomonas*, and bacteria with extended spectrum beta lactamases (ESBL)
- Intermediate: Targeted therapy against identified opportunistic pathogens
- Late: Standard treatment for common infections with added coverage against any resistant organisms from previous infections as well as treatment targeting recurrent CMV, *Cryptococcus*, and *P. jirovecii*

Other key issues: Hematopoietic stem cell transplantation patients are at the highest risk for infection during the period from transplant to neutrophil recovery. Empiric broad-spectrum antibiotics with coverage of resistant pathogens are needed until the immune system is reconstituted. These patients are also at risk for opportunistic pathogens for up to 3 years post-transplant.

323

Disease Description

Recipients of donor-derived tissues and organs represent a group at particularly high risk of infection because of their unique combination of risk factors. Chronic illness, both pre-transplant and post-transplant, results in more exposure to health care contexts in which pathogens—especially drug-resistant species—might be acquired. The transplant surgery itself compromises anatomical barriers to infection via indwelling venous and urinary catheters, endotracheal tubes, and, of course, surgical wounds.

Donor-derived tissues and organs may harbor infectious pathogens undetected during rapid pre-transplant evaluations. Most important, the immunosuppression necessary to prevent rejection of donor tissues increases the risk of infection by a variety of common and opportunistic pathogens. The relative importance of each of these factors is not static but rather waxes and wanes over time after transplantation. In addition, each type of transplanted organ bears unique infectious risks. Lastly, many of the pathogens typically seen in patients post-transplant have particular clinical presentations that can act as clues to their presence. Thus, triaging the likely causes of infection in the transplant patient is largely based on three variables: time from transplantation, type of organ transplanted, and the primary manifestation of infection.

Triaging by Post-Transplant Timing of Infection

The post-transplant period can be divided into three phases of infectious risk. It is important to note that the main factor underlying the division into these three phases is the degree to which a patient is immunosuppressed. Consequently, the timeline put forward here will be effectively reset after episodes of acute rejection that are followed by increased immunosuppression.[1] Thus, a careful history eliciting not only the *date of transplant* but also the *timing of episodes of rejection* is key.

Early Phase (less than 1 month post-transplant)

This period includes the transplant surgery and post-operative care when immunosuppression has not had its full effect on the patient. Most infections during this period fall into three categories:

1. **Surgery-related** *bacterial* infections predominate during this phase. These include pneumonia, UTIs, line-associated blood stream infections, and bacterial and fungal infections of surgical wounds.[2]
2. **Recurrent** infections can be reactivated by relative immunosuppression, especially viral pathogens like hepatitis B (HBV) and C (HCV) viruses as well as herpes simplex virus (HSV).[1] Latent M. tuberculosis can also reactivate at this time and is sometimes missed in pre-transplant screening.
3. **Donor-derived** pathogens can be transmitted in transplanted tissues, including drug-resistant bacteria, such as vancomycin-resistant *Enterococcus* (VRE), MRSA, and *Pseudomonas*. West Nile virus (WNV), HIV, HBV, HCV, *Trypanosoma cruzi* (ie, Chagas disease), and *Toxoplasma* can also originate from donors.[3]

Intermediate Phase (1 to 6 months post-transplant)

This is the period of peak immunosuppression, leading to the emergence of opportunistic infections. It is important to note that differing immunosuppressive regimens result in susceptibility to particular pathogens (Table 56.1). Key pathogens during this period include CMV and other herpes viruses, *P. jirovecii*,

Table 56.1 Common Pathogens Associated with Immunosuppressive Agents[a]

Immunosuppressive Agent	Common Pathogens
Corticosteroids, chronic	Pneumocystis, bacteria, molds, hepatitis B virus
Corticosteroids, bolus (graft rejection)	CMV, BK polyomavirus nephropathy (PVAN)
Azathioprine	Papillomavirus?
Mycophenolate mofetil	Early bacteria, late CMV?
Calcineurin inhibitors (CNI)	Viruses, gingival infections
Rapamycin	Pneumonitis (excess infections in combinations with CNIs)
T-lymphocyte depletion (agent specific)	Herpes virus activation, PVAN, late fungal and viral infections, PTLD, hepatitis C virus
B-lymphocyte depletion, plasmapheresis	Encapsulated bacteria, sepsis

Abbreviations: CMV, *Cytomegalovirus*; PTLD, post-transplant lymphoproliferative disorder.

[a]Modified from Van Burik JA, Freifeld AG. Infection in the severely immunocompromised host. In: Abeloff MD, Armitage JO, Niederhuber JE, et•al, eds. *Clinical Oncology*. 3rd ed. Philadelphia: Churchill Livingstone; 2004:942; and Fishman and Issa.[40]

Toxoplasma, Cryptococcus, Candida, Aspergillus, and endemic molds. Each of these is discussed in more detail following.

Late Phase (more than 6 months post-transplant)

Patients more than 6 months post-transplantation are likely to be on a reduced, stable immunosuppressive regimen. Along with the continued use of appropriate prophylactic antibiotics, this results in a reduction in opportunistic infections.[4] Most infections during this period are due to the following[1,4]:

1. **Community-acquired** pathogens, such as bacteria causing typical pneumonias or UTIs. Often both the *severity* and *duration* of these infections are increased in this population.
2. **Exposure-related** infections due to fungi (eg, *Aspergillus* spp., mucormycosis, and environmental molds), bacteria (eg, *Listeria, Rhodococcus*, and *Nocardia*), and parasites (eg, *Leishmania*).
3. **Opportunistic** infections, such as CMV, HSV, Varicella Zoster Virus (VZV), *Cryptococcus*, and *Pneumocystis* persisting from the intermediate phase.

Organ-Specific Considerations

Patients receiving lung and heart-lung transplants have the highest incidence of infections, followed by liver, heart, and kidney recipients.[5] The unique circumstances surrounding each type of transplanted organ predisposes the patient receiving them to particular pathogens and infections.

Lung

Lung transplant patients suffer from the highest frequency of infections, likely because of the exposure of the lung's large surface area to the environment, reduced cough reflex, impeded mucociliary clearance, and impaired lymphatic drainage.[6] This results in frequent pneumonias, with bacteria predominating (~80%). Additionally, community-acquired respiratory viruses (eg, respiratory syncytial virus, influenza, and parainfluenza) can be more serious in lung transplant patients where they are more likely to cause lower respiratory tract infections and increase the chances of rejection.[7] CMV pneumonitis, which can present without CMV viremia, is also a significant concern in this population.[6]

325

Liver

Bacteria are the most common cause of infection in liver transplant recipients, with incidences ranging from 35% to 70%.[8] *S. aureus* and enteric gram-negative bacteria predominate, with anaerobic infections occurring less frequently. Most infections occur in the first 2 months after transplantation, largely as a consequence of the mechanical complications of surgery: bile leaks often lead to peritonitis and intra-abdominal abscesses, whereas biliary strictures increase the risk of cholangitis. Note that Charcot's triad may be absent in the context of immunosuppression, making this an unreliable diagnostic adjunct in these patients.[5]

In addition to bacterial infections, liver transplant patients suffer from more fungal infections than other solid organ recipients, with incidences ranging from 20% to 30% of infections. *Candida* and *Aspergillus* species predominate, causing infection in the blood, sputum, bile, and the peritoneal cavity.[9] Lastly, viral hepatitides are a common cause of cirrhosis and the need for transplantation, and they can often be associated with post-transplant complications.[5] In particular, HCV—which has become the most common indication for liver transplantation—is associated with decreased graft function, shorter time to recurrence of cirrhosis, and increased mortality.[10]

Heart

The majority of infections in heart transplant patients are due to bacteria (~40%) and viruses (~40%), with fungi and rare heart-specific pathogens comprising the remainder.[11] The most common sites of primary infection leading to cardiac infection are the lungs, followed by the oral cavity, urinary tract, and skin. In addition, mediastinitis and chronic infections of sternal wounds—especially with *S. aureus* and *S. epidermidis*—can complicate the post-operative course.[5] Also, given their proclivity for cardiac and vascular tissue, infections with *Aspergillus, Toxoplasma, Trypanosoma cruzi, Nocardia*, and CMV are more frequently seen among heart transplant recipients.[5,11,12]

Kidney

UTIs predominate in renal transplant recipients. Although cystitis is common in this population, up to 13% of patients may develop pyelonephritis.[5] Recurrent episodes of infection are associated with stricture formation and loss of graft function. Renal transplant patients are also uniquely at risk for *BK virus* (BKV) infections, which can result in polyomavirus-associated nephropathy (PVAN) and hemorrhagic cystitis.[13] BKV is often present prior to transplant and resurfaces as immunosuppression increases. The only effective treatment for BKV flares is reduction of immunosuppression.

Diagnosis and Management of Specific Presentations

Wound Infection

Presentation: Induction of immunosuppression and the frequent use of post-transplant glucocorticoids put transplant patients at increased risk for wound infections and dehiscence. The presentation is typical and rarely serious in nature.[5] Typical pathogens are S. aureus and epidermidis, as well as Candida spp.

Diagnosis: Close inspection of all surgical wounds at the time of presentation is key. One should note the level of healing, erythema, drainage, dehiscence, and pain out of proportion to expectations post-surgically. Wound cultures are of variable utility in diagnosis.

Treatment: Coverage against gram-positive skin flora (including MRSA) with vancomycin. For surgeries involving gastrointestinal and genitourinary structures or the axillae, extended spectrum penicillins, second generation cephalosporins, or carbapenems can be added.[14]

Central Nervous System Infection

Presentation: Signs of meningitis or encephalitis should be thoroughly investigated in the transplant patient. Typical pathogens in this population include Listeria monocytogenes, Nocardia, Cryptococcus, Candida, Aspergillus, Toxoplasma, VZV, human herpes virus-6 (HHV-6), and the John Cunningham (JC) virus.[5] Most of these cause infection in the first 1 to 6 months post-transplant, with the notable exception of Cryptococcus, which can present later.

Diagnosis: Imaging of the head via computerized tomography (CT) or magnetic resonance imaging (MRI) with and without contrast should be performed. Lumbar puncture (LP) should be performed with cerebrospinal fluid (CSF) sent for bacterial, mycobacterial, and fungal culture; polymerase chain reaction (PCR) analysis for enteroviruses, CMV, Epstein-Barr virus (EBV), VZV, HSV, JC virus, and WNV; and antigen-based studies for Cryptococcus and T. pallidum based upon the presentation and duration of symptoms.[15] LP should not be performed if CT or MRI demonstrates space-occupying lesions causing mass-effect, as this could lead to brain herniation. Brain lesions may require brain biopsy for diagnosis and treatment.

Treatment: Definitive treatment should be guided by imaging and CSF analysis. Initial antimicrobial coverage for meningitis should include vancomycin (To cover MRSA and S. pneumoniae), ceftazidime or cefepime (To cover Pseudomonas, Neisseria, Haemophilus, and S. pneumoniae), ampicillin (To cover Listeria and S. agalactiae), and acyclovir (To cover HSV and VZV).[16] Patients with encephalitis should have similar coverage while awaiting CSF analysis with emphasis on acyclovir to cover HSV. Doxycycline should be added if rickettsial or ehrlichiainfections are suspected.[17]

Pneumonia

Presentation: Early pneumonias are often due to ventilator-associated bacteria, such as gram-negative bacilli, oral anaerobes, and S. aureus.[5] More than 30 days from transplantation, S. pneumoniae, Haemophilus influenzae, and less common organisms, such as CMV, respiratory viruses, M. tuberculosis, Nocardia, Aspergillus, Histoplasma capsulatum, Coccidioides species, and Pneumocystis are seen.[5] Bacterial pneumonias typically have an acute onset (3 days), productive cough, and focal infiltrate, whereas atypical or opportunistic pathogens often present more gradually (7 or more days) with a nonproductive cough and diffuse or nodular infiltrate on imaging.

Diagnosis: Sputum and blood should be cultured. Bronchoalveolar lavage (BAL) should be considered for patients not responding to therapy or presenting with atypical symptoms concerning for an opportunistic pathogen. Urine should be tested for the presence of S. pneumoniae and Legionella pneumophila antigens. Respiratory viral PCR-based diagnostic panels can be performed according to the season and clinical presentation.

Treatment: Typical pneumonias should be treated as hospital-acquired pneumonia (including ventilator-associated pneumonia and health care-associated pneumonia), with antibiotics covering typical bacterial pathogens (including the drug-resistant species MRSA and Pseudomonas) until culture-guided therapy can be instituted. Atypical causes of pneumonia should be treated according to guidelines after their diagnosis is proven unless suspicion is very high.[18]

Gastrointestinal Infections

Presentation: Intra-abdominal infections in liver transplant were discussed previously. Gastroenteritis and colitis are common presentations in the transplant patient. In addition to the common causes of these conditions, transplant patients appear to be particularly susceptible to salmonellosis and C. difficile colitis.[5] Acute hepatitis due to HBV, HCV, or CMV can be seen in these patients as well. Chronic diarrhea in the transplant patient can indicate CMV or a parasitic infection.

Diagnosis: Stool should be sent for culture, *C. difficile* toxin detection, examination for ova and parasites, and lactoferrin. PCR-based assays for HBV, HCV, and CMV should be sent if there is evidence of hepatitis. Note that viremia may be absent in CMV colitis.

Treatment: Diarrhea should be treated conservatively. *C. difficile* and CMV colitis should be treated if they are proven to be present.[19]

Opportunistic Pathogens in Transplant Patients

Cytomegalovirus and other Herpes Viruses

Presentation: CMV infection or reactivation is seen in 75% of solid organ transplant patients.[20] Primary infection is generally more severe than reactivation and occurs when an organ from a CMV positive donor (D+) is transplanted into a seronegative (R-) patient.[1] Of note, 5% of D-R- patients will develop primary CMV infection post-transplant.[20] CMV has both "direct effects" on the organs and tissues it infects as well as "indirect effects" secondary to the host immune response. Primary CMV infection often manifests as a flu or mononucleosis-like syndrome with fever, neutropenia, and occasional lymphadenopathy. The direct effects of CMV may manifest as pneumonitis, retinitis, hepatitis, pancreatitis, or gastroenteritis. Primary CMV infection should be suspected in all seronegative patients transplanted with an organ from a seropositive donor presenting with flu-like symptoms and signs of primary organ infection. Likewise, reactivation should be considered in seropositive patients presenting during periods of peak immunosuppression. Patients should be asked if they are currently or have previously taken prophylactic valganciclovir to prevent CMV infection or activation.

Diagnosis: Diagnosis of acute CMV infection in the transplant patient is made by testing for viremia with PCR-based assays or with pp65 antigen detection.[20] Of note, viremia may be absent in CMV chorioretinitis and gastritis/colitis. Evaluation with slit-lap examination and colonoscopy is necessary if these entities are suspected.[1] Diagnostic biopsies are usually of highest yield when taken from the transplanted organ or the clinically affected organ.[20]

Treatment: Acute CMV infection is treated with intravenous (IV) ganciclovir (5 mg/kg q12 hours).[20,21] Weekly viral loads should be followed so that conversion to oral valganciclovir can be timed with clearance of viremia. CMV resistance to treatment with ganciclovir is rare (2%–6% of patients with previous treatment) and is associated with the UL 97 mutation in the viral genome. Resistant CMV is treated with high-dose ganciclovir (up to 10 mg/kg) or foscarnet under the guidance of infectious disease specialists.[21] CMV retinitis can be treated with ganciclovir, cidofovir, or foscarnet; it often requires intravitreal therapy through injection or implant.[21]

Other Herpes Viruses: In addition to CMV, other members of the herpes virus family are known to both acutely infect or reactivate in immunocompromised hosts.[22,23] HSV reactivation is observed in roughly 60% of patients not taking prophylaxis and is associated with typical oral and genital lesions in most; it can cause keratitis, pneumonitis, and hepatitis.[24] EBV is also prevalent in transplant patients, with three-quarters of seronegative patients developing primary infection and one-third of seropositive patients developing reactivation.[5] In addition to causing the typical mononucleosis syndrome and occasional organ dysfunction (similar to CMV), EBV plays an important role in the development of post-transplant lymphoproliferative disorder, the most common malignant complication of organ transplantation.[25] Another malignancy strongly associated with immunosuppression and observed in transplant patients, Kaposi's sarcoma, is also caused by the human herpes virus 8.[5]

Pneumocystis jirovecii

Presentation: *P. jirovecii* (formerly *Pneumocystis carinii*) pneumonia, or PCP, is an important cause of respiratory compromise in immunocompromised individuals, including transplant patients. Transplant patients present differently than AIDS patients, with transplant patients developing symptoms sooner (3–5 days instead of 1–2 weeks) and occasionally presenting without fever.[26] Nevertheless, fever, dyspnea, and nonproductive cough are still common in the transplant patient.[26]

Diagnosis: Chest x-ray may be normal or demonstrate the presence of increased interstitial markings. Chest CT scans are more sensitive and often demonstrate diffuse, bilateral interstitial pneumonia. Induced sputum should be performed to demonstrate the presence of *Pneumocystis* by direct fluorescence.[26] This can be repeated to increase sensitivity. Patients unable to produce a sample on induced sputum should undergo BAL. Open biopsy should be restricted to instances where the previously mentioned methods are nondiagnostic or where concern for concomitant infection is present.[26]

Treatment: PCP is treated with high-dose trimethoprim-sulfamethoxazole for 21 days.[26] Prednisone (40 mg PO for 5–7 days) should be added when the pAO_2 is less than 70 mmHg and gradually tapered over 1 to 2 weeks.

Cryptococcus Species

Presentation: *Cryptococcus* is the third most common cause of fungal infection in transplant patients, typically causing pulmonary or CNS disease.[27] Pneumonia typically presents with fever and chest pain. Dyspnea, cough, and hemoptysis are seen less frequently.[28] Cryptococcal pneumonia can also lead to acute respiratory failure with poor prognosis.[27] Cryptococcal meningitis typically presents with fever, headache, and nuchal rigidity. It progresses to encephalitis with lethargy and confusion over time.[15]

Diagnosis: Cryptococcal antigens can be detected in the serum of 88% to 91% of transplant patients with meningitis.[27] CNS manifestations should prompt large-volume LP with measurement of opening and closing pressures, and CSF should be sent for fungal culture and cryptococcal antigen studies.[15,27] Blood and urine specimens should also be sent for culture to investigate disseminated infection.

Treatment: Meningoencephalitis and disseminated *Cryptococcus* are treated with induction therapy consisting of liposomal amphotericin B plus flucytosine for 14 days, followed by consolidation therapy consisting of 8 weeks of fluconazole.[27] Maintenance therapy is often recommended for 6 to 12 months following acute infection. Mild to moderate pulmonary cryptococcosis can be treated with oral fluconazole for 6 to 12 months, whereas severe disease should be treated like CNS or disseminated disease.[27]

Toxoplasma gondii

Presentation: Transplant patients can acquire primary infection with *Toxoplasma* or can experience reactivation of a latent infection.[29] Primary infection after ingestion of oocytes results in fever, lymphadenopathy, sore throat, and myalgia and can lead to myocarditis, pneumonitis, and nephritis.[30] Reactivation of latent infection is more commonly seen in transplant patients and usually presents as CNS disease. Patients present with persistent headache that is not responsive to analgesics and progresses to ataxia, lethargy, and encephalitis.[29]

Diagnosis: Serum should be tested for immunoglobulin M (IgM) and immunoglobulin G (IgG) antibodies against *Toxoplasma*. The presence of IgM ± IgG indicates acute infection, whereas IgG positivity without IgM indicates reactivation. CNS symptoms should be evaluated with CT or MRI, where the typical finding is multiple space-occupying lesions in the cerebrum and basal ganglia.[30]

Treatment: Transplant patients with IgG against *Toxoplasma* are usually given trimethoprim-sulfamethoxazole prophylaxis to prevent infection or reactivation.[29] Higher doses are used for prophylaxis in heart transplant patients and to treat active disease.[15]

Candida, Aspergillus, and Endemic Molds

Epidemiology: The vast majority of fungal infections occur within the first 6 months post-transplant. According to the transplant-associated infection network, the most common causes of fungal infections are *Candida* species (53%–56%), followed by *Aspergillus* species (19%) and endemic fungi and molds (14%).[31] Among all transplant-associated fungal infections, Candidiasis predominates in small bowel, pancreas, liver, heart, and kidney transplants in order of decreasing incidence. However, *Aspergillus* is more frequently the cause of fungal infections in lung transplant patients. Fungal infections are difficult to treat and are often disseminated at the time of diagnosis, resulting in a higher mortality rate than for bacterial sepsis.[32]

Diagnosis: Standard blood culture systems generally also assay for the presence of pathogenic fungi.[33] However, blood cultures may only be positive in 50% of autopsy-proven cases of Candidiasis and 10% of invasive Aspergillosis.[34] Positive blood cultures should prompt repeat blood cultures to rule out contamination. Communication with the microbiology laboratory about special concern for fungal infection can help ensure proper handling of specimens and increase the diagnostic yield. Biopsy for histopathologic diagnosis of organ-specific involvement is more invasive but increases diagnostic certainty beyond blood culture. Serum galactomannan levels offer a sensitivity of 73% and specificity of 81% for invasive *Aspergillus*, making this a useful test to help identify infection.[32] Serum β-glucan can also be used to identify the presence of a variety of fungi, but cross-reaction with surface glucans of bacteria like *Pseudomonas* limit the utility of this test in isolation. Suspected fungal sinusitis should prompt surgical evaluation by an ear, nose, and throat specialist.

Treatment: Empiric treatment in suspected fungal infection should be targeted against *Candida* species, with additional coverage for *Aspergillus* in high-risk populations (ie, lung and hematopoietic transplant patients as well as patients with previous *Aspergillus* infections).[32,35] Fluconazole is a generally well-tolerated antifungal with activity against most species of *Candida* and is an appropriate first-line therapy in stable patients.[32] Unstable patients, individuals with suspected *Candida glabrata* or *krusei* infections (based on local prevalences), and patients treated with fluconazole in the previous 30 days should be treated with echinocandins or voriconazole (limited coverage of *C. glabrata and krusei*). If broader coverage is needed, amphotericin B has excellent activity against most pathogenic fungi (though dose increases are required for *C. glabrata and krusei*). Voriconazole is the treatment of choice for *Aspergillus* and endemic molds, but the addition of echinocandins or amphotericin may be required in severe cases or in the context of slow response to voriconazole alone.[32] Mucormycosis should treated with amphotericin and debridement as indicated.[32] Indwelling hardware should be removed or replaced after documented fungemia.

Complications: Fungal endocarditis is a serious complication after fungemia in hosts with prosthetic heart valves, indwelling hardware, or valvular damage (eg, IV drug users and patients with a history of rheumatic fever).[35] Fungal endocarditis often requires surgical management for definitive treatment. Fungal endophthalmitis is a severe complication of fungemia. Slit lamp examination should be performed 1 week after the diagnosis of Candidemia. Fungal endophthalmitis is treated with a combination of systemic therapy and vitrectomy.[36]

Hematopoietic Stem Cell Transplant Infections

Hematopoietic stem cell transplantation (HSCT), also known as bone marrow transplantation (BMT), is used to treat a variety of illnesses, including leukemias and lymphomas, myeloma, aplastic anemia, sickle cell anemia, and autoimmune disorders.[37] Unlike solid organ transplantation, patients undergoing successful HSCT typically experience a period of profound immunodeficiency followed by reconstitution of the immune system and eventual return to immunocompetence. Thus, although the pathogens encountered by both patients are similar, the timing of highest infectious risk varies between the solid-organ and HSC transplant patients (Figure 56.1).

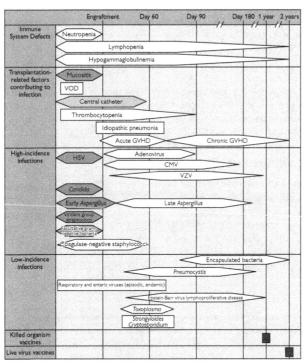

Figure 56.1 Phases of predictable opportunistic infections among patients undergoing hematopoietic stem cell transplantation (HSCT). Immune defects predisposing to infection are bordered by color (pink, neutropenia; blue, lymphopenia; green, hypogammaglobulinemia). Barrier defects predisposing to infection are shaded in color (yellow, mucosal breakdown; silver, skin breakdown.) Modified from Young J-AH, Weisdorf DJ. Infections in Recipients of Hematopoietic Cell Transplantation. 7th ed. Amsterdam, Netherlands: Elsevier Inc; 2010.
VOD, vasoocclusive disease; GVHD, graft versus host disease; HSV, herpes simplex virus; CMV, cytomegalovirus; VZV, varicella zoster virus.

Pre-Engraftment Infections

Patients preparing for BMT first undergo myeloablation, or removal of the native bone marrow, through a variety of cytotoxic regimens ± irradiation.[37] They are subsequently transfused with exogenous stem cells and monitored for up to 42 days for recovery of the bone marrow, a process termed "engraftment." The pre-engraftment period from myeloablation to recovery of the bone marrow is the period of highest infectious risk in HSCT patients. Their risk of infection during this period is greater than any period after solid organ transplantation because of the depletion of neutrophils in addition to their cell-mediated and humoral immune systems.[38]

Epidemiology: Bacterial infections predominate during this period, with oral gram-positive and enteric gram-negative bacteria translocating to the blood stream because of mechanical barrier defects, such as mucositis and typhlitis. Fungal infections, such as candidiasis and aspergillosis, are also common because of neutropenia. Prophylactic use of antibiotics and antifungals has reduced infections with typical pathogens, but this has shifted the spectrum toward drug-resistant species, including MRSA, VRE, and *Pseudomonas*. Antibiotic-induced *C. difficile* infection is also increasingly common. Despite immunodeficiency, patients will still typically present with a fever as well as rigors and other signs of systemic inflammatory syndrome.

Diagnosis: Blood, sputum, and urine should all be cultured, including cultures drawn from any indwelling venous catheters. Imaging of the chest should be performed to evaluate for occult pneumonia, especially of fungal origin. All indwelling lines should be examined for signs of infection and removed if the patient is severely ill. Diarrhea should be tested for *C. difficile* toxin.

Treatment: Initial coverage with piperacillin-tazobactam or cefepime is indicated for fever in the neutropenic patient.[39] Carbapenems can be used for patients with known histories of ESBL producing bacterial infections. Vancomycin should be added if signs of venous catheter, skin and soft tissue infection, pneumonia, or hemodynamic instability are present.[39]

Post-Engraftment Infections

This period extends from the time of engraftment (neutrophil recovery) to 100 days post-transplant. Patients who received allogeneic HSCT are at higher risk of infection than those who received autologous HSCT during this period.[38] This is because allogeneic HSCT patients are at higher risk for graft-versus-host disease, which can disrupt mechanical barriers to infection and increase the risk of bacterial and fungal infections. These patients are also at higher risk of CMV infection/reactivation. Late-onset aspergillosis and PCP can also occur during this period.[38]

Late Infections

This period extends from day 101 post-transplant until the time of reconstitution of the normal immune system, typically 1½ to 3 years after transplant. Recurrent VZV infection (ie, shingles), as well as infections due to encapsulated bacteria, invasive *Aspergillus*, and other tissue-invasive molds may occur during this period. CMV reactivation may still occur during this period.[38]

Suggested Readings and References

1. Fishman JA. Infection in solid-organ transplant recipients. N Engl J Med. 2007;357(25):2601–2614.
2. Snydman DR. Infection in solid organ transplantation. Transpl Infect Dis. 1999;1(1):21–28.
3. Fishman JA, Greenwald MA, Grossi PA. Transmission of infection with human allografts: essential considerations in donor screening. Clin Infect Dis. 2012;55(5):720–727.
4. San Juan R, Aguado JM, Lumbreras C, et al. Incidence, clinical characteristics and risk factors of late infection in solid organ transplant recipients: data from the RESITRA study group. Am J Transpl. 2007;7(4):964–971.
5. Dummer JS, Singh N. Infections in Solid Organ Transplant Recipients. 7th ed. Amsterdam, Netherlands: Elsevier Inc; 2010.
6. Burguete SR, Maselli DJ, Fernandez JF, Levine SM. Lung transplant infection. Wiley Online Library. Respirology. 2012;18(1). DOI: 10.1111/j.1440-1843.2012.02196.x
7. Billings JL, Hertz MI, Wendt CH. Community respiratory virus infections following lung transplantation. Wiley Online Library. Transpl Infect Dis. 2001;3(3). . ISSN 1398-2273
8. Winston DJ, Emmanouilides C, Busuttil RW. Infections in liver transplant recipients. Clin Infect Dis. 1995;21(5):1077–89.
9. Rabkin JM, Oroloff SL, Corless CL, et al. Association of fungal infection and increased mortality in liver transplant recipients. Am J Surg. 2000;179(5):426–430.
10. Forman LM, Lewis JD, Berlin JA, Feldman HI, Lucey MR. The association between hepatitis C infection and survival after orthotopic liver transplantation. Gastroenterology. 2002;122(4):889–896.
11. Montoya JG, Giraldo LF, Efron B, et al. Infectious complications among 620 consecutive heart transplant patients at Stanford University Medical Center. Clin Infect Dis. 2001;33(5):629–640.

12. Petri WA. Infections in heart transplant recipients. *Clin Infect Dis*. 1994;18(2):141–146, 147–148.

13. Karuthu S, Blumberg EA. Common infections in kidney transplant recipients. *Clin J Am Soc Nephrol*. 2012;7(12):2058–2070.

14. Stevens DL, Bisno AL, Chambers HF, et al. Practice guidelines for the diagnosis and management of skin and soft-tissue infections. *Clin Infect Dis*. 2014 Jul 15;59(2):147–159.

15. Zunt JR. Central nervous system infection during immunosuppression. *Neurol Clin*. 2002;20(1):1–22.

16. Tunkel AR, Hartman BJ, Kaplan SL, et al. Practice guidelines for the management of bacterial meningitis. *Clin Infect Dis*. 2004;39(9):1267–1284.

17. Tunkel AR, Glaser CA, Bloch KC, et al. The management of encephalitis: clinical practice guidelines by the Infectious Diseases Society of America. *Clin Infect Dis*. 2008;47(3):303–327.

18. American Thoracic Society, Infectious Diseases Society of America. Guidelines for the management of adults with hospital-acquired, ventilator-associated, and healthcare-associated pneumonia. *Am J Respir Crit Care Med*. 2005;171(4):388–416.

19. Ginsburg PM, Thuluvath PJ. Diarrhea in liver transplant recipients: etiology and management. Wiley Online Library. *Liver Transpl*. 2005;11(8). doi:10.1002/lt.20500.

20. Fishman JA, Emery V, Freeman R, et al. Cytomegalovirus in transplantation—challenging the status quo. *Clin Transpl*. 2007;21(2):149–158.

21. Preiksaitis JK, Brennan DC, Fishman J, Allen U. Canadian society of transplantation consensus workshop on cytomegalovirus management in solid organ transplantation final report. *Am J Transpl*. 2005;5(2):218–227.

22. Mendez JC, Dockrell DH, Espy MJ, et al. Human β-herpesvirus interactions in solid organ transplant recipients. *J Infect Dis*. 2001;183(2):179–184.

23. Razonable RR, Brown RA, Humar A, et al. Herpesvirus infections in solid organ transplant patients at high risk of primary cytomegalovirus disease. *J Infect Dis*. 2005;192(8):1331–1339.

24. Dummer JS, Thomas LD. *Risk Factors and Approaches to Infections in Transplant Recipients*. 7th ed. Amsterdam, Netherlands: Elsevier Inc; 2010.

25. Preiksaitis JK. New developments in the diagnosis and management of posttransplantation lymphoproliferative disorders in solid organ transplant recipients. *Clin Infect Dis*. 2004;39(7):1016–1023.

26. Martin SI, Fishman JA, the AST Infectious Diseases Community of Practice. Pneumocystis pneumonia in solid organ transplant recipients. *Am J Transplant*. 2009;9:S227–233.

27. Singh N, Dromer F, Perfect JR, Lortholary O. Cryptococcosis in solid organ transplant recipients: current state of the science. *Clin Infect Dis*. 2008; 47:1321–1327

28. Kerkering TM, Duma RJ, Shadomy S. The evolution of pulmonary cryptococcosis: clinical implications from a study of 41 patients with and without compromising host factors. *Ann Intern Med*. 1981;94(5):611–616.

29. Hill D, Dubey JP. Toxoplasma gondii: transmission, diagnosis and prevention. Wiley Online Library. *Clin Microbiol Infect*. 2002; Oct;8(10):634–640.

30. Martino R, Maertens J, Bretagne S, et al. Toxoplasmosis after hematopoietic stem cell transplantation. *Clin Infect Dis*. 2000; Nov;31(5):1188–1195.

31. Pappas PG, Alexander BD, Andes DR, et al. Invasive fungal infections among organ transplant recipients: results of the Transplant-Associated Infection Surveillance Network (TRANSNET). *Clin Infect Dis*. 2010;50(8). doi: 10.1086/651262.

32. Perlroth J, Choi B, Spellberg B. Nosocomial fungal infections: epidemiology, diagnosis, and treatment. *Med Mycol*. 2007;45(4):321–346.

33. Marcos JY, Pincus DH. Fungal diagnostics: review of commercially available methods. *Methods Mol Biol*. 2013;968:25–54.

34. Tuite NL, Lacey K. Overview of invasive fungal infections. *Methods Mol Biol*. 2013;968:1–23.

35. Segal BH. Current approaches to diagnosis and treatment of invasive aspergillosis. *Am J Respir Crit Care Med*. 2006;173(7):707–717.

36. Chen K-J, Wu W-C, Sun M-H, Lai C-C, Chao A-N. Endogenous fungal endophthalmitis: causative organisms, management strategies, and visual acuity outcomes. *Am J Ophthalmol*. 2012;154(1):213–214, author reply214.

37. Copelan EA. Hematopoietic stem-cell transplantation. *N Engl J Med*. 2006;354(17):1813–1826.

38. Young J-AH, Weisdorf DJ. *Infections in Recipients of Hematopoietic Cell Transplantation*. 7th ed. Amsterdam, Netherlands: Elsevier Inc; 2010.

39. Freifeld AG, Bow EJ, Sepkowitz KA, et al. Clinical practice guideline for the use of antimicrobial agents in neutropenic patients with cancer: 2010 update by the Infectious Diseases Society of America. *Clin Infect Dis*. 2011;52(4):e56–e93.

40. Fishman JA, Issa NC. Infection in organ transplantation: risk factors and evolving patterns of infection. *Infect Dis Clin North Am*. 2010;24(2):273–283.

Chapter 57

Infection in Travelers and Emigrants

Mark Tenforde

Summary Box

Disease Description: Annually, one billion people now travel internationally. Emergency physicians should be aware of pre-travel recommendations and prepared to diagnose and manage common travel-related infections.

Organisms: Common problems include systemic febrile illness, traveler's diarrhea, and dermatoses. The etiology and risk of each disease varies by region of travel and travel-related activities.

Treatment: This chapter discusses the diagnosis and management of common diseases in international travelers.

333

Disease Description

Introduction

Almost one billion people traveled internationally in 2011, a number expected to nearly double by 2030. The rate of increase in travel to low-income countries, many with a high burden of infectious disease, is outpacing growth in travel to developed countries.[1]

This chapter focuses on common travel-related health topics. Comprehensive resources include the World Health Organization (WHO's) *International Travel and Health* (the Green Book) and the US Centers for Disease Control and Prevention (CDC's) *Health Information for International Travel* (the Yellow Book).[2,3] The CDC website provides information on infectious disease risks and alerts by country of travel.[4]

Pre-Travel Consultation

Overview

Emergency physicians are a frequent source of pre-travel consultation. Travelers should visit a travel clinic at least 5 to 6 weeks prior to anticipated departure. This consultation provides an opportunity to review prior vaccinations and administer any further vaccines that are recommended for the patient's particular travel plans. It also provides the time necessary for postvaccination immunity to develop before the patient is at risk in their travel destination. Table 57.1 gives a list of additional vaccines recommended by the US Advisory Committee on Immunization Practices (ACIP) for adults traveling internationally. Travelers should be aware that proof of yellow fever vaccination is required for entry into many African and South American countries.

Travelers should consider bringing the following items for the prevention and management of infectious diseases based on region of travel and travel activities:

1) Malaria chemoprophylaxis
2) Mosquito nets and insecticide spray for fabrics and clothing
3) Antibiotics for common infections (travelers' diarrhea, respiratory infections, urinary tract infections, skin and soft tissue infections)
4) Antidiarrheal medications (eg, loperamide or diphenoxylate)
5) Water disinfectant
6) Antibacterial topical ointment
7) Antifungal powder
8) Condoms or other form of barrier contraception

Malaria Chemoprophylaxis

Malaria is caused by the protozoan species *Plasmodium falciparum, P. vivax, P. ovale,* and *P. malariae,* which are transmitted by the female *Anopheles* mosquito. *Plasmodium knowlesi,* which infects macaques, has also become an increasingly important cause of malaria in Southeast Asia.[5] An estimated 350 to 500 million infections and one million deaths occur annually. Along with parts of Eastern Europe, endemic areas include all of sub-Saharan Africa and much of Southeast Asia, Oceana, Central and South America, and the Caribbean.[6]

The *Anopheles* mosquito bites primarily from dusk to dawn. Travelers should bring pyrethroid-covered bed nets and apply pyrethroid spray to living quarters to reduce the risk of infection. Clothing should cover most of the body, and clothing and skin should be treated regularly with insect repellant (eg, diethyltoluamide-containing products). Clothing can be treated with permethrin for added protection.

Chemoprophylaxis should be taken before, during, and after travel, as it decreases both the risk of infection and the fatality rate for those infected.[7] Chemoprophylaxis is primarily targeted toward *Plasmodium falciparum, Plasmodium vivax,* and *P. ovale* that generate hypnozoites that are only susceptible to primaquine, so terminal prophylaxis with primaquine is used for travelers heavily exposed to these species.[8] Chemoprophylactic regimens are summarized in Table 57.2.

Post-Travel Evaluation

Fever

Assessment of fever includes evaluation of localizing signs or symptoms, areas of travel, preexisting health status, immunization status, and duration of fever. Life-threatening conditions, particularly malaria, must be promptly recognized. Box 57.1 includes tests for initial evaluation, based on availability of resources.

Causes of systemic febrile illness (fever without localizing symptoms) vary by region of travel. Malaria is the most commonly identified cause in sub-Saharan Africa, whereas Dengue is more often encountered

Table 57.1 Vaccination Recommendations for Adult Travelers

Vaccine	Recommendations	Immunization Schedule
Hepatitis A	• Travel to intermediate- to high-endemicity areas	• Dose at 0 and 6–12 months (Havrix or Vaqta hepatitis A vaccines) • Accelerated schedule available with Twinrix combined hepatitis A and B vaccine at 0, 7, and 21–30 days (with 12-month booster dose) • If unvaccinated, hepatitis A immunoglobulin should be administered before travel
Influenza	• High-risk individuals not vaccinated prior fall or winter traveling to the tropics, with a tourist group, or between April and September in the Southern Hemisphere	• Annual vaccination
Japanese Encephalitis	• Recommended if traveling ≥ 1 month in endemic area during transmission season (endemic in most Asian countries) • Consider if traveling < 1 month in endemic area during transmission season if traveling outside urban areas or traveling to an area with a current outbreak	• Ixiaro vaccine at 0 and 28 days completed ≥ 1 week before travel
Meningococcus	• Travel to the "African meningitis belt" (Senegal to Ethiopia) between December and June • Required for travelers to Mecca during the Hajj	• If ≤ 55 years, 1 dose Menactra or Menveo • For all adults, including those > 55 years, Menomune ≥ 7–10 days before travel • Revaccination every 3–5 years for at-risk travelers
Polio Vaccine (Inactivated)	• Travel to areas where polio is endemic (Afghanistan, Nigeria, Pakistan) or epidemic	• If > 8 weeks before travel, 3 doses IPV ≥ 4 weeks apart • If < 8 weeks but ≥ 4 weeks before travel, 2 doses IPV ≥ 4 weeks apart • If < 4 weeks before travel, 1 dose of IPV
Typhoid	• Travel to areas with high risk of transmission, particularly those with poor water hygiene standards and water supply facilities	• Oral (Ty21a) series of 4 capsules every other day completed ≥ 1 week before travel • Intramuscular (ViCPS) vaccine ≥ 14 days before travel • For oral (Ty21a) series, revaccination every 5 years; for injectable (ViCPS), booster every 2–3 years
Varicella	• Consideration for those without evidence of immunity at increased risk for exposure or transmission	• Two doses of varicella-containing vaccine if no evidence of immunity, 4–8 weeks apart
Yellow Fever	• Travelers to at-risk areas in South America or Africa	• Single dose of vaccine (YF-Vax) • Revaccination every 10 years

Abbreviations: ViCPS, Vi capsular polysaccharide; IPv, inactivated polio vaccine; Ty21a, Typhoid Vaccine Live Oral Ty21a; YF-Vax, Yellow Fever vaccine.

in the Caribbean and Southeast Asia. Table 57.3 includes the most common causes of systemic febrile illness in international travelers documented in GeoSentinal clinics between 1997 and 2004, broken down by region.[10]

Malaria, Dengue, and Mononucleosis

Malaria and dengue are discussed in chapter 52. Mononucleosis is more familiar to domestic practitioners and will not be discussed in this chapter.

Rickettsia

Fourteen species of tick-borne *Rickettsia* have been reported internationally.[11] Most species are confined to a limited geographic region based on endemicity of vector species. Typical clinical features include

Table 57.2 Malaria Chemoprophylaxis

Drug	Adult dosing	Interval and duration	Comment
Atovaquone-proguanil (Malarone)	1 tablet daily (250 mg atovaquone plus 100 mg proguanil)	Daily 1–2 days before travel through 7 days after leaving an endemic malaria area.	• Contraindicated in pregnant women or if creatinine clearance < 30 mL/minute • Generally well tolerated[9]
Doxycycline	100 mg daily	1–2 days before travel through 4 weeks after leaving malarious area	• Contraindicated in pregnant women or if allergy to tetracyclines • Risk of photosensitivity
Mefloquine	1 tablet (228 mg base) weekly	≥ 2 weeks before travel through 4 weeks after leaving malarious area	• Growing resistance in Southeast Asia • Risk of neuropsychiatric side effects • Contraindicated if known sensitivity to mefloquine, quinine, or quinidine; and if cardiac conduction abnormalities, active psychiatric disturbances, or seizure disorder
Choroquine	1 tablet (300 mg base) weekly	1–2 weeks before travel through 4 weeks after leaving malarious area	• P. falciparum sensitive in Caribbean and Central America west of Panama Canal
Primaquine	1 tablet (30 mg base) daily	• Primary prophylaxis: 1–2 days before travel through 7 days after leaving malarious area • Terminal prophylaxis: 14 days after leaving malarious area concurrently with primary prophylaxis medicine (if using Malarone, primaquine taken the last 7 days of Malarone use and for an additional 7 days)	• Used for chemoprophylaxis in areas with primarily P. vivax or terminal prophylaxis to prevent relapse with P. ovale or P. vivax • Must rule out G6PD deficiency before use

Abbreviation: G6PD, Glucose-6-Phosphate Dehydrogenase.

fever, headache, myalgias, and inoculation eschars. In international travelers, a majority of reported cases have been due to African tick bite fever or Mediterranean spotted fever.

Rickettsia africae, which parasitizes cattle and game, causes African tick bite fever and is found in sub-Saharan Africa and the French West Indies. Multiple inoculation eschars are often found, clustering of cases is common, and severe disease and death are rare. In about half of cases, a nonpruritic maculopapular or vesicular rash and regional lymphadenopathy are observed.[12]

Mediterranean spotted fever, transmitted by dog ticks, is endemic to the Mediterranean basin, Middle East, India, and parts of sub-Saharan Africa. Inoculation eschars are typically solitary, and a maculopapular rash is observed in most cases. In untreated cases, mortality rate may exceed 2%.[13]

Box 57.1 Tests for Evaluation of fever in the international traveler

Serial peripheral blood smears to evaluate for malaria

Complete blood count with differential cell count

Liver function tests

Urinalysis and urine, blood, and stool cultures

Chest x-ray

Rapid tests based on history and physical examination (eg, RNA viral load for acute human immunodeficiency virus infection, viral hepatitis, or leptospirosis serologic tests)

Adapted from US Center for Disease Control and Prevention. *Health Information for International Travel*. Atlanta, Georgia: CDC, 2012.

Cause	All Regions	Caribbean	Central America	South America	Sub-Saharan Africa	South Central Asia	Southeast Asia	Other or Multiple Regions
Specific pathogen identified	59	46	53	45	72	52	55	45
Malaria	35	6	13	13	62	14	13	23
Dengue	10	24	12	14	1	14	32	4
Mononucleosis (EBV or CMV)	3	7	7	8	1	2	3	6
Rickettsial infection	3	0	0	0	6	1	2	2
Salmonella typhus or S. paratyphi	3	2	2	2	1	14	3	2
No cause identified	41	54	47	55	28	48	45	55

Abbreviations: EBV, Epstein-Bar virus; CMV, cytomegalovirus.

A serum immunofluorescence assay (IFA) is the usual diagnostic tool used to confirm rickettsiosis; it does not help differentiate between species. Other diagnostic tests, including culture and polymerase chain reaction amplification, are available at a limited number of specialized centers. Doxycycline is the drug of choice for treatment at 100 mg oral administration or intravenous twice daily.[13]

Typhoid
Typhoid fever, caused by *Salmonella enterica*, is transmitted by food or water contaminated with urinary or fecal carriers.[14] It occurs internationally, but prevalence is highest in overcrowded areas with poor sanitation. Vaccination is only 60% to 70% effective in preventing infection.

After an asymptomatic period of 7 to 14 days, a nonspecific clinical syndrome develops, which includes escalating fevers, chills, and flu-like illness. Relative bradycardia, in which the pulse rate does not rise commensurately with temperature, is frequently observed. Abdominal tenderness, either diarrhea or constipation, and hepatosplenomegaly develop later. In a minority of cases, a blanching erythematous maculopapular rash ("rose spots") develops on the abdomen and trunk. Serious complications can develop, including encephalopathy, abdominal bleeding, or perforation from erosion of infected Peyer's patches with consequent sepsis and/or peritonitis. Prior vaccination does not eliminate the risk of infection.

Diagnostic workup includes cultures of blood, stool, urine, rash, or bone. Bone culture is the most sensitive but may take several days to become positive, so the decision to treat should be based on clinical criteria. Fluoroquinolones, azithromycin, 500 mg daily, or third-generation cephalosporins have shown good treatment efficacy, with parenteral fluoroquinolone used in severe disease.[14–17]

Other Travel-Related Infections
Leptospirosis
Leptospirosis, caused by *Leptospira* species of spirochetes, is transmitted by exposure to the infected urine of carrier mammals.[18] Although infection is more common in the tropics, the distribution of leptospirosis is worldwide.

Acute illness typically resembles a nonspecific flu-like illness (ie, fevers, chills, headache, myalgias, anorexia, nausea, and vomiting) lasting for about 1 week. Characteristic findings in leptospirosis include conjunctival suffusion and myalgias localized to the calves and lumbar region. After 3 to 4 days of remission, an immune phase of the illness often develops as the body produces antibodies; this presents as an undifferentiated febrile syndrome. Aseptic meningitis may also develop, characterized by increased cerebrospinal fluid opening pressures and lymphocytic pleocytosis. In 5% to 10% of cases, severe disease known as icteric leptospirosis, also known as Weil's disease, develops. At its extreme, it can involve jaundice, renal failure, and hemorrhage.

Diagnosis of acute leptospirosis is often difficult, given the nonspecific clinical findings. Confirmatory tests for leptospirosis include culture, serologic testing, or microscopic agglutination testing (MAT), which is the "gold standard." MAT is considered positive with either seroconversion or a fourfold increase in titers on serial testing at least 2 weeks apart.[19] Clinical trials have studied various antibiotics, including penicillin, doxycycline, and cephalosporins for the treatment of leptospirosis. Data is lacking on the clinical benefits of antibiotics, but they may decrease the length of stay in hospitalized patients.[20,21] Management is based on supportive care for complications of disease.

Rabies

Rabies cases occur worldwide. Common disease vectors include canines in Africa; canines and vampire bats in Latin America; and canines, mongooses, and jackals in Africa.[22]

Pre-travel vaccination is not recommended to the general public. Vaccination should be considered for limited populations, including rabies laboratory workers, cavers, and veterinarians traveling to epizootic areas. For post-exposure immunization, after cleaning the wound site, rabies immune globulin (20 IU/kg) is administered at day 0, preferably infiltrating around the site of the animal bite with the remainder intramuscular. Intramuscular vaccination (1 mL human diploid cell or purified chick embryo cell vaccine) is also administered at days 0, 3, 7, and 14.

After an incubation period of typically 1 to 3 months, disease is characterized by a prodromal phase with nonspecific symptoms, followed by a neurologic phase with agitation, confusion, pathognomonic aerophobia and hydrophobia, development of paralysis, and then coma followed by death. In a minority of cases, rabies can present as an ascending paralysis mimicking Guillain-Barre Syndrome. Diagnosis is based on a history of exposure and clinical presentation, although many cases are first diagnosed post-mortem. Only a handful of individuals have survived a rabies infection.[23]

Diarrheal Disease

Traveler's diarrhea affects an estimated 20% to 60% of people traveling to low-income countries. Diarrhea typically develops within the first few days of travel and follows a self-limited course, with resolution within 5 days of onset. In addition to unformed stool, signs and symptoms may include nausea, vomiting, abdominal pain, fever, and bloody stool. Dehydration can be a serious complication, especially in travelers at the extremes of age.

In most regions, bacterial infections account for the majority of cases, with enterotoxigenic E. coli the most common culprit. Different causes of infectious diarrhea and their relative frequencies are summarized in Table 57.4.

The cornerstone of treatment is hydration. For mild diarrhea, clean drinking water alone is usually adequate. For more severe disease, oral rehydration solutions are available at pharmacies in most

Table 57.4 Causes of Traveler's Diarrhea[a]

Pathogen	Estimated Frequency (%)
Bacterial	50–75
Enterotoxigenic E. coli	10–45
Enteraggregative E. coli	5–35
Campylobacter spp	5–25
Salmonella spp	0–15
Shigella spp	0–15
Bacteroides fragilis	0–10
Others	0–5
Viral	5–20
Norovirus spp	0–10
Rotavirus spp	0–5
Parasitic	0–10
Giardia intestinalis	0–5
Cryptosporidium spp	0–5
Cyclospora cayetanensis	< 1
Entamoeba histolytica	< 1
Acute food poisoning	0–5
No pathogen identified	10–50

Abbreviation: spp, multiple species.

[a]Adapted from Hill DR, Beeching NJ. Travelers' diarrhea. Curr Opin Infect Dis. 2010;23:481–487.

Table 57.5 Antibiotic Regimens for Traveler's Diarrhea	
Antibiotic	Adult Dose
Ciprofloxacin	500 mg BID for up to 3 days
Levofloxacin	500 mg daily up to 3 days
Norfloxacin	400 mg BID for up to 3 days
Ofloxacin	200 mg BID for up to 3 days
Azithromycin	1000 mg once
Rifaximin	200 mg TID for up to 3 days

Abbreviations: BID, twice a day; TID, three times a day.

low-income countries. Alternatively, a solution can be prepared by mixing one liter of clean drinking water with one-half teaspoon of salt, one-half teaspoon of baking soda, and four tablespoons of sugar.

Antibiotics should be reserved for moderate-to-severe diarrhea. Suggested regimens include those in Table 57.5.

Use of antimotility agents (eg, loperamide, diphenoxylate) may promote earlier resolution of symptoms but should only be used in conjunction with antibiotics.[24] Use is cautioned for suspected dysentery (acute bloody diarrhea) or in those with high fevers.

Most cases do not require physician consultation, with notable exceptions for dysentery, high fevers, moderate-to-severe dehydration, or duration of symptoms of more than 2 weeks. For diarrhea of greater than 2 weeks duration, parasites are the most likely cause; Giardia is by far the most likely offending organism.

Dermatoses

Dermatologic complaints are among the most common reasons for international travelers to seek medical attention. From a study of GeoSentinel clinics, the most common causes of skin conditions in international travelers are included in Box 57.2.

Cutaneous larva migrans, found in tropical climates in Asia, Africa, Latin America, and the Caribbean, is caused by canine and feline hookworms (most frequently *Ancylostoma braziliense* and *A. caninum*) that burrow through skin. The typical skin finding is a pruritic, serpiginous, linear, and erythematous lesion. Oral thiabendazole, albendazole, and ivermectin have good success in curing this disease.[25]

Tungiasis, found in Latin America, sub-Saharan Africa, and Central Asia, is caused by infection of the fertilized sand flea, *Tunga Penetrans*. Lesions are most often located on the feet, typically nodular with a brown-black central opening, and the source of localized pain and itching. Treatment involves removal of the flea.[26]

Box 57.2 Most common causes of dermatoses in international travelers
Arthropod (eg, insect bite with or without superinfection, dengue, and cutaneous leishmaniasis)
Pyodermas (eg, cellulitis, abscess, and erysipelas)
Soil related (eg, cutaneous larva migrans and tungiasis)
Animal bite
Allergy related
Human-to-human (eg, scabies, varicella, and syphilis)
Fungal
Endogenous (eg, HSV and zoster)
Trauma related
Water born

Adapted from Lederman ER, Weld LH, Elyazar IR, et al. Dermatologic conditions of the ill returned traveler: an analysis from the GeoSentinel Surveillance Network. *Int J Infect Dis*. 2008;12:593–602.

Summary

International travel generally requires appropriate preparation, including careful consideration of vaccinations and prophylaxis. For acute febrile illness, malaria and dengue are common culprits, but an organism is not identified in a significant number of patients. Traveler's diarrhea affects an estimated 20% to 60% of people traveling to low-income countries and usually develops within the first few days of travel, lasting only about 5 days. Rehydration is the cornerstone of management. Comprehensive travel resources include the WHO's *International Travel and Health* (the Green Book) and the US CDC's *Health Information for International Travel* (the Yellow Book).

Suggested Readings and References

1. World Tourism Organization. *UNWTO Tourism Highlights*. Madrid, Spain: World Tourism Organization; 2012.
2. World Health Organization. *International Travel and Health*. Geneva, Switzerland: World Health Organization; 2012.
3. US Centers for Disease Control and Prevention. *Health Information for International Travel*. Atlanta, Georgia: CDC; 2012.
4. Traveler's health: destinations. US Center for Disease Control and Prevention website. Atlanta, Georgia: 2012. http://wwwnc.cdc.gov/travel/destinations/list.htm). Accessed September 26, 2012.
5. Daneshvar C, Davis TM, Cox-Singh J, et al. Clinical and laboratory features of human Plasmodium knowlesi infection. *Clin Infect Dis*. 2009;49:852–860.
6. van Vugt M, van Beest A, Sicuri E, van Tulder M, Grobusch MP. Malaria treatment and prophylaxis in endemic and nonendemic countries: evidence on strategies and their cost-effectiveness. *Future Microbiol*. 2011;6:1485–1500.
7. Krause G, Schoneberg I, Altmann D, Stark K. Chemoprophylaxis and malaria death rates. *Emerg Infect Dis*. 2006;12:447–451.
8. Hill DR, Baird JK, Parise ME, Lewis LS, Ryan ET, Magill AJ. Primaquine: report from CDC expert meeting on malaria chemoprophylaxis I. *Am J Trop Med Hyg*. 2006;75:402–415.
9. Jacquerioz FA, Croft AM. Drugs for preventing malaria in travellers. *Cochrane Database Syst Rev*. 2009;(4): doi: 10.1002/14651858.
10. Leder K, Tong S, Weld L, et al. Illness in travelers visiting friends and relatives: a review of the GeoSentinel Surveillance Network. *Clin Infect Dis*. 2006;43:1185–1193.
11. Other tick-borne spotted fever rickettsial infections. US Centers for Disease Control and Prevention website. Atlanta, Georgia: 2012. http://www.cdc.gov/otherspottedfever/). Accessed September 26, 2012.
12. Raoult D, Fournier PE, Fenollar F, et al. Rickettsia africae, a tick-borne pathogen in travelers to sub-Saharan Africa. *N Engl J Med*. 2001;344:1504–1510.
13. House HR, Ehlers JP. Travel-related infections. *Emerg Med Clin North Am*. 2008;26:499, 516, x.
14. Parry CM, Hien TT, Dougan G, White NJ, Farrar JJ. Typhoid fever. *N Engl J Med*. 2002;347:1770–1782.
15. Effa EE, Lassi ZS, Critchley JA, et al. Fluoroquinolones for treating typhoid and paratyphoid fever (enteric fever). *Cochrane Database Syst Rev*. 2011;(10): doi: 10.1002/14651858.
16. Effa EE, Bukirwa H. Azithromycin for treating uncomplicated typhoid and paratyphoid fever (enteric fever). *Cochrane Database Syst Rev*. 2008;(4):CD006083.
17. Crump JA, Mintz ED. Global trends in typhoid and paratyphoid Fever. *Clin Infect Dis*. 2010;50:241–246.
18. Bharti AR, Nally JE, Ricaldi JN, et al. Leptospirosis: a zoonotic disease of global importance. *Lancet Infect Dis*. 2003;3:757–771.
19. Marchiori E, Lourenco S, Setubal S, Zanetti G, Gasparetto TD, Hochhegger B. Clinical and imaging manifestations of hemorrhagic pulmonary leptospirosis: a state-of-the-art review. *Lung*. 2011;189:1–9.
20. Brett-Major DM, Coldren R. Antibiotics for leptospirosis. *Cochrane Database Syst Rev*. 2012;2:CD008264.
21. Vinetz JM. A mountain out of a molehill: do we treat acute leptospirosis, and if so, with what? *Clin Infect Dis*. 2003;36:1514–1515.
22. Takayama N. Rabies: a preventable but incurable disease. *J Infect Chemother*. 2008;14:8–14.
23. Willoughby REJr, Tieves KS, Hoffman GM, et al. Survival after treatment of rabies with induction of coma. *N Engl J Med*. 2005;352:2508–2514.
24. Riddle MS, Arnold S, Tribble DR. Effect of adjunctive loperamide in combination with antibiotics on treatment outcomes in traveler's diarrhea: a systematic review and meta-analysis. *Clin Infect Dis*. 2008;47:1007–1014.
25. Patel S, Sethi A. Imported tropical diseases. *Dermatol Ther*. 2009;22:538–549.
26. Veraldi S, Valsecchi M. Imported tungiasis: a report of 19 cases and review of the literature. *Int J Dermatol*. 2007;46:1061–1066.

Chapter 58

Infection in the Intravenous Drug User

Caren Euster

Summary Box

Disease Description: Infections in patients with a history of injection drug use (IDU) can affect multiple systems. The most commonly affected include the skin (eg, abscess), heart (eg, endocarditis), lung (eg, pneumonia), kidney, and brain (eg, septic emboli secondary to endocarditis). Systemic infections can also occur.

Organisms: Common: Human immunodeficiency virus (HIV), hepatitis B and C, *Staphylococcus aureus*, and *Streptococcus viridans*. Possible: *Clostridium, Tuberculosis* (TB), Tetanus, *Bacillus anthracis*.

Treatment:
  Oral First line:
  Skin/soft tissue: Trimethoprim/sulfamethoxazole double strength (DS) one tab PO q12 hours; clindamycin 300 mg PO q6 hours or 450 mg PO q8 hours
  Pneumonia: Azithromycin 500 mg PO on day 1, 250 mg PO on days 2 through 5; oral quinolones
  Oral Second line: Doxycycline 100 mg PO BID
  Parenteral: Vancomycin 15 mg/kg q12 hours, broad-spectrum antibiotics for systemic infections

Other Key Issues: Tuberculosis, fungal infections, tetanus, botulism, necrotizing fasciitis, osteomyelitis, acute viral infections, and toxin-mediated reactions are seen.

Disease Description

Injection drug abuse has spread worldwide and is increasing among young adults and adolescents. This chapter focuses on the management of acute infectious consequences of injection drug use (IDU), including skin and soft tissue infections, endocarditis, and systemic infections. The approach will be divided into local (injection site) infections, infections distant to the injection site, systemic infections, complications of primary infections, modifying factors, and infections associated with the IDU patient's lifestyle.

Organisms

A wide variety of organisms may be involved but are dominated by organisms of the patient's own skin flora. Infectious organisms also derive from drug-related paraphernalia, the drug itself, or agents mixed with the drug. The most common bacterial organisms are *Staphylococcus aureus* and *Streptococcus* species, but many other organisms have been reported, including *Clostridium botulinum, Clostridium tetani,* and *Bacillus anthracis*. Oral pathogens, such as *Eikenella, Fusobacterium*, and *Peptostreptococcus* species, are also seen. *Pseudomonas* has been reported due to contaminated water used in drug preparation. Viral infections, such as HIV, generally present less acutely or are found as part of the workup of an acute bacterial infection.

Injection Site Infections

Injection site infections often present as an abscess or cellulitis, both of which can present with skin erythema at or nearby the injection site. Cellulitis is an infection of the dermis and subcutaneous tissue and is typically characterized by a spreading erythema at the surface of the skin. The most common organisms tend to be *Staphylococcus* and *Streptococcus* species, especially S. *pyogenes* and S. *aureus*. Although cellulitis may extend to deeper structures, an abscess tends to expand in all directions and may progress more deeply toward soft tissue. In addition, an abscess resulting from IDU may actually begin deep to the skin, depending on where in the needle tract the bacteria were inoculated. As an abscess progresses, it may become fluctuant with increasing pain.

Lymphangitis, an inflammatory response of the lymphatic vessels, is characterized by an ascending, painful red line on the skin. It may occur with an abscess, cellulitis, or both. Fever and malaise may also develop. Large areas of induration in the abdomen, buttocks, and thighs may overlie deep abscesses that are not palpable at the surface. The primary organisms seen in abscess are methicillin-resistant S. *aureus* (MRSA) and methicillin-sensitive S. *aureus* (MSSA). Group A Streptococcal and Clostridial abscesses are also seen. In patients who appear ill or have significant pain, necrotizing fasciitis and toxic shock syndrome must be considered. Other less common organisms include C. *botulinum*, C. *tetani*, and B. *anthracis*.

Ultrasound may be useful in detecting deep abscesses. Incision and drainage should be performed on fluctuant abscesses, and careful attention should be paid to disrupting any loculations that may exist and inhibit abscess drainage. In general, abscesses should be packed and allowed to close by secondary intention.

Labs and systemic antibiotics should be considered if there is fever or extensive cellulitis. The initial choice of oral antibiotics should be guided by local resistance, but generally accepted empiric treatments include trimethoprim/sulfamethoxazole DS PO BID for 7 to 10 days, clindamycin 300 mg IV q6, 8, or 12 hours, or doxycycline 100 mg PO BID (if not precluded by allergy or risk of pregnancy). Isolated abscesses without other signs of systemic infection or cellulitis can be treated with incision and drainage only.

Infections Distal to the Injection Site

Other complications related to intravenous drug use occur as a result of bacterial infection, including endocarditis, bacterial toxins, severe local infection, or systemic infection. Viral infections may also cause systemic symptoms but often present less acutely. However, viral infections may increase susceptibility to and complicate bacterial infections.

The combination of fever, chest pain, dyspnea, and hemoptysis may represent endocarditis. Right-sided heart valve involvement is more common than left-sided, but left-sided may have worse outcomes. Right-sided infection may lack traditional Duke criteria for left-sided endocarditis, such as a loud murmur, Roth Spots, and Janeway lesions. Right heart involvement is often associated with pleuritic chest pain dyspnea and shortness of breath. Pulmonary infiltrates can be seen due to septic emboli. Left-sided endocarditis can produce complications, such as systemic emboli to kidneys, brain, and skin (4,5).

TB is also a concern in IV drug users, as other TB risk factors may be present, such as crowding and poor living conditions. Fever may also be associated with the acute viral infections HIV, Hepatitis B, and Hepatitis C. Other noninfectious causes of symptoms should also be considered, such as acute drug reaction to cocaine, amphetamines, cotton filters, and withdrawal (3, 4, 5).

Fever

The febrile patient should be pan cultured (three sets of blood cultures), sputum cultured, and, if applicable, wound cultures should be included as well as urine culture. Other studies include chest x-ray and basic labs, such as complete blood count, comprehensive metabolic panel, and urinalysis.

Ultrasound may show a cardiac vegetation; the atrial side of the tricuspid valve is the most commonly involved area.

Initially, there may be no culture results to go by, so empiric therapy with broad-spectrum antibiotics with MRSA coverage should be started.

Abdominal Pain

Causes of abdominal pain include acute viral hepatitis, septic emboli to the kidneys, and opioid withdrawal. Direct bacterial infections of abdominal organs are less commonly reported. It appears that abdominal pain in patients with IDU are more likely to occur as a complication of drug abuse, including mesenteric ischemia or infarction that may be related to cocaine abuse.

Altered Mental Status

Causes of altered mental status in patients with IDU include the same etiologies as in the patient who does not have a history of IDU, but certain infections may be more likely. Patients with IDU are at higher risk for primary central nervous system (CNS) infection, septic emboli, or local extension of infection to the CNS. Other considerations include noninfectious causes, such as drug intoxication, metabolic derangement, trauma, and seizures. Infectious considerations should include leukoencephalopathy in the immunosuppressed patient (eg, John Cunningham virus),(3) and Clostridial infections as discussed previously, such as botulism, tetanus, gangrene, and sepsis.(6,8,9)

Botulism may occur due to environmental contamination of wounds (ie, "Wound Botulism"). Symptoms include slurred speech, blurred vision, and descending paralysis. Given that this is a rare diagnosis and that IDU is a risk factor, it must be considered in high-risk patients, as early diagnosis may prevent mortality. Antitoxin and supportive care are the only treatments.

Tetanus is uncommon in the developed world but has presented in patients with IDU. Even if a patient has been vaccinated, immunity wanes over time if not periodically updated with a tetanus booster vaccination every 10 years. Presentation includes muscle spasms, trismus, respiratory difficulty, and, eventually, severe autonomic instability including both hypertension and hypotension. Wound debridement can help to decrease the number or local organisms. Administration of tetanus immune globulin 3,000 to 6,000 units intramuscularly can help to lessen the severity of illness. Morphine can be used for sedation and pain; in severe cases, neuromuscular blockers have been used. Short acting beta blockers, clonidine, and ace inhibitors have been found helpful for severe hypertension. Metronidazole 500 mg IV q6 hours for 7 to 10 days should be considered. Other antibiotic choices include penicillin 20 million units/day in divided doses q4 hours, clindamycin, chloramphenicol, or tetracycline.

Back/Bone pain

Consideration must be given to vertebral osteomyelitis, epidural abscess, localized osteomyelitis due to local extension, and septic joint. Consultation with surgery is indicated to help determine the timing of antibiotics, as cultures will likely be required to guide therapy. As S. Aureus is a common cause, initial therapy should be directed toward this organism (eg, vancomycin). However, infections near the groin, such as at the hip, may include gram-negative organisms.

Lifestyle-Related

Often, the patient with a history of IDU will not have routine, preventative, or primary care, as some of these individuals may be so occupied with drug seeking that they will not establish or use primary care even if it is available to them. They will therefore present to the emergency department with a variety of relatively minor complaints. If not addressed in the emergency department, these will go untreated. Notable diseases to consider include:

Skin rash: cellulitis, impetigo, syphilis, scabies, and drug reactions to medications, especially those that may be used for IDU-related diseases are often present.

Sexually Transmitted Diseases: Gonorrhea and chlamydia are common and can often be treated empirically (Centers for Disease Control and Prevention Guidelines) in areas of high prevalence. Syphilis must also be considered, especially if there is a rash, or evidence of other sexually transmitted diseases. Syphilis is treated with penicillin 20 million units/day given intravenously in equally divided doses every 4 hours for 7 to 10 days.

Modifying Factors

Previous HIV, malnutrition, and co-addictions, such as alcohol, may alter presentation and add to severity. The addiction itself may compromise compliance. The desire not to undergo withdrawal symptoms may complicate a patient's willingness to undergo inpatient treatment. Certain medicationsm, such as buprenorphine or methadone, may be provided to hospitalized patients to help encourage them to stay and complete courses of therapy. If a patient still refuses to stay, oral regimens can be considered in extreme cases, even in endocarditis; but the success of such treatment regimens remains unclear.

Emerging issues

Anthrax has been reported in Germany, France, and Denmark as of 2012.(11) Leishmaniasis has been found in patients with IDU in Spain.(12)

Occupational exposure is always a risk for those doing procedures on patients with a history of IDU. Adherence to universal precautions, including eye protection in addition to other contact precautions is recommended when performing any procedures in such patients. If any occupational exposure were to occur, such as being splashed by body fluids or stuck by a needle, hospital infection control should be notified for post-exposure management.

As the presentation and course of infections in IV drug users is so varied, a chart is provided for concise guidance (see Table 58.1). Antibiotic recommendations should be tailored to local resistance patterns.

Table 58.1 Summary Table for Clinical Presentations, Diagnostic Considerations, and Antibiotic Choices[a]

Clinical Presentation	Diagnostic Tests	Possible Diagnosis	Initial Therapy & Oral Antibiotics	Initial Therapy IV
Skin and soft tissue	Ultrasound Gram Stain Culture	Abscess MRSA MSSA *Streptococcus*	Incision and drainage; Suspected MRSA: Bactrim 6–10 mg/kg q8–12 h; clindamycin, 300 mg q6 h or 450 mg q8 h; doxycycline/minocycline 100 mg q12 h; MSSA suspected: dicloxacillin 500 mg QID or cephalexin 500 mg QID for 10 days	MRSA suspected: clindamycin 600 mg IV q6–8 h or vancomycin 15 mg/kg q12 h if clindamycin resistance suspected; teicoplanin 6 mg/kg q12 h x 3, then 6 mg/kg q24 h; linezolid 600 mg q12 h, daptomycin 4 mg/kg q24 h
Localized extremity pain,Back pain, Joint pain, Sternal pain	Plain x-rays of limb or back, Consider CT or MRI with contrast, Bone Biopsy: not part of ED workup	Cellulitis or abscess as previously; Septic Thrombophlebitis; arthritis, bursitis, or tenosynovitis; also consider oral pathogens.	Localized infection as previously; Augmentin 875 mg q12 h; PCN allergy: clindamycin and quinolone	May need admission for surgical drainage and/or biopsy before antibiotics; if given empirically, consider: ampicillin-sulbactam 1.5–3 g q6 h, piperacillin-tazobactam 3.375 mg q4–6 h, ticarcillin-clavulanate 3.1 g q4–6 h, cefipime 1–2 g q12 h; If MRSA suspected, vancomycin or teicoplanin as previously

Table 58.1 Continued

Clinical Presentation	Diagnostic Tests	Possible Diagnosis	Initial Therapy & Oral Antibiotics	Initial Therapy IV
Fever, Fever and cough	Chest x-ray Blood Cultures CBC, ESR, CRP Echocardiogram Oxygen saturations	Endocarditis R > L, CHF, Pneumonia, Septic Pulmonary Emboli, Bacteremia, Valvular Disease, Valvular Vegetations, Drug Withdrawal, Cotton Fever	Oral therapy rarely considered if endocarditis suspected. Would not consider without expert ID consultation	Stabilize patient if needed; IV antibiotics directed toward MRSA and MSSA; if endocarditis suspected: vancomycin plus gentamycin or nafcillin/oxacil-lin plus gentamycin, also consider gram negatives, clostridia (anaerobes), and fungal coverage
Anorexia, Nausea, Malaise, Night sweats (cough)	HIV serology Blood cultures Chest x-ray Sputum for AFB Liver function testing including PT/PTT	Viral: HIV, Hepatitis B & C; Tuberculosis; Consider endocarditis, fungal, septic emboli	Isolation if TB suspected; Outpatient management if mild disease	Supportive for viral in the acute setting; refer for definitive treatment of HIV and hepatitis
Abdominal pain	As previously; also consider pelvic exam, renal or pelvic ultrasound, MRI for splenic lesions; Lactate	Hepatitis PID Septic Emboli: renal, splenic, mesenteric	Treat for STDs; Emboli will need parenteral treatment.	Workup will guide therapeutic decisions.
Headache, Altered mental status, Blurred vision, Slurred speech, Muscle weakness, Muscle rigidity, Descending paralysis	Head CT Scan CBC BMP PT/PTT May need LP with Fungal Cultures Drug Screen	CNS lesions, Septic emboli, Meningitis, Bacterial Toxins (Wound Botulism), Drug effect		Empiric treatment for meningitis; if botulism: give botulinum antitoxin, debride wound, and contact local health department for antitoxin; if tetanus: tetanus immune globulin 3,000–6,000 units; metronidazole first line; erythromycin, clindamycin, chloramphenicol, or tetracycline are second line; neuromuscular blockade; respiratory support; ICU

Table 58.1 Continued

Clinical Presentation	Diagnostic Tests	Possible Diagnosis	Initial Therapy & Oral Antibiotics	Initial Therapy IV
Unusual organisms: necrotic ulcer, black wound	High index of suspicion for inadequate Immunizations, (Non–US) Illness out of proportion for presentation	Tetanus Gangrene (Clostridia) Toxic Shock (Streptococcus) Anthrax		As previously; notify hospital lab of suspected organism; Notify local health department or CDC (1–800–CDC–Info)

Abbreviations: CT, computed tomography; MRI, magnetic resonance imaging; ED, emergency department; CBC, complete blood count; ESR, erythrocyte sedimentation rate ; CRP, C-reactive protein; HIV, human immunodeficiency virus; AFB, acid-fast bacilli; PT/PTT, prothrombin time/partial thromboplastin time; LP, lumbar puncture; MRSA, methicillin-resistant *Staphylococcus aureus*; MSSA, methicillin-sensitive *Staphylococcus aureus*; Endocarditis R > L, right greater than left; CHF, congestive heart failure; PID, pelvic inflammatory disease; CNS, central nervous system; h, hours; QID, four times a day; PCN, penicillin; ID, infectious disease; TB, tuberculosis; STD, sexually transmitted disease; IV, intravenous; ICU, intensive care unit; CDC, Centers for Disease Control and Prevention.

ᵃAdapted from Gordon RJ. Bacterial infections in drug users. *N Engl J Med.* 2005;353:1945–1954; and Tintanelli JE, Kelen GD, Stapczynski S. *Emergency Medicine: A Comprehensive Study Guide.* American College of Emergency Physicians. 6th ed. New York, NY: McGraw-Hill; 2006.

Suggested Readings and References

1. Chatterjee S, Tempalski B, Pouget E, Cooper HLF, Cleland CF, Friedman SR. Changes in the behavior of injection drug use among adolescents and young adults in large U.S. metropolitan areas. *AIDS Behav.* 2011;15(7):1570–1578.

2. Gordon RJ. Bacterial infections in drug users. *N Engl J Med.* 2005;353:1945–1954.

3. Tintanelli JE, Kelen GD, Stapczynski S. *Emergency Medicine: A Comprehensive Study Guide.* American College of Emergency Physicians. 6th ed. New York, NY: McGraw-Hill; 2006.

4. Berdusco EP, Steiner IP. Acute bacterial endocarditis in intravenous drug users; case presentation and review. *Israeli J Emerg Med.* 2004;4(2).

5. Moss R, Munt B. Injection drug use and right sided endocarditis heart. *Heart.* 2003;89(5): 577–581.

6. Health Protection Agency, Health Protection Agency Scotland, National Public Service for Wales, CDSC Northern Ireland, CRDHB. *Shooting Up: Infections among Injecting drug users in the United Kingdom.*

7. Botulism. Centers for Disease Control and Prevention website. URL. October 2012. Accessed .

8. Trujillo MH et al. Impact of intensive care management on the prognosis of tetanus: analysis of 641 cases. *Chest.* 1987;92(1):63–65.

9. Cook TM, Protheroe RT, Handel JM. Tetanus: a review of the literature. *Br J Anaesth.* 2001;87(3):477–487.

10. Burningham MD, Walter FG, Haber J, Ekins BR. Wound botulism. *Ann Emerg Med.* 1994;24(6):1184–1187.

11. European Monitoring Centre for Drugs and Drug Addiction. Joint ECDC and EMCDDA Rapid Risk Assessment. Anthrax cases among injecting drug users: Germany, June-July 2012. Update July 13, 2012.

12. Pineda JA, Martin Sanchez J, Macias J, Morillas F. Leishmania spp in injecting drug users. *Lancet* 2002;360(9337):950–951.

Chapter 59

Infection in the Pregnant Patient

Vanessa Vasquez

Summary Box

Disease Description: Infections in pregnancy can result in significant complications for both the mother and fetus and can increase the risk of preterm labor.

Organisms: Gram-positive and gram-negative bacteria, viruses

Treatment:
- Airway, breathing, and circulation management
- Careful fluid resuscitation
- Early administration of appropriately targeted antibiotics:
  - Urinary tract infection (UTI): nitrofurantoin 100 mg every 12 hours for 5 days, amoxicillin 500 mg every 12 hours for 3 to 7 days, amoxicillin-clavulanate 500 mg every 12 hours for 3 to 7 days, cephalexin 500 mg every 12 hours for 3 to 7 days, or fosfomycin as a single 3 g dose.
  - Influenza: oseltamivir 75 mg BID for 7 to 10 days
  - Pneumonia and acute chest syndrome: azithromycin 500 mg daily for 5 to 7 days, with the addition of ceftriaxone1–2 g IM or IV q24 h in severe cases.
  - Herpes simplex virus (HSV): acyclovir 400 mg PO TID for 7–10 days or 10–15 mg/ kg IV q8 hours

Other Key Issues: Prophylaxis, vaccination, high degree of suspicion, and early intervention can help improve morbidity and mortality

Although infections represent a serious medical threat at any point, infections during pregnancy can cause significant acute and chronic complications to both mother and fetus. Fever in a pregnant woman should raise concern not only for infection but also for its associated risk of preterm birth due to release of prostaglandins and cytokines that stimulate uterine contractility. Infection can be passed to the neonate hematogenously or ascend from the genital tract, increasing the risk of spontaneous abortion, physical malformations, stillbirth, preterm labor, and maternal death. Treatment of infections during pregnancy creates a unique problem, as many antimicrobials cross the placenta and may carry a teratogenic risk.

Although most pregnant patients with concern for infection present to the emergency department with specific complaints related to the organ system that is involved, there are important historical questions that should uniformly be asked. These include history of uterine tenderness, leakage of vaginal fluid, exposure to or symptoms of sexually transmitted infection, previous preterm labor, history of pregnancy complications, and a thorough social history. The following infections present special risks and concerns for pregnant women and should be treated promptly and appropriately to reduce the risk of harm to mother and fetus.

UTI and Asymptomatic Bacteria

UTI, including cystitis, pyelonephritis, and asymptomatic bacteriuria (a positive urine culture in a patient without urinary symptoms), are very common during pregnancy. Bacteriuria occurs in 2% to 7% of pregnant women and is thought to occur more frequently due to dilated to smooth muscle relaxation and ureteral dilation that facilitate migration of bacteria from the urethra to the bladder. Bacteriuria has been associated with preterm birth and perinatal mortality. Routine surveillance screening with a clean catch urine culture should be done routinely at the beginning of the second trimester. Women with positive cultures benefit from treatment, and the following regimens are appropriate: nitrofurantoin 100 mg every 12 hours for 5 days, amoxicillin 500 mg every 12 hours for 3 to 7 days, amoxicillin-clavulanate 500 mg every 12 hours for 3 to 7 days, cephalexin 500 mg every 12 hours for 3 to 7 days, or fosfomycin as a single 3 g dose. Because 30% of women have a persistent infection after treatment, follow-up cultures are indicated, and consideration of monthly urine cultures should be entertained. Up to 40% of patients with asymptomatic bacteriuria develop asymptomatic UTI, and this risk can be reduced by 70% to 80% if bacteriuria is appropriately treated.(1)

A total of 1% to 2% of pregnant women will develop acute cystitis and should be treated similarly to those with asymptomatic bacteriuria. Patients with pyelonephritis typically present with flank pain, fever, and nausea with vomiting. Women in their second trimester are at the highest risk for developing pyelonephritis. Because 20% of pregnant women with pyelonephritis develop sepsis, it is an indication for hospitalization for IV antibiotics. Second- or third-generation cephalosporins (eg, ceftriaxone 1 g IV or IM q24 hours until afebrile for 48 hours) are considered first-line therapy and can be transitioned to oral antibiotics after the patient has been afebrile for 48 hours to complete a 14 day course. Fluoroquinolones and aminoglycosides should be avoided in pregnancy, unless indicated by the bacterial resistance pattern.

Respiratory Infections

Pregnant women have many changes in their respiratory physiology, including increased tidal volume, decreased functional residual capacity, and increased oxygen consumption. These changes place pregnant women with respiratory infections at higher risk for hypoxia and acidosis. Additionally, pregnant women are predisposed to developing pulmonary edema and aspiration.

Because 90% of upper respiratory infections are viral in etiology, pregnant patients should generally be treated with reassurance and minimal intervention. Humidified air, acetaminophen, and oral fluids can be offered for supportive care. Because influenza is associated with increased morbidity and mortality during pregnancy, pregnant women should be vaccinated, and acute infection should be treated with oseltamivir 75 mg BID for 7 to 10 days.

Although pneumonia is not more common in pregnant women, it is associated with maternal and fetal morbidity. Chest radiograph should be performed on any patient with consistent symptoms, as the low radiation exposure has not been associated with abortion, congenital abnormalities, low birth weight, or perinatal morbidity. Pneumonia can be treated with azithromycin 500 mg daily for 5 to 7 days. Ceftriaxone can be used in more severe cases. Clindamycin, penicillins, beta lactams, and aminoglycosides can also be considered. Doxycycline, clarithromycin, and fluoroquinolones should uniformly be avoided.

Human Parvovirus B19

Parvovirus B19 is a virus that replicates in erythroid progenitor cells and leads to inhibition of erythropoiesis, occasionally resulting in severe aplastic anemia. It is transmitted via respiratory droplets, and those at highest risk tend to be health care workers or those in close contact with young children. This infection is common in children and described as a limited febrile illness followed days later by a lacey erythematous rash on the face that spreads to the trunk and extremities. Clinical manifestations in adults vary from asymptomatic to a flu-like syndrome with a milder rash. There is an increased risk of polyarthralgia and synovitis in adults compared to children. Parvovirus B19 infection during pregnancy can be much more serious, resulting in the risk of nonimmune hydrops fetalis, miscarriage, and intrauterine fetal death.(2)

Approximately 25% to 45% of women of childbearing age are nonimmune to parvovirus B19, and, if infected during pregnancy, are at risk of transmitting the virus to the fetus. Transplacental, also described as "vertical" transmission, occurs in one-third to one-half of the cases. The risk of fetal complications is thought to be highest in infections that occur before 22 weeks gestation.(3,4) Complications include severe fetal anemia, thrombocytopenia, nonimmune hydrops fetalis, and fetal death. Hydrops fetalis is diagnosed by ultrasound of the fetus and is defined by the presence of two or more abnormal fetal fluid collections, such as ascites, pleural effusion, pericardial effusion, skin edema, or polyhydramnios (3).

Pregnant women who are exposed to parvovirus or who have symptoms consistent with parvovirus infection should have serological testing for antibody detection. An immunoglobulin M titer can be detected 7 to 10 days after symptomatic infection. Amniotic fluid polymerase chain reaction (PCR) can be sent if there is a high clinical suspicion. If a woman is found to have acute infection during pregnancy, she should be monitored by serial doppler ultrasound examinations. If signs of severe anemia or hydrops develop, emergent referral to a tertiary center for intrauterine transfusion is indicated.(5,6)

Pregnant women should avoid contact with individuals with known parvovirus infection and should be educated on its clinical manifestations. Meticulous hygiene, such as handwashing, is also recommended.(7)

Herpes Simplex Virus (HSV)

Approximately 50 million people in the United States have genital herpes, including HSV type 1 (HSV-1) and HSV type 2 (HSV-2).(8) Genital HSV is clinically classified into three categories: primary infection, nonprimary first episode, and recurrent infection. In pregnancy, HSV can be transmitted to the fetus, typically during labor and delivery, by direct contact between the neonate and infected genital mucosa. Although rare, transplacental transmission can also occur. Neonatal HSV is associated with serious morbidity and mortality. Its clinical manifestations are divided into three classifications: disease localized to skin, eye, and mouth; disease involving the central nervous system; and disseminated disease involving multiple organs.(9,10) Up to 25% of neonates with HSV infection have disseminated disease, with a 30% fatality rate despite appropriate antiviral therapy.

Primary HSV genital infection occurs when a person without immunity to either HSV-1 or HSV-2 is infected for the first time. Classically, this initial presentation is severe, causing systemic symptoms, such as fever, malaise, and dysuria, and multiple painful genital ulcers. Nonprimary first-episode HSV infection is the first occurrence of genital HSV-1 infection in a patient with preexisting HSV-2 antibodies or vice versa. Typically, the symptoms are milder than primary genital infection.

Recurrent genital infection occurs when there is reactivation of genital HSV. Recurrent disease is usually associated with fewer genital lesions and few systemic symptoms. HSV can be transmitted during sexual intercourse by direct contact with active ulcers or released from skin that does not appear to have any lesions, also called viral shedding. Viral shedding is more common and occurs for a longer period of time after the primary infection; therefore, the risk of neonatal infection is much higher in women with primary infection near the time of delivery. Women presenting with genital ulcers during pregnancy should be tested for type-specific serology (antibodies to either HSV-1 or HSV-2) and have a virus-specific assay (viral culture and or HSV antigen detection) sent from a swab of an open ulcer.(9)

Pregnant women with primary HSV infections or nonprimary first-episode HSV infection should be offered treatment, as it decreases symptoms and duration of active lesions and reduces asymptomatic viral shedding. Systemic antiviral therapy with acyclovir 400 mg PO TID for 7–10 days is appropriate. Patients with a history of recurrent HSV should be placed on suppressive antiviral therapy with acyclovir 400 mg PO TID at 36 weeks gestation through delivery to reduce the risk of active lesions and viral shedding. Prior to 36 weeks gestation, pregnant patients with recurrent HSV should be started on antiviral therapy acyclovir 400 mg PO TID or 800 mg PO BID for 5 days within the first 24 hours of initial symptoms. Acyclovir, valacyclovir, and famciclovir are all Food and Drug Administration pregnancy category B medications. There are no reports of adverse effects or teratogenicity in newborns of women using acyclovir during pregnancy.(9,11)

According the American College of Obstetrics and Gynecology, women with active lesions or prodromal symptoms at the time of labor and delivery should be offered cesarean delivery to decrease the risk of transmission to the fetus. Cesarean delivery does not prevent all vertically transmitted HSV neonatal infections, but substantially lowers the risk compared to infants delivered vaginally. Cesarean delivery is not recommended for women with a history of HSV without active genital lesions or prodromal symptoms. Routine testing for HSV prior to delivery in asymptomatic patients with recurrent disease is also not recommended.

Varicella-zoster virus (VZV)

VZV is a herpesvirus that predominantly causes a moderate febrile illness in unvaccinated children, but infection in adults and pregnant women is associated with serious morbidity and mortality. VZV presents in two forms, including primary varicella infection and herpes zoster. Primary varicella infection, also known as chickenpox, presents with a prodrome of fever, malaise, and anorexia followed 24 hours later by a characteristic diffuse, pruritic vesicular rash. Herpes zoster, also known as shingles, is caused by the reactivation of latent VZV and presents with a unilateral dermatomal rash and neuritis.(12) Most of the US population is primarily infected or vaccinated against VZV during childhood or adolescence; however, primary infection during pregnancy can cause much more severe maternal disease and fetal complications, such as death and congenital abnormalities.(13)

VZV is transmitted by aerosolized droplets from nasopharyngeal mucosa of infected persons or direct contact with vesicle fluid. Although the transmission rate is lower in zoster compared to chickenpox, all patients with VZV are considered infectious 2 days prior to the onset of the rash until all skin lesions have completely crusted over. Zoster during pregnancy is not associated with a higher risk of maternal or fetal complications.(14)

Primary varicella infection in pregnant women typically presents as moderate to severe flu-like infection, followed by a vesicular skin eruption on the face and trunk that spreads to the extremities. The most common maternal complication of primary infection is varicella pneumonia, appearing 3 to 5 days after the onset of the rash. Generally, varicella pneumonia presents with chest pain, tachypnea, dyspnea, and fever with diffuse nodular infiltrates on chest x-ray. It may be complicated by hypoxia and respiratory failure.(15)

Maternal varicella infection can be transmitted to the fetus across the placenta and can cause congenital varicella syndrome, characterized by low birth weight, microcephaly, hydrocephalus, ophthalmic lesions, hypoplasia, gastrointestinal abnormalities, and cutaneous scars. The highest risk for congenital varicella syndrome is with maternal infection occurring before 20 weeks gestation. The mortality rate associated with congenital varicella syndrome in the first months of life is 30%.(13) If maternal varicella infection occurs just before or after delivery, the newborn is at greatest risk for neonatal VZV, which is also associated with serious morbidity and mortality. Peripartum infection can be devastating to the neonate because protective maternal antibody titers may not be adequate, and therefore the neonate is at a higher risk of developing disseminated disease.(16)

Although maternal varicella is a clinical diagnosis and does not require laboratory testing, if the presentation is not clear, diagnosis can be confirmed by testing vesicular fluid with PCR or immunofluorescence. Pregnant women with varicella infection and any respiratory symptom should have a chest x-ray to evaluate for pneumonia. Pregnant women with a primary varicella infection should be treated with acyclovir 20 mg/kg PO 4 times daily or 800 mg PO 5 times per day for 5 days. Severe maternal varicella infection or patients with varicella pneumonia should be admitted for intravenous acyclovir 10–15 mg/kg IV q8 hours.(17,18)

Women exposed to VZV during pregnancy should have serologic testing within 24 hours of exposure and should be treated prophylactically if seronegative for VZV immunoglobulin G. Exposure is defined as direct contact with varicella/zoster noncrusted lesions, face to face contact two days prior to the onset of the rash, or face to face proximity longer than 5 minutes or sharing a hospital room or household with a person with noncrusted lesions. Prophylactic treatment consists of an investigational varicella zoster immune globulin (VariZIG). VariZIG confers passive immunity and reduces the severity of maternal infection; however, there is not sufficient data on the prevention of congenital varicella syndrome. The dosage of VariZIG is 125 units/10 kg body weight given IM and ideally should be administered within 96 hours but up to 10 days following exposure. After administration, these patients should be monitored for symptoms of varicella, which, if present, should be placed on antiviral treatment.(13,18,19,20)

The varicella vaccine, VARIVAX, is a live attenuated vaccine and is the main method of preventing varicella infection and its complications in women with no history of previous infection. The varicella vaccine is contraindicated during pregnancy, and women should refrain from becoming pregnant for 1 month after immunization.(13)

Sexually Transmitted Diseases in Pregnancy: Gonorrhea, Chlamydia, Trichomonas

Sexually transmitted diseases in pregnancy are common and can cause morbidity in the patient and fetus. Gonorrhea in pregnant women is typically localized to the lower genital tract, presenting as cervicitis, urethritis, and infection in the Bartholin and Skene's glands. It is often accompanied by chlamydia, and patients should be treated for both infections simultaneously. Uncomplicated gonorrhea infection of the cervix, urethra, or rectum can be treated with ceftriaxone 250 mg IM once plus Azithromycin 1 g PO once or cefixime 400 mg PO once plus azithromycin 1g PO once. Azithromycin also is effective for the treatment of chlamydia. Women allergic to penicillin should be treated with azithromycin 2 g orally as a single dose. Doxycycline should be avoided in pregnancy.(21,22)

Chlamydia trachomatis is an obligate intracellular bacterium that usually is asymptomatic in pregnancy but can present as urethritis, Bartholin gland infection, or cervicitis. The preferred treatment for chlamydial infection in pregnancy is azithromycin 1 g PO or amoxicillin 500 mg TID for 7 days. Doxycycline and fluoroquinolones should be avoided in pregnancy. Follow-up cultures 3 to 4 weeks after appropriate treatment should be done to document infection resolution.(21)

Pelvic inflammatory disease (PID) is less common in pregnancy. However, if PID is suspected, patients should be admitted to the hospital and OB-GYN should be consulted due to the high risk of maternal complications and preterm delivery (22).

Trichomonas vaginalis is a flagellated protozoan that causes vaginitis. Although it can increase the risk of premature rupture of membranes and preterm delivery, treatment has not been shown to decrease these complications. Treatment is therefore only recommended for symptomatic T. vaginalis with metronidazole 2 g PO once or 500 mg PO BID for 5 to 7 days.(21,23). Metronidazole crosses the placenta. Although some clinicians avoid its use in the first trimester due to the theoretical risk of teratogenicity, it has not been associated with any specific birth defects (24).

Bacterial vaginosis (BV) is a common cause of vaginal discharge due to the loss of normal lactobacilli, leading to an overgrowth of vaginal anaerobes. BV is not a sexually transmitted disease but is more common in women with multiple partners or who douche regularly. Symptomatic BV in pregnant women should be treated with metronidazole 500 mg PO BID for 7 days, Metronidazole 250 mg PO TID for 7 days, clindamycin 300 mg PO BID for 7 days, or 2% clindamycin cream (one applicator dose inserted vaginally at bedtime) for 7 days. BV increases the risk of preterm delivery, but it is unclear if treatment reduces this risk.(21,23,25).

Human immunodeficiency virus (HIV)

Management of HIV-infected pregnant women has evolved over the last two decades, and the current risk of perinatal transmission in the United States is estimated to be less than 2%.(26) It is recommended that all pregnant women take antiretroviral (ARV) medication during pregnancy, regardless of their cluster of differentiation 4 count or viral load, in order to reduce the risk of transmission to the fetus. The risk of HIV transmission is directly correlated with the patient's viral load and complexity of their HIV treatment regimen. In a prospective cohort study, patients on a three-drug regimen with non-detectable viral load had a 1% risk of transmission versus more than 20% risk in patients not on ARV therapy or with a viral load of > 30,000 copies/mL.(26,27)

In women who are ARV naïve, a regimen of zidovudine plus lamivudine plus lopinavir/ritonavir or atanzanavir/ritonavir is recommended. Generally, treatment may be deferred after the first trimester to reduce the teratogenic risk but should begin before 28 weeks gestation to increase the likelihood that the patient has a fully suppressed viral load at the time of delivery. Patients who are already on a treatment regimen should have drug resistance testing to allow for optimal treatment with full viral suppression. Post-exposure prophylaxis for the neonate is also recommended to further reduce risk from exposure of infected blood via fetal circulation or during delivery. Current guidelines recommend that infants receive zidovudine dosed for gestational age within 6 to 12 hours of delivery and for 6 weeks thereafter.

Suggested Readings and References

1. Nicolle LE, Bradley S, Colgan R, et al. Infectious Diseases Society of America guidelines for the diagnosis and treatment of asymptomatic bacteriuria in adults. Clin Infect Dis. 2005;40:643.
2. Young NS, Brown KE. Parvovirus B19. N Engl J Med. 2004;350(6):586–597.
3. Dijkmans AC, de Jong EP, Dijkmans BA, et al. Parvovirus B19 in pregnancy: prenatal diagnosis and management of fetal complications. Curr Opin Obstet Gynecol. 2012;24(2):95–101.
4. Broliden K, Tolfvenstam T, Norbeck O. Clinical aspects of parvovirus B19 infection. J Intern Med. 2006;260(4):285–304.
5. McCarter-Spaulding D. Parvovirus B19 in pregnancy. J Obstet Gynecol Neonatal Nurs. 2002;31(1):107–112.
6. American College of Obstetrics and Gynecologists. ACOG practice bulletin. Perinatal viral and parasitic infections. Number 20, September 2000. Int J Gynecol Obstet. 2002;76:95–107.
7. Seng C, Watkins P, Morse D, et al. Parvovirus B19 outbreak on adult ward. Epidemiol Infect. 1995;113:345.
8. Xu F, Sternberg MR, Kottiri BJ, et al. Trends in herpes simplex virus 1and 2 seroprevalence in the United States. JAMA. 2006;296:964.
9. ACOG Practice Bulletin, clinical management guideline for obstetrician-gynecologists. Number 82, June 2007.

10. Corey L, Wald A. Maternal and neonatal herpes simplex virus infections. *N Engl J Med.* 2009;361:13.

11. Briggs GG, Freeman RK, Yaffe, SJ. Acyclovir. *Drugs in Pregnancy and Lactation.* 8th ed. e-book; 2013.

12. Strauss SE, Ostrove JM, Inchauspe G, et al. Varicella-zoster virus infections. *Ann Intern Med.* 1988;108:221.

13. Lamont RF, Sobel JD, Carrington D, et al. Varicella-zoster virus (chickenpox) infection in pregnancy. *BJOG.* 2011;118(10):1155–1162.

14. Ender G, Miller E, Cradock-Watson J, et al. Consequences of varicella and herpes zoster in pregnancy: prospective study of 1739 cases. *Lancet.* 1994;343:1548.

15. Gnann JW Jr. Varicella-zoster virus: atypical presentations and unusual complications in women seropositive for varicella-zoster virus. *J Infect Dis.* 1994;170:991.

16. Prober CG, Gershon AA, Grose C, et al. Consensus: varicella-zoster infections in pregnancy and the perinatal period. *Pediatr Infect Dis J.* 1990;9:865.

17. Smego RAJr, Asperilla MO. Use of acyclovir for varicella pneumonia during pregnancy. *Obstet Gynecol.* 1991;78:1112.

18. Satin Andrew J, Stohl H. Perinatal infections. In: Hurt JK, Guile MW, Bienstock JL, Fox HE, eds. *Johns Hopkins Manual of Gynecology and Obstetrics.* 4th ed. Philadelphia, PA: Lippincott Williams & Wilkins; 2011.

19. Centers of Disease Control and Prevention (CDC). FDA approval of an extended period for administering VariZIG for postexposure prophylaxis of varicella. *MMWR Morb Mortal Weekly Rep.* 2012:61:212.

20. VariZIG for prophylaxis after exposure to varicella. *Med Lett Drugs Ther.* 2006:48:69.

21. Centers for Disease Control and Prevention. Sexually transmitted diseases treatment guidelines, 2010. *MMWR Morb Mortal Weekly Rep.* 2010;59:12.

22. Cunningham FG, Leveno KJ, Bloom SL, Hauth JC, Rouse DJ, Spong CY. Sexually transmitted diseases. In: Cunningham FG, Leveno KJ, Bloom SL, Hauth JC, Rouse DJ, Spong CY, eds. *Williams Obstetrics.* 23rd ed. New York, NY: McGraw-Hill; 2010:chapter 59.

23. Guile Matthew W, Keller J. Infections of the genital tract. In: Hurt JK, Guile MW, Bienstock JL, Fox HE, eds. *Johns Hopkins Manual of Gynecology and Obstetrics.* 4th ed. Philadelphia: PA: Lippincott Williams & Wilkins; 2011.

24. Caro-Paton T, Carvajal A, Martin de Diego I, et al. Is metronidazole teratogenic? a meta-analysis. *Br J Clin Pharmacol.* 1997;44:179.

25. ACOG Practice Bulletin, clinical management guideline for obstetrician-gynecologists: vaginitis. Number 72, May 2006.

26. Cooper ER, Charurat M, Mofenson L, et al. Combination antiretroviral strategies for the treatment of pregnant HIV-1-infected women and prevention of perinatal IV-1 transmission. *J Acquir Immune Defic Syndr.* 2002;29:484.

27. Siegfried N, van der Merwe L, Brocklehurst P, Sint TT. Antiretrovirals for reducing the risk of mother-to-child transmission of HIV infection. *Cochrane Database Sys Rev.* 2011;XX:CD003510.

Chapter 60

Infection in the Patient with Sickle Cell Anemia

Raymond Young

Disease Description
- Patients with sickle cell anemia are considered immunocompromised because of functional hypo or asplenism.
- Certain infections, including pneumonia, acute chest crisis, osteomyelitis, bacteremia, and meningitis, should be considerations when evaluating a patient with sickle cell anemia.

Organisms:
- Gram-positive and gram-negative bacteria, viruses

Treatment:
- Airway, breathing, and circulation management
- Aggressive fluid resuscitation
- Early administration of appropriately targeted antibiotics
  - Pneumonia and Acute Chest Syndrome (ACS)—cefotaxime (1–2 g intravenous [IV] q6–8 hours) or ceftriaxone (1–2 g intramuscularly [IM] or IV q24 hours [up to 4 g max per day]) as well as a 7-day course of oral or parenteral macrolide such as azithromycin.
  - Osteomyelitis—ceftazidime (2 g IV q12 hours) and highly effective bone penetrating fluoroquinolones (levofloxacin, 750 mg IV or oral administration [PO] once daily) are agents of choice for gram-negative bacteria (Oxacillin, 2 g IV q4 hours, or Vancomycin, 15 mg/kg IV q12 hours [± rifampin, 600 mg PO once daily] for *staphylococcus* infections).

Other Key Issues:
- Prophylaxis, vaccination, high degree of suspicion, and early intervention can help improve morbidity and mortality

Sickle cell anemia is characterized by an abnormality of the 6th amino acid in the β chain in hemoglobin synthesis. This allows polymerization of the red blood cells (RBC) in states of low oxygen tension leading to painful vaso-occlusive crisis as well as infarcts in various organs. Most individuals with sickle cell anemia are functionally asplenic by adolescence, which can occur as early as 2 years of age. This immunocompromised state leads to frequent infections of the skin, respiratory tract, bone, central nervous system (CNS), and blood. The life span of patients with sickle cell anemia has increased with the advent of vaccinations and prophylactic antibiotics. Infectious complications remain one of the leading causes of death, especially in young children. The more serious infections and their respective management are discussed in this chapter.

Pneumonia and Acute Chest Syndrome (ACS)

When approaching a sickle cell patient with suspected bacterial pneumonia, an important consideration is the ACS. ACS is one of the most common causes of death in these patients. It is defined by a new radiodensity accompanied by either fever, tachypnea, hypoxia, or chest pain and is often hard to distinguish from pneumonia. The etiology of ACS is thought to be vaso-occlusions within the pulmonary microvasculature that are either triggered by infection or hypoventilation or as a direct effect from fat emboli. In all likelihood, a combination of insults—including hypoxia, infection, fat emboli, inflammation, or acidosis—are the underlying causes of ACS. In one large study of ACS, more than 50% of cases were found to have an infectious agent—with *Chlamydia pneumoniae, Mycoplasma pneumoniae*, and viruses accounting for greater than 30% of isolates—and *Pneumococcal* and *Haemophilus influenzae* accounting for less than 10% of isolates.[1]

Presenting symptoms of bacterial pneumonia resemble that of ACS and are similar to non-sickle cell patients with community-acquired pneumonia (CAP). Symptoms can include fever, rigors, dyspnea, cough, chest pain, and tachypnea.

Blood and sputum cultures should be obtained in all patients with sickle cell anemia who present with signs and symptoms consistent with pneumonia or ACS. Although often nondiagnostic if an infectious etiology can be found, it can spare evolution or duration of the ACS episode and reduce respiratory deterioration. Chest radiographs may demonstrate multilobar or unilobar infiltrates.

Management should include antibiotics to cover *S. pneumoniae, Chlamydia pneumoniae*, and *mycoplasma* with consideration of legionella coverage. Therapy involves a 7-day course of a 3rd-generation parenteral cephalosporin such as cefotaxime (1–2 g IV q6–8 hours) or ceftriaxone (1–2 g IM or IV q24 hours [up to 4 g max per day]) as well as a 7-day course of oral or parenteral macrolide such as azithromycin. Ceftriaxone should be used with caution in children due to reports of hemolysis.[2] Supportive care should include efforts to avoid hypoxemia with oxygen therapy, IV hydration to decrease sickling, and transfusions as needed for deteriorating respiratory status.

Osteomyelitis

The prevalence of osteomyelitis in sickle cell patients is variable and may be as high as 60%. Analogous to the often indistinguishable presenting features of CAP and ACS, osteomyelitis in sickle cell populations may be difficult to differentiate from an acute vaso-occlusive crisis (VOC) and bony infarcts.

Impaired splenic function to clear encapsulated organisms and repeated bony infarcts that act as reservoirs for proliferating blood-borne bacteria contribute to the development of osteomyelitis. The most common organism is *Salmonella*, which, during the incubation phase, requires phagocytosis with subsequent colonization in reticuloendothelial organs such as the spleen, liver, and bone marrow. Other organisms that trigger osteomyelitis in the sickle cell population include enteric gram-negative bacteria followed by *Staphylococcus aureus*, which only accounts for about 25% of cases. Conversely, *S. aureus* is noted as the number one cause in non-sickle cell patients

Clinically, the presentation of osteomyelitis in sickle cell patients mimics the presenting features of VOC; hence, a high index of suspicion is warranted. High fevers, leukocytosis, and localized pain particularly in long bones that is unresponsive and persists despite traditional management of a VOC are the key clinical features. Blood cultures are useful but may be negative due to the initiation of antibiotics for VOC with fever; a positive bone culture via aspiration or biopsy is diagnostic. Plain radiographs and bone scans seldom differentiate VOC from osteomyelitis; magnetic resonance imaging (MRI) with Gadolinium increases the diagnostic yield but does not have a 100% sensitivity in distinguishing the two.[3]

Management should include debridement or drainage of infected necrotic tissue followed by a 2 to 6 week course of parenteral antibiotics based on the culture and sensitivity. Empiric treatment for suspected cases should include coverage for *Salmonella*, enteric gram-negative organisms, and *Staphylococcus*. Once the organism is identified, 3rd-generation cephalosporins such as ceftazidime (2 g IV q12 hours) and highly effective bone penetrating fluoroquinolones (levofloxacin, 750 mg IV or PO once daily) are agents of choice for gram-negative bacteria; and Oxacillin (2g IV q4 hours) or Vancomycin (15 mg/kg IV q12 hours [± rifampin, 600 mg PO once daily]) for *Staphylococcus* infections. In well-controlled cases, oral fluoroquinolones may be considered because of the effective oral bioavailability and excellent bone penetration.

Bacteremia

Although less common in adults, blood stream infection can have catastrophic consequences in the sickle cell population, with mortality reaching as high as 50%. The theme of impaired immunity due to functional asplenia remains; however, patients are also at risk of blood-borne infections due to indwelling devices such as vascular catheters and orthopedic hardware. In one study, there was a high association of bacteremia with bone-joint infections.[4]

Hospital-acquired etiologic organisms include *Staphylococcus* and gram-negative Enterobateriaceae; community-acquired organisms include *Streptococcus, E. Coli, Salmonella*, and *Haemophilus Influenzae* type B in children. Diagnosis is similar to non-sickle cell patients and includes blood cultures and traditional systemic inflammatory response syndrome criteria with a focus on infection.

Despite the marked reduction in streptococcal infections with widespread *Pneumococcal* vaccinations and prophylactic antibiotics, strep infections, especially in children, have been strongly associated with the development of meningitic extension. Empiric antibiotics should cover *pneumococcus* and *Haemophilus* with extension to cover *Salmonella* and other gram-negative enteric infections.[2]

Meningitis

Bacterial Meningitis is rare in adults; however, patients who have not received appropriate *Haemophilus influenzae* Type B and *Pneumococcal* vaccinations remain at risk for CNS extension, which has significant mortality. Risk factors for the development of bacterial meningitis in addition to impaired host defenses include exposure to persons with meningococcal infection, cerebrospinal fluid (CSF) leaks, or recent upper respiratory infection (URI) associated with ear infections.

In a series of case reports of adult sickle cell patients with confirmed meningitis, all had high fevers averaging 39.8°C (103.7°F), weakness, leukocytosis greater than 30 000, and 75% had nuchal rigidity.[5]

Lumbar puncture demonstrating lower than normal CSF glucose concentrations, increased CSF protein, pleocytosis, and microbacteriologic evidence of an organism similar to findings in non-sickle cell disease patients remain key.

Toxic children presenting with signs of CNS infections should be treated with antibiotics promptly prior to imaging or labs. Empiric antibiotics for all patients should cover *Streptococcus, Haemophilus*, and *Neisseria Meningitidis*; and therapy should be for 2 to 4 weeks.

Parvovirus B19/Transient Red Cell aplasia

Parvovirus B19, a respiratory-transmitted, single stranded DNA virus, is a common childhood infection, with 26% of children (non-sickle cell and sickle cell) seropositivity by age 5 and 64% by adulthood. Parvovirus B19 is well known for three different presenting clinical manifestations; but it should be noted that in the general population, most B19 parvovirus infections are asymptomatic. One of the most common manifestations of Parvovirus B 19 infection is erythema infectiosum, or fifth disease, a rash illness of childhood that results in "Slapped cheek" rash in toddlers. The infection can also affect adults, especially middle-aged women, resulting in an inflammatory arthropathy, resembling rheumatoid arthritis. The third clinical manifestation is a transient red cell aplasia in the patients who have a high demand for erythropoiesis, such as those patients with sickle cell anemia. Transient red cell aplasia has a noted prevalence of 65% to 80% of those patients infected with Parvovirus B19.[6]

The normal RBC lifespan is 120 days; however, in the sickle cell population, it is markedly reduced. The addition of a viral infection such as Parvovirus B19, which has direct cytotoxic effects of erythroid precursors, can lead to profound anemia.

Patients with sickle cell disease who are acutely infected with Parvovirus B19 may present with headache, fatigue, dyspnea, and worsening anemia from baseline that that is preceded by a viral URI or gastroenteritis. The appearance of a rash is rare.

Diagnostically reticulocytopenia, less than 1%, generally begins 5 days post-exposure and continues for 7 to 10 days. Serum levels of elevated Parvovirus B19 immunoglobulin M (IgM) have a sensitivity approaching 90% and a 99% specificity and helps confirm the diagnosis. Parvovirus B19 polymerase chain reaction (PCR) may be helpful, especially in those who may not mount antibody response. Occasionally leukopenia and thrombocytopenia can occur.

Most children infected recover from red cell aplasia spontaneously and have lifelong immunity. Transfusions are indicated for symptomatic anemia and in those who have recurrent disease or have other concomitant causes of immunodeficiencies such as human immunodeficiency virus, lymphop-roliferative malignancies, or those receiving concomitant chemotherapy IV immune globulin can be considered.

Key Considerations

In view of the fact that that sickle cell patients have a predisposition to infections with devastating consequences, primary prevention is key. The 23-valent polysaccharide *Pneumococcal* vaccination should be administered at age 2 and ages 3 to 5 years after the first dose in children with sickle cell disease, whereas the protein conjugated vaccine is recommended in all infants. Adult patients should continue to receive *Pneumococcal* vaccinations every 5 years. *Haemophilus Influenzae* type B vaccinations should also be administered in childhood as scheduled. Prophylactic penicillins for invasive streptococcal infection have proven to be the hallmark for prevention. Current recommendations include administration of penicillin

---

Summary Box 60.1 Bacterial Pneumonia

- Often indistinguishable from acute chest syndrome
- Patients present with fever, cough, tachypnea, chest pain, and dyspnea
- Blood and sputum cultures helpful when positive
- Organisms:
  - Chlamydia Pneumoniae, *Mycoplasma Pneumoniae*, and less often *Pneumococcal* and *Haemophilus*
- 7-day course of 3rd-generation IV Cephalosporin **and** PO or IV Macrolide or fluoroquinolone

Osteomyelitis

- May mimic acute vaso-occlusive crisis and bony infarcts
- Prolonged pain particularly in long bones not responsive to traditional acute crisis management
- Organisms:
  - *Salmonella* and other enteric gram negatives Microcystins; *Staphylococcus Aureus* seen in only 25%
- MRI with Gad may help diagnosis but not 100%; bone aspiration or biopsy essential for diagnosis and therapy
- Empiric coverage includes 3rd-generation IV cephalosporin for gram negatives and Vancomycin for *Staph* until organism identified, followed by 2 to 6 week course after source control with debridement or drainage. Oral fluoroquinolone may be considered if organism sensitive and there is good source control.

Bacteremia

- Less common, but mortality as high as 50%.
- Associated with indwelling catheters and bone-joint infections
- Organisms
  - *Salmonella, Haemophilus*, and *Streptococcus*
- Empirically cover for the *Streptococcus, Haemophilus, Salmonella*, and other gram-negative enteric organisms

Meninigitis

- Risk factors include non-immunization, CSF leaks and URI with ear involvement in children
- Organisms
  - *Streptococcus, Haemophilus, Neisseria Meningitidis*
- Therapy should be tailored to the preceding organisms empirically with narrowing based on culture data

Transient Red Cell Aplasia

- Most people are seropositive by late adulthood
- Organism
  - Parvovirus B19, which has a direct cytotoxic effect on erythroid precursors
- Reticulocytopenia is characteristic; Parvovirus B19 IgM is diagnostic and PCR can be considered in those who do not mount an immune response
- Treatment is supportive, simple transfusions for symptomatic anemia

V potassium 125 twice a day from newborn to 3 years of age with a doubling of the dose from ages 3 to 5 (see summary Box 60.1).

Suggested Readings and References

1. Poncz M, Kane E, Gill FM. Acute chest syndrome in sickle cell disease: etiology and clinical correlates. *J Pediatr*. 1985;107(6):861–866.
2. National Institutes of Health, National Heart, Lung, and Blood Institute, Division of Blood Diseases and Resources. *The Management of Sickle Cell Disease*. 4th ed. Bethesda, MD: NIH; 2002:02–2117.
3. Almeida A, Roberts I. Bone involvement in sickle cell disease. *Br J Haematol*. 2005;129(4):482–490.
4. Zarrouk V, Habibi A, Zahar JR, et al. Bloodstream infection in adults with sickle cell disease: association with venous catheters, Staphylococcus aureus, and bone-joint infections. *Medicine*. 2006;85(1):43–48.
5. Olopoenia L, Frederick W, Greaves W, Adams R, Addo FE, Castro O. Pneumococcal sepsis and meningitis in adults with sickle cell disease. *South Med J*. 1990;83(9):1002–1004.
6. Booth C, Inusa B, Obaro SK. Infection in sickle cell disease: a review. *Int J Infect Dis*. 2010;14(1):e2–e12.
7. Yang Q, Olney RS. Sickle hemoglobin (Hb S) allele and sickle cell disease. *Am J Epidemiol*. 2000;151(9):839–845.
8. Bennett OM, Namnyak SS. Bone and joint manifestations of sickle cell anaemia. *J Bone Joint Surg*. 1990;72(3):494–499.
9. Goyal M, Donoghue A, Schwab S, Hasbrouck N, Khojasteh S, Osterhoudt K. Severe hemolytic crisis after ceftriaxone administration. *Pediatr Emerg Care*. 2011;27(4):322–323.

Fever of Unknown Origin

Annie Antar

Summary Box

Disease Description: Classic fever of unknown origin (FUO) describes a febrile illness lasting 3 or more weeks with several temperatures of $\geq 38.3°C$ and with no diagnosis after investigation during three outpatient visits or 3 days of hospitalization.

Organisms: The differential is large, but FUO can be a result of infection, neoplasia, connective tissue disease, or other noninfectious inflammatory diseases, granulomatous disease, or miscellaneous febrile illnesses.

Treatment: Unless the patient is neutropenic or unstable, treatment is not advised until a diagnosis is made.

Disease Description

Fever of unknown origin (FUO) meets *all* three of the following criteria:

1. Temperatures of ≥ 38.3°C (≥ 101°F) on several occasions,
2. fevers occurring for more than 3 weeks, and
3. no diagnosis after appropriate evaluation during three outpatient visits, 3 days in the hospital, or 1 week of invasive ambulatory investigation.

FUO is now classified into **four groups**: (1) nosocomial FUO: acute care patients hospitalized with FUO who were not incubating or displaying signs of infection on admission and who have an uncertain diagnosis after 3 or more days of appropriate evaluation, including cultures that have been incubating 2 or more days; (2) neutropenic FUO: FUO in a patient with a current absolute neutrophil count (ANC) < 500 or an ANC expected to be < 500 within 2 days who has an uncertain diagnosis after 3 or more days of appropriate evaluation, including cultures that have been incubating 2 or more days; (3) human immunodeficiency virus (HIV)-associated FUO: FUO in a patient known to have HIV infection with fevers greater than 4 weeks as an outpatient or 3 or more days as an inpatient and with an uncertain diagnosis after 3 or more days of appropriate evaluation, including cultures that have been incubating 2 or more days; and (4) classic FUO: all other FUO patients, which is the entity focused on in this chapter.

Epidemiology: No studies have determined the exact incidence and prevalence of FUO in recent years in the United States.

Typical Disease Course: The course of FUO varies widely depending on the underlying etiology. The long-term prognosis of FUO that remains undiagnosed despite intensive investigation is good, with one prospective study finding an attributable mortality of 3.2% at 5 years.

Diagnostic Considerations

The patients who meet the preceding criteria for classic FUO fall into five general categories of illness: infection, neoplasia, connective tissue or other noninfectious inflammatory disease, granulomatous disease, or miscellaneous febrile illnesses.

Diagnostic Tests

Standard initial workup of FUO should begin with a thorough history, including any history of prior or current infections, neoplasms, or inflammatory diseases; prior hospitalizations, surgeries, procedures, or prostheses; prior or current medications and supplements; sick contacts; sexual contacts; animal contacts; drug and dietary history; travel and outdoors exposure history; occupational and professional history; family history; and psychiatric history. Serial physical examinations and interval histories should follow. A reasonable initial diagnostic workup, guided by and modified after thorough and repeated histories and physical exams, is in Table 61.1.

Table 61.1 Initial Diagnostic Workup for FUO		
Microbiologic	Laboratory	Imaging
3 blood cultures	CBC with differential	CXR
UA and urine culture	CMP	Abdominal/pelvic imaging by US or CT
Sputum culture	Peripheral smear	
Stool culture	ESR/CRP	
Culture from any other amenable body site	CK	
HIV	LDH	
RPR or treponemal test	SPEP	
PPD or interferon gamma release assay	ANA	
CMV, EBV	RF	
	Serum to be stored for future testing (eg, trending antibody titers)	

Abbreviations: FUO, fever of unknown origin; CBC, complete blood count; CXR, chest x-ray; UA, urinalysis; CMP, comprehensive metabolic panel; US, ultrasound; CT, computed tomography; ESR, erythrocyte sedimentation rate; CRP, C-reactive protein; CK, creatine kinase; HIV, human immunodeficiency virus; LDH, lactate dehydrogenase; RPR, rapid plasma reagin; SPEP, Serum protein electrophoresis; PPD, purified protein derivative; ANA, antinuclear antibody; CMV, cytomegalovirus; EBV, Epstein-Barr virus; RF, rheumatoid factor.

Further investigation should be guided by the results of this initial diagnostic workup. In the absence of other diagnostic clues, a 2009 systematic review of eight studies has shown that if either erythrocyte sedimentation rate (ESR) or C-reactive protein is elevated, FDG-PET (especially when combined with computed tomography) can help localize malignancy, inflammation, or infection in over one-third of patients. Other imaging options that are cheaper but less sensitive and specific include nuclear scintigraphy with ^{67}Gallium-citrate and ^{111}Indium labeled leukocytes.

The next steps to take in an undiagnosed patient with FUO should again be guided by the patient's history and physical exam and could include any of the following in Table 61.2.

Supervised temperature taking or simultaneous urine and body temperatures can be undertaken if there is a concern for factitious disorder.

Organisms/Differential Diagnosis

The differential diagnosis for FUO is one of the most extensive in medicine.

Granulomatous diseases that can cause FUO include granulomatous hepatitis (which can occur with normal liver function tests), Crohn's disease, and sarcoidosis. Other causes of FUO are drug fever (which can have any pattern of fever), gout, hematomas, aortic dissection, pulmonary embolus, hemoglobinopathies, post-myocardial infarction syndrome, subacute thyroiditis, tissue infarction or necrosis, adrenal insufficiency, Fabry disease, hereditary periodic fever syndromes like familial Mediterranean fever, factitious disorder, and other rarer disorders. Finally, thermoregulation can be disrupted centrally by tumor, stroke, disease, encephalitis, or hypothalamic dysfunction as well as peripherally by hyperthyroidism or pheochromocytoma. The differential may change depending on the patient's travel and exposure history. After exhaustive diagnostic investigation, 7% to 50% of cases of FUO are never diagnosed.

Table 61.2 Subsequent Diagnostic Workup of FUO if Initial Testing Is Nondiagnostic

Microbiologic	Laboratory	Imaging
Thick and thin blood smears for parasites (eg, *Plasmodium*)	Tumor antigens (eg, PSA, CA-125, CEA)	CT of chest, abdomen, and pelvis with IV and PO contrast
Fungal and mycobacterial blood cultures	Fe, transferrin, TIBC, MCHC, B12, folate	Fundoscopic, sinus, and dental imaging
2-week evaluation of blood cultures for HACEK and slow-growing pathogens	Flow cytometry and cytopathology	Echocardiogram for endocarditis (bacterial and nonbacterial thrombotic), pericarditis, or atrial myxoma
Induced sputum or bronchoscopy with BAL	Serum cryoglobulins	Small bowel follow-through or colonoscopy
Needle aspiration of any other abnormal fluid collection	Serum immunoglobulins	Arteriography if suspected systemic necrotizing vasculitis
Hepatitis C antibodies	C3/C4	Bone scan to look for metastases
LP with PCRs	ANA	
STD Panel		
Urine cultures for *Mycobacteria*, fungi, and CMV	ANCA	
Serologic studies for *Salmonella*, *Brucella*, and *Rickettsia*	Cortisol	
Re-evaluation of relevant tissue taken during surgery	Amylase	
	Uric Acid	
	TSH	
	ACE	
	Paracentesis for ascitic fluid	
	Liver biopsy	
	Bone marrow biopsy	
	Temporal artery biopsy in patients over the age of 55	

Abbreviations: PSA, prostate specific antigen; CA-125, cancer antigen 125; CEA, carcinoembryonic antigen; CT, computed tomography; IV, intravenous; PO, by mouth; Fe, iron; TIBC, total iron binding capacity; MCHC, mean corpuscular hemoglobin concentration; B12, cobalamin; HACEK, please copy from previous chapter on endocarditis; BAL, bronchoscopic alveolar lavage; C3/C4, complement molecules 3 and 4; LP, lumbar puncture; PCRs, polymerase chain reactions; ANA, anti-nuclear antibody; STD, sexually transmitted diseases; CMV, cytomegalovirus; ANCA, anti-neutrophil cytoplasmic antibody; TSH, thyroid stimulating hormone; ACE, angiotensin converting enzyme.

Treatment

If a patient is having vital sign instability or neutropenia, they should be treated immediately with appropriate antibiotic coverage. The Infectious Diseases Society of America has published guidelines on treatment with antimicrobials in the setting of neutropenic fever. However, in a clinically stable patient, treatment should not commence until a diagnosis is found or the condition of the patient changes, as treatment itself may decrease the chances of correctly diagnosing the patient. Empiric *M. tuberculosis* treatment in appropriate patients with negative testing can be considered if there is a strong clinical suspicion or in an area where *M. tuberculosis* is prevalent. Glucocorticoids should be avoided unless infection has been ruled out or unless inflammatory disease is probable and debilitating, as they may mask symptoms and delay diagnosis. Nonsteroidal anti-inflammatory drugs may be given if the preceding investigations have not yielded a diagnosis. In undiagnosed patients, as mentioned previously, prognosis is good. Factors that may tip the balance in favor of treating rather than waiting would include patients who are frail and elderly, cirrhotic, asplenic, immunosuppressed, or have had recent exotic travel.

Suggested Readings and References

1. Bleeker-Rovers CP, Vos FJ, de Kleijn EM, et al. A prospective multicenter study on fever of unknown origin: the yield of a structured diagnostic protocol. *Medicine*. 2007;86:26–38.

2. Bleeker-Rovers CP, van der Meer JW, Oyen WJ. Fever of unknown origin. *Semin Nucl Med*. 2009;39:81–87.

3. Durack DT, Street AC. Fever of unknown origin—reexamined and redefined. *Curr Clin Top Infect Dis*. 1991;11:35–51.

4. Gelfand JA, Callahan MV. Fever of unknown origin. *Harrison's Principles of Internal Medicine*, ed. Fauci AS, Braunwald E, Kasper DL, et al. New York, NY: McGraw Hill Medical; 2008:130–134.

5. Iikuni Y, Okada J, Kondo H, Kashiwazaki S. Current fever of unknown origin 1982–1992. *Intern Med*. 1994;33:67–73.

6. Knockaert DC, Dujardin KS, Bobbaers HJ. Long-term follow-up of patients with undiagnosed fever of unknown origin. *Arch Intern Med*. 1996;156:618–620.

7. Varghese GM, Trowbridge P, Doherty T. Investigating and managing pyrexia of unknown origin in adults. *BMJ*. 2010;341:c5470.

Bioterrorism

Chapter 62

Anthrax

Rebecca Smith

Summary Box

Disease Description: Symptoms depend upon the route of spore exposure: cutaneous, ingestion, or inhalational. Symptoms range from a black eschar with surrounding edema to fever, nausea, vomiting, abdominal pain, gastrointestinal hemorrhage, cough, respiratory distress, sepsis, and death.

Organism: *Bacillus anthracis*
  Treatment:
  Cutaneous or post-exposure prophylaxis:
    First line: Ciprofloxacin 500 mg PO q12 hours (10–15 mg/kg)* for 60 days or
    doxycycline 100 mg PO q12 hours (2.2 mg/kg)* for 60 days
    Second line: Amoxicillin 500 mg PO q8 hours (80 mg/kg/day, divided TID)* x 60 days
  Inhalational:
    Ciprofloxacin 400 mg IV q12 hours (10–15 mg/kg)* for 60 days or
    doxycycline 100 mg IV q12 hours (2.2 mg/kg)* PLUS one or two additional antimicrobials with activity against *B. anthracis* (see "Treatment" following)

Other Key Issues: Personal protective equipment and patient decontamination are important before addressing a potential exposure. Mass casualty incidents will likely cause a strain on resources and appropriate triage will be crucial.

*Pediatric dosing in parentheses

Disease Description

Epidemiology

Anthrax spores are found in the soil in many parts of the world and usually cause disease in grazing animals. Human disease is typically seen in farmers, ranchers, and workers handling animal carcasses, hides, hair, and bones. In biologic warfare or terrorism, aerosolization of the spores has been considered an effective route of mass dissemination.

Presenting Features and Disease Course

Clinical presentation depends upon the route of exposure: cutaneous, ingestion, or inhalation.

Cutaneous: Spores gain access to the skin via abrasions on the skin and form a black eschar with significant surrounding edema as well as vesicles at the site of skin entry. Most eschars heal spontaneously, but 10% to 20% of untreated cases can progress to sepsis and death. Figure 62.1 shows an initial anthrax skin lesion with surrounding vesicles and its evolution into a thick, black eschar (Figure 62.2).

Ingestion: Patients present with nausea, vomiting, abdominal pain, fever, and mucosal ulcers that can lead to gastrointestinal hemorrhage, perforation, sepsis, and death. Mortality is high.

Inhalational (aka Woolsorters' disease): The incubation period after inhalation of spores is 1 to 6 days. *B. anthracis* spores are inhaled, taken up by pulmonary macrophages, and carried into the lymphatic system. The spores germinate within the macrophages, producing active *B. anthracis* bacilli. The bacilli replicate and induce an immunologic reaction that causes a characteristic swelling of the mediastinal lymph nodes. Symptoms include fever, malaise, fatigue, nonproductive cough, and chest discomfort. Patients can rapidly develop severe respiratory distress with dyspnea, diaphoresis, stridor, cyanosis, bacteremia, shock, metastatic infection (meningitis in 50% of cases), and death within 24 to 36 hours. Historically, once a patient was symptomatic, mortality was 100% despite treatment with antibiotics. However, 50% of patients with inhalational anthrax due to the 2001 anthrax attacks in the United States recovered with early hospitalization, aggressive supportive care, and antibiotic therapy.

Diagnostic Considerations

In comparison to a flu-like illness, a patient with inhalational anthrax is more likely to have nausea or vomiting, tachycardia, elevated transaminases, hyponatremia, elevated hematocrit, hypoalbuminemia, and normal white blood counts. A patient with a flu-like illness is more likely to have myalgias, headache, and nasal symptoms.

Diagnostic Tests: All patients suspected of any form of anthrax should be placed on continuous cardiac and pulmonary monitoring. Chest radiographs and computed tomography scans of patients with inhalational anthrax often show a widened mediastinum (shown in Figure 62.3) and pulmonary effusions. Imaging may also show pulmonary infiltrates. Toxic or ill-appearing patients should receive a complete panel of blood tests, including an arterial blood gas, complete blood count, comprehensive metabolic panel, disseminated intravascular coagulation screening panel, serologies, blood cultures with antibiotic

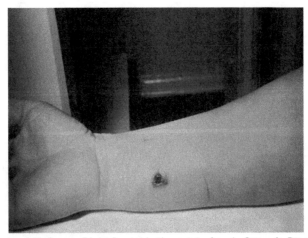

Figure 62.1 Anthrax, skin of right forearm, 7th day. Reprinted with permission from the Centers for Disease Control.

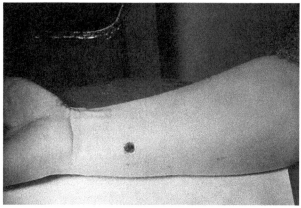

Figure 62.2 Anthrax, skin of right forearm, 12th day. Photo by Arthur E. Kaye. Reprinted with permission from the Centers for Disease Control.

sensitivities, and gram stain. Lab personnel should be made aware of the suspected pathogen so that they may take the proper precautions.

Organism

Microbiology
Bacillus anthracis is a gram-positive rod that is aerobic, nonmotile, and spore-forming. It grows readily on routine culture media and can be cultured from blood, sputum, or plural fluid. *B. anthracis* spores are present in soil, water, air, and vegetation.

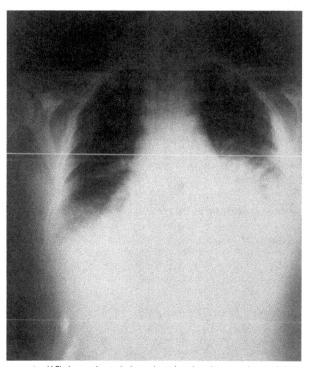

Figure 62.3 This anteroposterior (AP) chest radiograph showed a widened mediastinum due to inhalation anthrax, and was taken 22 hours before death. CDC / Dr. P.S. Brachman.

Life Cycle and Pathogenesis

Herbivores (eg, sheep, goats, cattle, and horses) either inhale *B. anthracis* spores or ingest spores as they graze. The heat and carbon dioxide within these herbivores activates the dormant spore, yielding active bacilli. These bacilli can then be contracted by humans via consumption of infected animal products or by way of a vector, such as blood-feeding insects. Bacilli are present in the excretions (ie, urine, feces, and saliva) and carcasses of infected herbivores, and they form spores upon exposure to oxygen.

Human infection with these spores in the environment or infected animal products (eg, animal hides) occurs via ingestion, inhalation, or skin defects. *B. anthracis* spores germinate in the tissue at the site of entry, and bacteria then multiply. They are engulfed by macrophages in which they produce the anthrax toxin that consists of 3 parts: (1) a protective antigen; (2) an edema factor, which is an adenylate cyclase; and (3) a lethal factor. All of these factors work together to kill white blood cells and deplete the host's immune system.

Treatment

First-line Recommendations

The two most important things to remember with any potential biologic weapon exposure are personal protective equipment and decontamination. It is important to note that most biologic weapon agents (**except anthrax spores**) are degraded in sunlight and by desiccation and will not survive in the environment for more than 1 to 2 days. By the time patients present several days after exposure, the disease is usually fatal.

There is no evidence of person-to-person transmission of anthrax. Removal of clothing and decontamination with soap and water will remove 99.99% of contaminants. This is something that can be done in patients' homes to reduce strain on medical resources. If there are any visible contaminants (eg, powders, spores) on a patient's clothes or skin, they should be removed with water irrigation, sterilization of the skin with a sporicidal/bactericidal solution (such as 0.5% sodium hypochlorite, a 1:10 dilution of household bleach), and a final water rinse. In the hospital setting, patients should remove their clothes and place them in sealed and labeled plastic bags, then wash their hands and shower thoroughly with soap and water.

The mainstay of antibiotic therapy is ciprofloxacin and doxycycline administered orally or parenterally, depending on the type of anthrax infection suspected. For **cutaneous anthrax or post-exposure prophylaxis**, give ciprofloxacin 500 mg (10–15 mg/kg in children) by mouth q12 hours or doxycycline 100 mg (2.2 mg/kg in children) by mouth q12 hours. For **anthrax ingestion** or **inhalational anthrax**, give ciprofloxacin 400 mg (10–15 mg/kg in children) IV q12 hours or doxycycline 100 mg (2.2 mg/kg in children) IV q12 h PLUS one or two additional antimicrobials with activity against *B. anthracis*, such as clindamycin, vancomycin, imipenem, meropenem, chloramphenicol, penicillin, ampicillin, rifampin, and clarithromycin. IV treatment can be changed to oral treatment when the patient is clinically stable. The duration of therapy for all suspected bioterrorism attacks is 60 days to adequately cover for delayed development of inhalational anthrax.

If a patient has developed **anthrax meningitis**, the following combination therapy is recommended: vancomycin 22.5 mg/kg IV q12 hours PLUS ciprofloxacin 400 mg IV q8 hours PLUS rifampin 600 mg IV q24 hours.

Second-line Recommendations and Third-line recommendations

Amoxicillin 500 mg by mouth TID (80 mg/kg/day PO, divided every 8 hours in children), may be given for cutaneous anthrax or post-exposure prophylaxis if a patient cannot tolerate other drugs.

Evolving or emerging treatment developments and considerations

There is a vaccine called *anthrax vaccine adsorbed* that is used in the United States for people who may have occupational exposure to *B. anthracis* bacilli or spores, including military and lab personnel. The vaccine is associated with up to a 20% incidence of mild local skin reaction and up to a 1.5% incidence of self-limited systemic symptoms. Vaccine dosing is 0.5 mL subcutaneously at zero, 2, and 4 weeks as well as at 6, 12, and 18 months. Yearly boosters are also required. After confirmed exposure, the vaccine should be given as soon as possible, then at 2 and 4 weeks, and in conjunction with post-exposure prophylaxis.

Other Key Issues

In the event of mass casualty incidents, resources are likely to become strained and will need to be rationed. Cardiopulmonary monitoring may not be available for all patients and should be reserved for patients with a high suspicion of inhalational anthrax.

Suggested Readings and References

1. Bioterrorism in *2011–2012 Antibiotic Guidelines: Treatment and Recommendations for Adult Inpatients*. Baltimore, MD: The Johns Hopkins Hospital Antimicrobial Stewardship Program; 2011.
2. Goering RV, ed. Anthrax. In: *Mims' Medical Microbiology*. 5th ed. Philadelphia, PA: Saunders; 2012. http://www.mdconsult.com Accessed October 17, 2012.
3. Mason RJ, Murray JF, eds. Other less common causes of pneumonia. In: *Murray and Nadel's Textbook of Respiratory Medicine*. 5th ed. Philadelphia, PA: Saunders; 2010. http://www.mdconsult.com. Accessed October 17, 2012.
4. Mehmet, D. Anthrax. In: Cohen J, Powderly WG, eds. *Infectious Diseases*. 3rd ed. Philadelphia, PA: Mosby; 2010. http://www.mdconsult.com Accessed October 17, 2012.
5. Suchard JR. Biological warfare agents. In: Wolfson AB, ed. *Harwood and Nuss' Clinical Practice of Emergency Medicine*. 5th ed. Philadelphia, PA: Lippincott Williams & Wilkins; 2010:1531–1536.

Chapter 63

Smallpox

Rebecca Smith

Summary Box

Disease Description: Symptoms include fever and a progressive papular rash that becomes vesicular and then pustular. A systemic inflammatory response syndrome (SIRS) leads to septic shock and death in 30% of cases.

Organism: *Variola major* and *Variola minor*

Treatment:
   First line: Aggressive supportive care and smallpox vaccine within 4 days
   Second line: Cidofovir 3 to 5 mg/kg IV

Other Key Issues: Any suspected case of smallpox should be considered a biologic attack because the virus has been eradicated. The Department of Public Health and Centers for Disease Control and Prevention (CDC) must be contacted immediately. Patients are extremely contagious and must be placed on contact, droplet, and airborne precautions in a negative pressure room.

Disease Description

Epidemiology

Naturally occurring smallpox was eradicated by a global vaccination campaign in the 1960s and 1970s. The last documented case was in Somalia in December of 1979. However, there are stocks of the virus in labs in the United States and Russia. A large portion of today's population has not been vaccinated, and the degree of immunity conferred by remote vaccination is not clear. Thus, smallpox is a significant threat as a potential biologic weapon.

Presenting Features and Clinical Course

The smallpox virus has a 12- to 14-day incubation period. Initial symptoms include fever, malaise, rigors, vomiting, and prostration with headache and backache. The first lesions to appear are oral mucosal lesions that allow shedding of the virus into the saliva. On day 2 or 3, a papular rash develops on the face and spreads to the extremities, involving the palms and soles. The fever continues as the rash becomes vesicular and then both pustular and umbilicated (see Figure 63.1). The pustules scab over in the 3rd week of the disease and eventually separate, leaving pitted and hypopigmented scars. The disease can progress to SIRS and septic shock, often with secondary bacterial infection. Mortality is up to 30% and usually occurs during the second week of the illness.

Diagnostic Considerations

The differential for smallpox is wide and includes many viral syndromes, drug reactions, and respiratory illnesses. However, the following specific characteristics can help narrow the differential diagnosis toward smallpox: synchronous lesions, umbilicated appearance in the pustular stage, early involvement of palms and soles, and centrifugal distribution of the eruption.

Diagnostic Tests

The diagnosis of smallpox is predominately based on clinical features. However, definitive diagnosis can be confirmed from blood samples, lesion contents, or scrapings from crusts that are analyzed using electron microscopy, viral antigen immunohistochemistry, and polymerase chain reaction. *Variola* can also be isolated from such samples. All lab work and culturing of *Varicella* should take place in the CDC's designated lab due to its high contagiousness. Ill patients should have a broad set of lab work sent, including complete blood count, comprehensive metabolic panel, arterial blood gas, blood cultures, and vesicular fluid cultures.

Imaging is nonspecific, but chest radiographs show diffuse alveolar opacities from an inflammatory response associated with the primary infection. Lobar opacities are seen and mostly associated with secondary bacterial pneumonia.

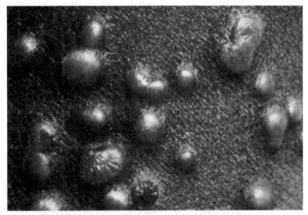

Figure 63.1 This is from the Public Health Image Library Small Pox image ID#2553. The figure is from the Centers for Disease Control and Prevention Public Health Image Library/Dr. Paul B. Dean.

Organisms

Microbiology
Variola major and *Variola minor*, the viruses that causes smallpox, are large DNA-bearing *Orthopoxviruses* with a host range limited to humans. It is a member of the Poxviridae family. Transmission occurs via inhalation of droplets or aerosols but may also occur through contaminated sheets, clothing, or fomites.

Treatment

First-Line Recommendations
The two foremost considerations with any potential biologic weapon exposure are personal protective equipment and decontamination. Patients should be placed on droplet precautions with a negative pressure isolation room, and all providers should wear N95 masks or a powered air purifying respirator. The virus is highly contagious and is communicable from the onset of the exanthem (generally 1 or 2 days prior to the rash) until all of the scabs have separated. Patients are felt to be most contagious during the 1st week of the rash due to high titers of replicating virus in the oropharynx at that time. If there are any visible contaminants (eg, powders, spores) on a patient's clothes or skin, patients should remove their clothes and place them in sealed and labeled plastic bags, wash their hands, and shower thoroughly with soap and water.

The mainstay of treatment for smallpox infection is aggressive supportive therapy. If a patient is exposed to smallpox, he should receive the smallpox vaccine within 4 days of exposure. Pre-exposure and post-exposure vaccination is recommended if it has been greater than 3 years since the patient's last vaccination. Complications of the smallpox vaccine can be serious and include encephalitis and progressive *Vaccinia* (a rare and often fatal event that occurs after vaccination with small pox vaccine). Post-vaccinal encephalitis occurs in three out of every one million people vaccinated. A total of 40% of cases are fatal, and some survivors are left with permanent neurologic sequelae. Progressive *Vaccinia* usually occurs in immunocompromised individuals and is treated with *Vaccinia* immune globulin 0.6 mg/kg im or IV once. *Vaccinia* immune globulin can only be obtained from the CDC.

If someone has been exposed to smallpox but exhibits no clinical evidence of disease, it is recommended that they be placed in isolation for 17 days and observed for the development of fever or rash. This can occur in the hospital setting or at home.

Evolving Treatment Developments and Considerations
The antiviral drug cidofovir, if administered early after exposure, may be beneficial in preventing the development of the disease. However, it has not been proven to be more effective than post-exposure vaccination.

Other Key Issues to Consider

In the event of mass casualty incidents, resources are likely to become strained and will need to be rationed. Cardiopulmonary monitoring may not be available for all patients and should be reserved for patients with a high suspicion of inhalational anthrax. Single-patient negative pressure isolation rooms could easily run out, so patients may need to be placed in rooms in groups.

The suspicion of a single smallpox case should lead to immediate notification of local public health authorities and the hospital epidemiologist. Because the disease does not exist in nature, the occurrence of even a single case of smallpox should be considered the result of a bioterrorist attack until proven otherwise. An epidemiologic investigation would be essential for determining the perimeter of the initial release so that tracking and quarantine of those exposed could be completed.

Suggested Readings and References

1. *Bioterrorism in 2011–2012 Antibiotic Guidelines: Treatment and Recommendations for Adult Inpatients.* Baltimore, MD: The Johns Hopkins Hospital Antimicrobial Stewardship Program; 2011.
2. *Smallpox: investigational vaccinia immune globulin (VIG) information.* Centers for Disease Control and Prevention website, 2009. http://www.bt.cdc.gov.ezproxy.welch.jhmi.edu/agent/smallpox/vaccination/vig.asp. Accessed October 18, 2012.

3. Cohen J, Powderly WG, eds. Smallpox. In: *Infectious Diseases*. 3rd ed. Philadelphia, PA: Mosby; 2010. http://www.mdconsult.com on Accessed October 18, 2012.

4. Goering RV, ed. Smallpox. In: *Mims' Medical Microbiology*. 5fth ed. Philadelphia, PA: Saunders; 2012. http://www.mdconsult.com on Accessed October 17, 2012.

5. Mason RJ, Murray JF, eds. CDC Category A Agents. In: *Mason: Murray and Nadel's Textbook of Respiratory Medicine*. 5th ed. Philadelphia, PA: Saunders; 2010. http://www.mdconsult.com Accessed October 17, 2012.

6. Suchard JR. Biological warfare agents. In: Wolfson AB, ed. *Harwood and Nuss' Clinical Practice of Emergency Medicine*. 5th ed. Philadelphia, PA: Lippincott Williams & Wilkins; 2010: 1531–1536.

Chapter 64

Botulism

Monica Mix

Summary Box

Disease Description: Botulism is a symmetric, descending, flaccid paralysis caused by exposure to botulinum toxin.

Organism: *Clostridium botulinum*
   Treatment: Botulinum antitoxin, supportive care

Other Key Issues:
- Botulinum toxin is a category A biological agent for bioterrorism.
- Botulinum toxin is the most potent naturally occurring toxin.
- Botulinum toxin is the first biologic toxin licensed as a drug for treating human disease.

Disease Description

Epidemiology

Botulism is a disease characterized by a symmetric, flaccid, descending paralysis, which is caused by the botulinum toxin. There are four naturally occurring forms of botulism in addition to two forms that require intentional manipulation of the toxin by humans. The four naturally occurring syndromes include foodborne botulism, infant botulism, adult intestinal botulism, and wound botulism. The intentionally altered forms of botulism are inhalational and iatrogenic botulism. All six forms are rare, with fewer than 200 total cases of botulism reported annually in the United States.

Among these cases, infant botulism is the most common. This syndrome occurs almost exclusively in infants less than 12 months of age and accounts for approximately 80 to 100 cases of botulism per year within the United States. Infant botulism results from the colonization of the intestinal tract by C. botulinum, which subsequently produces botulinum toxin in situ. Although ingestion of honey has been identified as a risk factor for the development of infant botulism, less than 20% of cases nationally are thought to be related to the ingestion of honey. The highest rates of botulism are noted in California and in the region surrounding Philadelphia, Pennsylvania, likely due to the prevalence of C. botulinum in the soil of those regions.

Foodborne botulism is the next most common form of botulism. It results from the ingestion of food contaminated with preformed botulinum toxin. Although the total number of cases varies annually, approximately 20 to 25 cases are reported per year. As the toxin requires very specific conditions, including an anaerobic environment, pH greater than 4.5, low salt and sugar content, and a temperature between 4 and 121°C, the vast majority of foodborne botulism cases in the United States are related to the consumption of home-canned foods. These cases are typically sporadic, although occasional small outbreaks of two to four individuals and very rare outbreaks of larger magnitude have been noted.

Wound botulism is rare, although an increasing number of cases have been reported in the United States over the last two decades. Wound botulism is due to the colonization of a wound with C. botulinum spores with subsequent germination and in situ production of the toxin within the wound. This form of botulism occurs almost exclusively among injection drug users and, for unknown reasons, has been particularly common among users of a specific preparation of heroin dubbed "black tar heroin."

Adult intestinal botulism is also rare. Like infant botulism, it results from colonization of the gastrointestinal tract with C. botulinum with subsequent toxin production. As most adults have gastrointestinal flora that seem to outcompete Clostridium without difficulty, the few known cases of adult intestinal botulism have occurred in patients with anatomical or functional bowel abnormalities, often in association with antimicrobial exposure that provided an environmental niche for C. botulinum.

The two artificially occurring forms of botulism: inhalational and iatrogenic. Each is associated with only a handful of known cases. Inhaled botulism, which results from the inhalation of aerosolized botulinum toxin, has been described only once in 1962 when three German lab workers accidentally inhaled botulinum toxin while disposing of animal carcasses that had been coated with the toxin for research purposes. Iatrogenic botulism, resulting from the injection of botulinum toxin for medicinal or cosmetic purposes, has occurred in only a few cases, most notably among four individuals in Florida in 2004 who received injected botulism for cosmetic purposes from an unlicensed provider.

Although botulinum toxin can be absorbed through mucosal surfaces, the eyes, and non-intact skin, no case of person-to-person transmission has ever been reported.

Presenting Features

In all six forms of botulism, the presenting symptoms include acute-onset, symmetric cranial nerve palsies with the subsequent development of a symmetric, descending, flaccid paralysis of the voluntary muscles. Due to cranial nerve palsies, affected individuals often first present with blurry vision, diplopia, ptosis, expressionless facies, a weakened and slurred voice, and an inability to suck or swallow. These bulbar palsies are often remembered as "the 4 D's," which are diplopia, dysarthria, dysphonia, and dysphagia. Due to the cranial nerve palsies, affected individuals may appear lethargic or confused. However, the toxin does not penetrate the brain parenchyma, so no true cognitive or sensory deficits are noted. Also, affected individuals remain afebrile unless they have an additional infection.

Of note, individuals affected by food-borne botulism may experience nausea, vomiting, abdominal pain, and diarrhea. These symptoms are not thought to be due to botulinum toxin but instead due to other contaminants in the spoiled food.

Diagnostic Considerations

The differential diagnosis of botulism includes Guillain-Barré syndrome (GBS), myasthenia gravis (MG), Lambert-Eaton syndrome, stroke syndromes, intoxication, and tick paralysis. Distinguishing botulism from these other diagnoses requires a careful history as well as a variety of diagnostic tests. Of note, routine laboratory values as well as cerebrospinal fluid studies and brain imaging are unremarkable in botulism. In contrast to botulism, the paralysis in GBS is typically ascending in nature (though variants like the Miller-Fischer syndrome can present with isolated eye muscle weakness and ataxia), and lumbar puncture will typically reveal elevated protein with a normal cell count (ie, cytoalbuminologic dissociation). In GBS, there may be a preceding history of a diarrheal or respiratory illness.

Those affected by MG tend to show muscle fatigability with repeated contraction, such as sustaining an upward gaze, so that muscles become weaker with sustained use but improve with rest. This is in contrast to botulism, which affects muscles more homogenously during times of both light and strenuous activity (and possibly precluding movement altogether). Muscles that tend to be affected by MG include ocular, facial, bulbar, and even respiratory muscles in addition to voluntary muscles throughout the body. A Tensilon test (administer edrophonium to increase muscle strength) should be strongly positive and autoantibodies may be present.

Lambert-Eaton syndrome can present similarly to MG with dysphagia, dysarthria, and trouble chewing. Unlike MG and botulism, the weakness in Lambert-Eaton syndrome favors the limbs and usually spares the eyes (ie, no diplopia or ptosis). Unlike MG, the weakness in Lambert-Eaton syndrome tends to improve with repeated activity. As with botulism, Lambert Eaton syndrome can present with autonomic dysregulation, including dry mouth, constipation, anhidrosis, blurred vision, and orthostatic hypotension. Lambert-Eaton syndrome often occurs in individuals with malignancy, especially small-cell carcinoma of the lung, and is considered a paraneoplastic syndrome.

In contrast to botulism, stroke syndromes usually result in asymmetric findings and abnormal neurologic imaging. Intoxication is often deduced by history or laboratory findings. Tick paralysis may be distinguished from botulism by the presence of an attached tick followed resolution of symptoms after tick removal. If an experienced electromyography (EMG) operator is available, EMG may be particularly helpful in distinguishing between botulism, GBS, and MG.

Typical Disease Course

Depending on the amount of botulinum toxin absorbed into the system, the extent of paralysis and the speed of progression varies significantly among affected individuals. Affected individuals may have paralysis of only a few cranial nerves or may have complete paralysis with subsequent respiratory arrest and death. Similarly, symptoms may progress over hours or days. Mildly affected individuals may develop only the bulbar palsies described previously. However, others will develop flaccid, descending, symmetric paralysis of the voluntary muscles with progressive involvement of the neck, shoulders, upper extremities, diaphragm, and lower extremities. Respiratory compromise can result from either an inability to protect the airway (secondary to pharyngeal muscle paralysis) or from paralysis of the diaphragm and accessory muscles of respiration. Of note, due to their paralysis, patients typically do not appear dyspneic or distressed even as respiratory arrest becomes imminent.

As noted previously, patients with botulism may also present with autonomic symptoms, including dry mouth, anhidrosis, orthostatic hypotension, blurred vision, and constipation. Progressively disappearing deep tendon reflexes can also be seen. Vital signs typically remain normal despite this autonomic dysregulation; vital sign perturbations should instead prompt consideration of possible orthostatic vital sign changes or vital sign changes due to respiratory impairment. Although hypotension is possible, most patients remain normotensive, likely due to the opposing effects of the vagal blockade and peripheral vasodilatation. Sensory or cognitive involvement is not typical of botulism. As recovery is dependent on the regeneration of new motor axons to reinnervate muscle fibers, full recovery can take weeks to months.

Complications

Complications due to botulism involve respiratory compromise from pharyngeal muscle paralysis or inadequate tidal volumes from paralysis of the diaphragm and accessory muscles of respiration. When mechanical ventilation is not available, respiratory arrest is the most common reason for death. Due to pharyngeal muscle paralysis, affected patients are also at high risk for aspiration and secondary infections.

Diagnostic Tests

Diagnostic testing for botulism is extremely limited within the United States. Testing is only available at the Centers for Disease Control and Prevention (CDC) and through a limited number of public health departments. Testing may be completed on samples obtained from the serum, gastric aspirates, stool, and, in the case of wound botulism, from wound debridement. As the presence of antitoxin nullifies the results, all samples must be obtained prior to the administration of botulinum antitoxin. Notably, due to the significant constipation associated with botulism, a sterile water enema is often required to obtain a stool sample.

The testing itself is resource intensive, requiring a mouse bioassay that tests for the presence of the toxin and delineates the subtype of toxin present. Once the laboratory receives specimens, results of the mouse bioassay typically take 24 to 48 hours. Alternatively, *C. botulinum* may be cultured anaerobically from stools and gastric specimens. However, these cultures usually take 7 to 10 days to result, and confirmation of toxin production requires the mouse bioassay.

Organisms

Microbiology

Botulinum toxin is produced by *C. botulinum*, a group of distinct organisms that are classified together due to their production of the botulinum toxin. All of these organisms are anaerobic, spore-forming, gram-positive bacilli that are found ubiquitously in soil. There are seven distinct types of botulinum neurotoxin produced by *C. botulinum*, named A, B, C, D, E, F, and G. Human cases are caused by toxins A, B, E, and, in very rare circumstances, F. Each of these subtypes contains a zinc proteinase that prevents vesicles containing acetylcholine from fusing with the terminal membrane of presynaptic motor neurons, thereby irreversibly preventing release of acetylcholine into the neuromuscular junction. This results in neuromuscular blockade and paralysis. Botulinum toxins are also among the most potent known with lethal doses for type A estimated at 0.09 to 0.15 μg intravenous or intramuscular, 0.7 to 0.9 μg inhalationally, and 70 μg oral administration.

Life Cycle

Under stress, *C. botulinum* forms spores that are hardy and able to survive standard cooking and food processing measures. These spores are routinely ingested and excreted by humans. In most cases, no germination or toxin production occurs during this process. However, under the right circumstances, including an anaerobic milieu, pH > 4.5, and low salt and sugar content, germination can occur, followed by toxin production. These conditions most commonly occur during home canning, leading to the close association of food-borne botulism with home-canned foods. Similar germination and toxin production can occur in the intestinal tracts of infants (where a full host of normal gastrointestinal flora has not yet developed), in adults with significantly altered gastrointestinal flora, and in the anaerobic milieu of some abscesses—which leads to infant botulism, adult intestinal botulism, and wound botulism, respectively.

Treatment

The treatment for botulism is botulinum antitoxin. There is an equine-derived formulation used in adults and a human-source formulation used in infants. The former is available from the CDC via state and local health departments, and the latter is available only from the California Department of Health. As the antitoxin halts the progression of paralysis but does not reverse existing paralysis, it should be given as soon as possible after a clinical diagnosis of botulism is made, preferably within 24 hours of symptom onset. As diagnostic testing typically requires at least 24 to 48 hours to result, the antitoxin should be given prior to laboratory confirmation of the diagnosis. The major side effect noted is hypersensitivity reaction. Accordingly, it is recommended that patients be given a small challenge dose of antitoxin prior to receiving a full dose and that epinephrine and diphenhydramine be on hand during the administration of both doses.

Even more important than the antitoxin in improving the outcomes of affected individuals is early diagnosis and excellent supportive care, typically in an intensive-care setting. Affected patients should be monitored closely for signs of impending respiratory failure, including loss of cough and gag reflexes as well as decreasing vital capacity and inspiratory force. Early, controlled intubation and initiation of mechanical ventilation is recommended if these signs are noted. In addition, affected individuals typically require fluid and nutritional support as well as measures to prevent and treat secondary infections. Because full recovery can take weeks to months, affected individuals often require extensive rehabilitation after discharge.

With early detection and intense supportive care, the mortality rate of botulism has declined from approximately 60% to 70% in the early twentieth century to a current rate of 3% to 5%. Of note, although botulinum antitoxin appears to effectively decrease the length of hospital stay, its use has not had a significant impact on mortality rate.

Other Key Issues

Whereas botulism is the first biologic toxin licensed as a drug for treatment of human diseases, botulism has also received a great deal of attention as a possible biological weapon and a tool of bioterrorism. This is due to its high potency and its lethality in the absence of supportive care in addition to the prolonged need for intensive care among affected individuals. It has been estimated by multiple sources that approximately one gram of evenly aerosolized botulinum toxin could kill over one million people. Accordingly, it is categorized as a category A biological agent. Every case of botulism should be considered a public health emergency and should be reported emergently to the state health department. In addition, clinicians should be aware that the CDC and the state health departments of California and Alaska maintain 24-hour clinical consult services that can be reached via phone at all times.

Suggested Readings and References

1. Arnon SS, Schechter R, Inglesby TV, et al. Botulinum toxin as a biological weapon: medical and public health management. *JAMA*. 2001;285(8):1059–1070.
2. Centers for Disease Control and Prevention: Botulism in the United States, 1899–1996. Handbook for Epidemiologists, Clinicians, and Laboratory Workers. Atlanta, GA: Centers for Disease Control and Prevention; 1998.
3. Dhaked RK, Singh MK, Singh P, Gupta P. Botulinum toxin: bioweapon and magic drug. *Indian J Med Res*. 2010;132:489–503.
4. Shukla HD, Sharma SK. Clostridium botulinum: a bug with beauty and weapon. *Crit Rev Microbiol*. 2005;31:11–18.
5. Sobel J. Botulism. *Clin Infect Dis*. 2005;41:1167–1173.

Chapter 65

Plague

Trisha Anest, and David Scordino

Summary Box

Disease Description: Zoonosis with three clinical forms: Bubonic Plague, Septicemia Plague, and Pneumonic Plague

Organisms: *Yersinia pestis* is a facultative anaerobe and a gram negative coccobacillus.

Treatment:
  First line: Streptomycin or gentamicin
  Second line: Doxycycline, ciprofloxacin, or chloramphenicol
  Parenteral therapy is recommended initially with transition to oral therapy after clinical improvement.

Other Key Issues: Used as biological weapon

Disease Description

Few diseases have impacted human history and culture like the plague. It has been credited with the fall of great empires, inspired literature and art, and shaped the way we view disease. It is because of this complex and tragic history that plague continues to inspire terror in the form of biological weaponry and has helped shape modern sanitation, antibiotics, and public health efforts.[2,5]

Epidemiology

Plague persists today, although with few cases and infrequent outbreaks around the globe. The United States has a large zoonotic reservoir; but on average, only seven human cases are reported each year. This small number is due to the rural, largely uninhabited area where these reservoirs are found.[1,3] The majority of these cases are the bubonic form.[1]

Presenting Features

Plague has three distinct clinical forms. Bubonic plague is the most common form and may resemble many viral syndromes with vague complaints of fevers, chills, headaches, and weakness. The distinct feature of bubonic plague is buboes, which are painfully swollen lymph nodes that are tender to palpation. Buboes are formed by bacteria multiplying within lymph nodes near the entry point of the bacterium into the bloodstream.[1,3]

Septicemic plague represents a systemic form of the illness. In addition to the vague symptoms of bubonic plague, patients often develop abdominal pain and shock in addition to bleeding into skin and internal organs. Tissue manifestations may be dramatic, with fingers, toes, or other areas turning black and necrotic. Septicemic plague may be a primary form of plague or develop from untreated bubonic plague.[1,3]

Unlike the bubonic and septicemic forms of plague, which are transmitted by flea bites or the handling of infected animals, pneumonic plague is easily transmitted from human to human by the inhalation of infectious droplets. Pneumonic plague can also develop when bubonic or septicemic plague is untreated and spreads to the lungs. In addition to vague symptoms of fevers and chills, headache, and weakness, this form presents with respiratory symptoms of a productive cough, chest pain, and shortness of breath. The resulting pneumonia is often lethal, resulting in respiratory failure and shock.[1,3]

Diagnostic Considerations

Plague can present in a similar manner to many less serious infections, such as viral syndromes; therefore, a high clinical suspicion is required to make the diagnosis. Large numbers of previously healthy individuals suddenly presenting with symptoms of severe pneumonia and sepsis should prompt suspicion for a biologic agent. Due to the limited number of cases, rapid diagnostic tests are not widely available. Initial studies should include blood and sputum cultures as well as lymph node aspirates from buboes. Appropriate health departments should be notified immediately for suspicious cases and any patients with symptoms of pneumonic plague should be placed under droplet isolation precautions.[1,2]

Typical Disease Course

Buboes appear after an incubation period of 2 to 6 days. These are often painful, limiting range of motion, and are usually found in the groin, axilla, or cervical lymph nodes. If untreated, bacteria quickly invade the blood stream, leading to septicemic plague and possibly pneumonic plague if the lungs become infected. Without appropriate antibiotic therapy, symptoms rapidly progress to death within 2 to 6 days.[1,5]

Complications

Overall mortality from plague in the United States has decreased in the in post-antibiotic era from 66% (1900–1941) to 16% (1942–2010), with further decrease in recent years to 11% (1990–2010). Current mortality estimates for each form of plague are 13% for bubonic, 28% for septicemic, and 36% for pneumonic, reflecting the need for early treatment to prevent progression to the more lethal forms of the disease.[1]

Diagnostic Tests

Blood cultures should be sent for analysis. Organisms may not be seen in blood smears until septicemia develops but may still be positive by culture. Any buboes should be aspirated and sent for microscopic evaluation and culture. Sputum cultures should be sent on any patients with respiratory symptoms, including bronchial/tracheal washings if possible.[1]

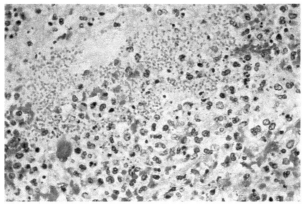

Figure 65.1 Photomicrograph of Giemsa stained lung tissue from a patient with fatal human plague, revealing pneumonia, and an abundance of Y. pestis organisms. Reprinted with permission from the Centers for Disease Control.

Yersinia Pestis may be observed on microscopic examination as ovoid, gram-negative organisms. Wright or Wayson stains are utilized to highlight the bipolar staining pattern, described as a "safety pin" appearance.[3,4] (See Figure 65.1.) If plague is suspected despite negative culture results, serological testing such as enzyme-linked immunosorbent assay should be performed early in the illness followed by a convalescent sample at 4 to 6 weeks after disease onset.[1] It is important to protect staff from exposure to plague from these microbiologic samples by properly labeling samples as high risk and handling samples in a biosafety cabinet.[3]

Organism

Microbiology
Yersinia pestis is a facultative anaerobe and a gram negative coccobacillus.[5]

Primary and Secondary Organisms
Plague is transmitted by fleas. It cycles in communities of small rodents, such as squirrels, prairie dogs, chipmunks, mice, moles, and rabbits.

Life Cycle
When fleas bite a host, they deposit the bacterium in the blood. The bacterium invades lymphatic tissues; as tissues and organs are destroyed, more bacteria spill into the blood stream, leading to septicemia. When the host dies from the infection, the fleas leave in search of a new host and, thus, continue to transmit the disease. Any animal or human that visits areas where host animals have died is at risk of being infected by a flea bite and developing bubonic or septicemic plague. Most cases in the United States occur in the rural or semirural areas of the Western United States, but this cycle can cause large outbreaks in urban settings when rats become infected hosts. The last urban outbreak in the United States occurred in Los Angeles from 1924 to 1925.[1,5] See Figure 65.2.

The most concerning form of transmission is through respiratory droplets. Pneumonic plague can be transmitted by direct and close contact with an infected host, resulting in human to human transmission or animal to human transmission. This form of exposure results in the most deadly form of plague, pneumonic plague.[1,3]

Treatment
Treatment should be started as soon as plague is suspected. Centers for Disease Control and Prevention guidelines recommend initial intramuscular or intravenous antibiotic administration with transition to an oral regimen only after clinical improvement. The recommended course is 10 days or 2 days after fever has subsided.[1]

Other Key Issues to Consider

Bioterrorism
Plague as a biological weapon is not a modern concept. During the siege of Caffa in 1345, plague-infected corpses were catapulted over the city walls in an attempt to infect the inhabitants. Modern technology has led to concerns that an aerosolized form of the plague could be utilized in a bioterrorist

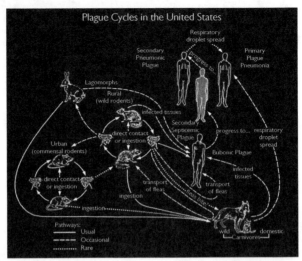

Plague Cycles in the United States

Figure 65.2 This diagram depicts the modalities of transfer between various hosts of Yersinia pestis bacteria, which are the cause of bubonic plague in the United States. Plague may involve a wide variety of mammal species, including rodents, rabbits, wild and domestic carnivores, and humans. Many hosts, such as humans, carnivores, and perhaps rabbits, are considered to be dead-end hosts because the disease almost never passes from infected individuals to other members of the same population. Other mammalian species act as amplification hosts for Y. pestis, and once one animal within a population is infected, the likelihood is high that other animals within that population will also become infected. In some instances, Y. pestis apparently circulates within populations of certain rodent species causing very little overt disease or mortality. Among other species, such as prairie dogs and rock squirrels, widespread mortality occurs among infected animals. Reprinted with permission from Centers for Disease Control.

attack, leading to widespread pneumonic plague. Symptom onset would be expected 2 to 4 days after exposure. Symptoms resemble a rapidly progressive, severe pneumonia with cough, fever, and dyspnea progressing to death within 2 to 6 days without antibiotic therapy. In the last 50 years, 4 out of 7 cases of pneumonic plague in the United States have resulted in death. Although large studies are lacking, mortality appears to be reduced when antibiotic therapy is started within 24 hours of symptom onset. Therefore, once there is suspicion for an outbreak of pneumonic plague, anyone with fever or cough in the area of exposure should be immediately treated with antibiotics as outlined in Table 65.1.[2]

There was a vaccine (no longer manufactured), which was effective against the bubonic form of the plague but did not offer protection against pneumonic plague. Research is ongoing for a vaccine that would be effective against pneumonic plague, as this is the form most likely to be utilized as a biological

Table 65.1 Treatment Guidelines[a]

	Adults	Children	Pregnant Women
Preferred Therapy	• Streptomycin 1g IM BID • Gentamicin 5 mg/kg IM or IV daily • Gentamicin 2 mg/kg loading dose IM or IV, followed by 1.7 mg/kg IM or IV TID	• Streptomycin 15 mg/kg IM BID (max 2 g daily) • Gentamicin 2.5 mg/kg IM or IV TID	• Gentamicin 5 mg/kg IM or IV daily • Gentamicin 2 mg/kg loading dose IM or IV, followed by 1.7 mg/kg IM or IV TID
Alternative Therapy	• Doxycycline 200 mg IV daily • Doxycycline 100 mg IV BID • Ciprofloxacin 400mg IV BID • Chloramphenicol 25 mg/kg IV QID	• > 45 kg: use adult dosing of Doxycycline • < 45 kg: Doxycycline 2.2 mg/kg IV BID (max 200 mg daily) • Ciprofloxacin 15 mg/kg BID (max 1 g daily) • Chloramphenicol 25 mg/kg QID (max 4 g daily)	• Doxycycline 200 mg IV daily • Doxycycline 100 mg IV BID • Ciprofloxacin 400 mg IV BID

Abbreviations: IM, intramuscular; BID, twice a day; IV, intravenous; TID, three times a day; QID, four times a day.
[a]Adapted from Inglesby TV, Dennis DT, Henderson DA, et al. Plague as a biological weapon. *JAMA*. 2000;283(17):2281–2290.

Table 65.2 Prophylaxis Guidelines		
	Adults (Including Pregnant Women)	Children
Preferred Regimens	• Doxycycline 100 mg PO BID • Ciprofloxacin 500 mg PO BID	• > 45 kg: use adult dosing of Doxycycline • < 45 kg: Doxycycline 2.2 mg/kg PO BID
Alternative Regimens	• Chloramphenicol 25 mg/kg PO QID	• Chloramphenicol 25 mg/kg PO QID

Abbreviations: PO, oral administration; BID, twice a day; QID, four times a day.
aAdapted from Inglesby TV, Dennis DT, Henderson DA, et al. Plague as a biological weapon. *JAMA*. 2000;283(17):2281–2290.

weapon. Until a vaccine is developed, the current post-exposure prophylaxis recommendations apply to anyone who has had contact with a patient with untreated pneumonic plague (Table 65.2). All drug regimens are recommended for a 7 day course.[2,3]

Suggested Readings and References

1. Plague. Resources for Clinicians. Diagnosis. Centers for Disease Control and Prevention website. http://www.cdc.gov/plague/healthcare/clinicians.html. Accessed
2. Inglesby TV, Dennis DT, Henderson DA, et al. Plague as a biological weapon. *JAMA*. 2000;283(17):2281–2290.
3. Prentice MB, Rahalison L. Plague. Lance. 2007;369:1196–1207.
4. Oyston P, Williamson ED. Modern advance against plague. *Advances in Applied Microbiology*. Amsterdam, Netherlands: Elsevier; 2012:209–241.
5. Abbott RC, Rocke TE. *Plague*. Reston, Virginia: US Geological Survey; 2012.

Chapter 66

Viral Hemorrhagic Fevers (Ebola, Lassa, Hantavirus)

Marcos Schechter

For dengue fever please see chapter 52.

Disease Description: Viral hemorrhagic fever (VHF) results from a variety of viral diseases unified by the following features: fever, capillary leak, and coagulation defects. Thrombocytopenia is a common laboratory finding. Clinical differentiation of the VHF is difficult. Although most of these diseases do not occur naturally in the United States, some of these viruses are considered viable agents for bioterrorism. See Box 66.1 for Ebola virus disease summary based on Centers for Disease Control and Prevention (CDC) data.

Organisms: The enveloped, single-stranded RNA viruses that cause VHF belong to four different virus families: Arenaviridae (eg, Lassa fever virus), Bunyaviridae (eg, Rift Valley fever), Filoviridae (Marburg and Ebola viruses), and Flaviviridae (eg, yellow fever virus).

Treatment: No standard treatment has been approved for these diseases, but some experts advocate for starting ribavirin when a VHF is suspected. This agent may be effective against both arenaviridae and bunyaviridae but not against filoviridae and flaviviridae. Ribavirin should be given intravenously when possible, but this formulation is of limited availability. An oral formulation is more commonly available. Of note, ribavirin is classified as pregnancy category X drug. Post-exposure prophylaxis (PEP) is indicated in some cases. Whereas the care is mostly supportive, investigational therapies are available for some conditions. Appropriate isolation measures and immediate reporting to the public health department are imperative.

Other Key Issues: The Special Pathogens Branch of the CDC in Atlanta, GA (404–639–1115), and/or the USAMRIID in Fort Detrick in Frederick, MD (301–619–2833), should be contacted for expert advice on diagnosis and management of most of these conditions.

There are five Ebola virus species within the genus *Ebolavirus*, including four that cause Ebola virus disease (EVD) in humans. Human outbreaks are thought to occur as a result of direct contact with an infected animal or its body fluids. Human to human transmission occurs via direct contact with blood, body fluids, or the skin of EVD patients, including from persons who have died of EVD. According to the CDC, the incubation period for Ebola is thought to be 2 to 21 days, with an average of 8 to 10 days. Symptoms include fever, severe headache, muscle pain, weakness, fatigue, diarrhea, vomiting, abdominal (stomach) pain, and unexplained hemorrhage (bleeding or bruising). The CDC defines a person under investigation as someone with fever or subjective fevers or symptoms as described previously AND an epidemiologic risk factor within the 21 days before thee onset of symptoms. Ebola virus can only be detected in the blood after symptom onset and can take up to 3 days to develop detectable levels. ELISA, PCR, and virus isolation are often used to confirm diagnosis. Treatment consists of intravenous fluid therapy to maintain adequate blood pressure with careful attention on electrolytes and supplemental oxygenation. Experimental vaccines are under development. It is unclear if patients who recover from Ebola and have antibodies can become infected with other strains of Ebola.

Disease Description

The Viral Hemorrhagic Fevers (VHF) is a large group of diseases. This chapter focuses on conditions that have occurred in the United States due to domestic transmission or due to returning travelers; the viruses considered are category A biological agents (Box 66.2).[1] For a broader review of these diseases, please refer to the consensus statement from Working Group in Civilian Biodefense published in the *Journal of the American Medical Association*.[2]

These viruses cause an acute onset illness except in the case of Arenaviridae, which tends to have a more gradual onset. These viruses can affect any organ system, and clinical manifestations are varied and nonspecific. Fever, headache, and myalgia are almost universal. Most diseases are associated with a rash or flushing. Conjunctivitis, pharyngitis, and pulse-temperature dissociation are commonly described, but the presence or absence of these findings should not be used to narrow the differential diagnosis. Clinical features typical of specific diseases are described following if they have been reported in the literature.

Capillary leak syndrome (leading to anasarca) and disseminated intravascular coagulation (with or without overt bleeding) are common manifestations of severe disease. Central nervous system manifestations usually predict poor outcomes. Leukopenia with a left shift is a common laboratory finding, together with thrombocytopenia and hemoconcentration. Elevated liver enzymes are common, and jaundice can be seen with almost all these infections but is typical for yellow fever and for Rift Valley fever. Renal injury due to circulatory shock and proteinuria are also common.

The incubation period for these pathogens ranges from 2 to 21 days. Mortality rates can be as high as 90% (for Marburg virus infection), whereas mortality rates for Dengue can be as low as 0.10% when the disease is appropriately managed. Higher mortality has been described in pregnant women and neonatal populations. Fetal mortality is also thought to be high.

Organisms

Arenaviridae (focus on Lassa fever)

Not all viruses in the Arenaviridae family cause VHF. The Lassa fever virus does produce a VHF and is probably the most important virus in this family given its large number of cases in West Africa and the fact that that one case of imported Lassa fever occurred in the United States in 2004.[3] There are different strains of Lassa virus, and the genetic distance correlates with the geographical distance of the regions where each strain is found. *Mastomys natalensis*, a rodent, is the reservoir of the Lassa fever virus.

These are RNA viruses that are zoonotic and have rodents as hosts. Transmission occurs by contact with rodent excretions either through ingestion or contact with mucosa or non-intact skin. Aerosolized rodent urine and saliva are also infectious. Person-to-person spread has been documented in Lassa virus infection, both by direct contact with bodily fluids and by airborne transmission. It is important to know that the Lassa fever virus can be isolated in the blood, stool, urine, vomitus, semen, and saliva of infected patients; viral shedding can persist for 30 days or more. Nosocomial outbreaks of Lassa fever have occurred in West Africa.

Box 66.2 Bioterrorism Agents Classification

Category A

Agents that

- can be easily disseminated or transmitted from person to person;
- result in high mortality rates and have the potential for major public health impact;
- might cause public panic and social disruption; and
- require special action for public health preparedness

Category B

Agents that

- are moderately easy to disseminate;
- result in moderate morbidity rates and low mortality rates; and
- require specific enhancements of CDC's diagnostic capacity and enhanced disease surveillance.

Category C

These agents are emerging pathogens that could be engineered for mass dissemination in the future because of

- availability;
- ease of production and dissemination; and
- potential for high morbidity and mortality rates and major health impact

http://www.bt.cdc.gov/agent/agentlist-category.asp#catdef

Lassa fever is endemic in West Africa, and it is estimated that 100,000 to 300,000 people are infected yearly in this region. The mortality is higher during epidemics and can reach 50%. The incubation period is of 5 to 16 days. Symptom onset tends to be more gradual when compared to other VHF. Cervical lymphadenopathy and exudative pharyngitis are typical but not universal. Capillary leak syndrome ensues in the later stages of disease, which can lead to anasarca due to third spacing. Hemorrhagic manifestations can occur but are less common when compared to other VHF. The convalescence period can be associated with pericarditis and an array of neurological manifestations. Temporary or permanent deafness is not uncommon.[4]

Diagnostic tests

Indirect fluorescent-antibody (IFA) assay had been the traditional method of detection in endemic countries. This test has been replaced by an enzyme-linked immunosorbent assay (ELISA) that detects a viral antigen and an immunoglobulin M antibody due to the low specificity of the IFA assay. Polymerase chain reaction (PCR) is the gold standard, but it is not widely available in endemic areas, and strain variation makes the use of this method technically challenging.

Treatment

Ribavirin was effective for the treatment of Lassa fever in small trials. It is also used for PEP.[5]

Bunyaviridae (brief review)

The bunyaviridae include the *Hantaviruses* and the Rift Valley fever virus. Hemorrhagic fever with renal syndrome is almost exclusively seen in Europe and Asia. The Seoul strain can be found in the United States, but there are very few reports of clinical disease. A small outbreak involving three patients occurred in the city of Balitmore.[6] *Hantavirus* pulmonary syndrome occurs in the Americas. This disease is not classified as a VHF.

The Rift Valley fever virus occurs in sub-Saharan Africa and in West Africa. Transmission occurs via mosquito bites and by close contact with infected mammals. Bodily fluids are also infectious. Transmission through aerosolized particles is possible, making this virus a potential agent for bioterrorism. The incidence of Rift Valley fever peaks in the rainy season. This disease can cause manifestations typical of other VHF viruses and can also have ocular manifestations. Vision loss secondary to retinitis occurs in 1% to 10% of affected patients. Ribavirin is efficient in animal models. It is worth noting that several genera of mosquitoes in the United States have the capacity to act as vectors for the Rift Valley fever virus.

Filoviridae (Ebola and Marburg)

Disease Description

The Marburg and the Ebola virus are the two known Filoviridae. Both are category A biological agents. Although these are rare diseases, the frequency of outbreaks has been increasing over the past two decades. The 2014 West Africa Ebola epidemic, the largest in history and the first Ebola epidemic, has at the time of this publication nearly 26,000 cases with over 10,000 deaths. Multiple countries were involved, including Sierra Leone, Liberia, and Guinea. The Democratic Republic of Congo had a separate outbreak in 2014 that was contained.

The number of non-human primates affected by Filoviridae has also been increasing. The increased incidence of disease in non-human primates is linked to a number of outbreaks because the ingestion of infected non-human primates is one of main modes of transmission. Experimental data suggests these viruses can initiate infection by ingestion, inhalation, or inoculation through skin breaks. Person-to-person transmission is thought to occur via contact with infected bodily fluids, including blood, vomitus, urine, feces, and probably sweat. Although aerosolized filoviridae are infectious in experimental models, person-to-person transmission through respiratory routes seems to be very uncommon during outbreaks.

Exposure to bats is thought to be the mechanism of initiation of at least two outbreaks of Marburg virus and of one case that occurred in a traveler returning to the United States from Uganda to Colorado in 2008.[7] Nosocomial transmission also occurs both by exposure to bodily secretions and by use of infected material (eg, unsterilized syringes). The virus is able to persist in the testes, an immune privileged site, and one case of sexual transmission was described during the 1967 Marburg outbreak.

Conjunctival injection and dark discoloration of the soft palate are common physical findings. Although not pathognomic nor universal, a non-pruritic maculopapular rash limited to the upper extremities occurring during the 1st week of disease is a distinctive feature. Overt bleeding is only common in dying patients when gastrointestinal and genitourinary hemorrhage can occur. It is important to note that bleeding can be absent, even in fatal cases. Thus, lack of a hemorrhagic manifestation does not exclude an infection by a filovirus. The most common hemorrhagic manifestations are conjunctival hemorrhage, easy bruising, and impaired clot formation at venipuncture sites.

Jaundice and hepatomegaly due to hepatic necrosis are also seen. Abdominal pain is a common symptom and can be secondary to both hepatic necrosis and pancreatitis. Patients either die of septic shock and multiple organ failure or improve 10 to 12 days after disease onset. Mortality varies from 20% to 90%. Recrudescence of fever should raise suspicion for a bacterial superinfection or, less likely, localized viral persistence. The convalescent period is marked by extreme weakness. Sloughing of the skin and hair loss are commonly seen. There is no data on imaging. Studies in non-human primates infected by aerosolized virus suggest that chest x-ray infiltrates are unlikely to occur. Given the lack of information, abnormalities on chest imaging should broaden the differential diagnosis but should not be used to exclude an infection by a Filovirus. For a literature review of the clinical and laboratorial features of filoviral infections, please refer to Kortepeter et al.[8]

Diagnostic tests

Most patients that are acutely ill have high concentrations of virus in the blood as measured by PCR assay. Antigen detection by ELISA is another rapid diagnostic method. These tests are thought to be 100% sensitive in patients who are sick. The performance of these tests in asymptomatic patients incubating the virus is not known.

Organism

It is thought that all Marburg viruses belong to a single species, whereas there are five species of Ebola viruses, namely, Zaire, Sudan, Ivory Coast, Bundibugyo, and Reston. The Reston virus occurs in the Philippines and seems to cause asymptomatic infection in humans.

The reservoir for both Filoviridae is unknown. Infection in non-human primates is often fatal, which is not compatible with being a reservoir for a microorganism. Exposure to bats has been linked to development of disease caused by Filoviridae, and Marburg virus was recovered from fruit bats in Uganda. This data is suggestive, but not conclusive, for the role of bats on being the reservoir for Filoviridae.

Treatment

Care is supportive. No antiviral drug, including ribavirin, has activity against these viruses. Therapy with biologic agents has never been shown to be efficient. Trials are lacking, and there are no US Food and Drug Administration approved agents for PEP. An experimental vaccine using vesicular stomatitis virus expressing glycoproteins from either Marburg or Ebola virus is efficient in animal models.

Flaviviridae (brief review)

The yellow fever virus is considered as category C biological agent by the CDC, and the last outbreak in the United States occurred in 1905. This disease occurs in South America and sub-Saharan Africa. It is transmitted by mosquitoes of the genera *Aedes*, which are present in the United States. Only nine cases of yellow fever in unimmunized travelers have been reported in the United States and in Europe between the years of 1970 and 2002. Travelers returning from endemic regions should be questioned about vaccination status in the case of suspected yellow fever. The vaccine is protective in 90% of the patients within 10 days of receiving vaccination, and this rate increases to around 100% within 3 to 4 weeks after vaccination. Therefore, vaccination prior to travel to endemic areas is considered effective prevention.

Reemergence of yellow fever in the United States, as seen with dengue fever, may be due to the increased population of *Aedes aegypti* in the country. Yellow fever is a biphasic disease. The so called "period of infection," which is the first clinical phase of this disease, usually lasts 3 to 4 days. Symptoms are not specific. The period of infection is followed by a "period of remission," when fever and other symptoms remit. Approximately 15% of the patients enter the last phase of disease known as the "period of intoxication." Systemic inflammatory response syndrome ensues, and patients can develop multiorgan failure. Hepatic involvement is common, with aspartate transaminase usually higher than alanine transaminase and jaundice (hence the name yellow fever). Hepatic necrosis leads to a bleeding diathesis with hemorrhage from multiple sites. Mortality rate for patients that progress to the period of intoxication is 20% to 50%.

Suggested Readings and References

1. http://emergency.cdc.gov/agent/agentlist-category.asp Accessed October 30, 2012.
2. Borio L, et al. Hemorrhagic fever viruses as biological weapons: medical and public health management *JAMA*. 2002;287(18):2391–2405.
3. CDC. Imported Lassa fever—New Jersey, 2004. *MMWR Morb Mortal Wkly Rep*. 2004;53(38):894.
4. Ogbu O, et al. Lassa fever in West African sub-region: an overview. *J Vector Borne Dis*. 2007;44:1–11.
5. Bausch DG, et al. Review of the literature and proposed guidelines for the use of oral ribavirin as postexposure prophylaxis for Lassa fever. *Clin Infect Dis*. 2010; 51(12):1435–1441. Epub November 8, 2010.
6. Glass GE, et al. Domestic cases of hemorrhagic fever with renal syndrome in the United States. *Nephron*. 1994;68(1):48.
7. CDC. Imported case of Marburg hemorrhagic fever—Colorado, 2008. *MMWR Morb Mortal Wkly Rep*. 2009;58(49):1377.
8. Kortepeter MG, et al. Basic clinical and laboratory features of filoviral hemorrhagic fever. *J Infect Dis*. 2011;204(Supp 3):S810–816.

Tularemia

Alida Gertz

Summary Box

Disease Description: Tularemia, caused by the gram-negative coccobacillus *Francisella tularensis*, is an extremely infectious bacterial zoonosis (requiring as few as 10 organisms to cause infection). Although naturally occurring in North America and Eurasia, tularemia was also extensively developed as a biological weapon during the 1900s. Symptoms depend on site of exposure; presenting symptoms can be nonspecific and may include fever, lymphadenopathy, ulcer or papule, and nausea/vomiting. Pneumonia, pneumonitis, chest pain, bloody sputum, and respiratory distress can also occur with inhalation. Natural transmission generally occurs via small mammals, such as rabbits or arthropod bites. If used as a biological weapon, aerosolized *tularensis* would be the most likely route of transmission.

Organisms:
   Francisella tularensis

Treatment:
   Contained Casualty: (Treat for 10 days)
   Adults: Streptomycin 1g IM BID or gentamicin 5 mg/kg IM or IV daily
   Children: Streptomycin 15 mg/kg IM BID (do not exceed 2 g/day) or gentamicin 2.5 mg/kg IM or IV TID
   Mass Casualty and Post-Exposure Prophylaxis: (Treat for 14–21 days)
   Adults: Doxycycline 100 mg PO BID or ciprofloxacin 500 mg PO BID
   Children: Ciprofloxacin 15 mg/kg PO BID or doxycycline (≥ 45kg → give 100 mg PO BID; < 45 kg → give 2.2 mg/kg PO BID)

Disease Description

Epidemiology

Tularemia is a rare disease with the highest reported annual incidence in 1939 and a steady decline since. Currently, the annual incidence in the United States is estimated to be in the range of 100 to 200, although it is also felt that the disease is highly underreported. Case fatality rates are variable and depend on the specific subspecies and type of infection; on average, case fatality rates are estimated to be 1% to 2%. In the pre-antibiotics era, rates as high as 50% were recorded due to more severe complications, such as pneumonia.

Tularemia occurs throughout Eurasia and North America, with the majority of US cases reported in South Central and Western states; however, cases have been reported in every state in the United States except Hawaii. The former Soviet Union as well as the Scandinavian and Baltic regions have reported the most cases in Europe, whereas China and Japan have the highest incidences in Asia. In North America, Europe, states of the Russian Federation, China, and Japan, tularemia is endemic. Furthermore, there is evidence that F. tularensis can persist in the local environment for years after an initial outbreak.

In the United States, most cases of tularemia occur in rural areas and are associated with insect bites, inhalation, the handling of rodents or small animals, or the ingestion of contaminated food or water. In humans, the main source of infection was previously rabbits. More recently, infections have most often been associated with arthropod bites. Farmers, veterinarians, and foresters are at a higher risk of infection due to their occupations.

Diagnosis

If the diagnosis of tularemia is suspected, laboratory personnel should be notified immediately due to the risk of occupational infection from lab cultures. Blood, secretions, and/or samples or swabs of any tissue thought to be affected should be collected. If the diagnosis is suspected, special culture mediums can be used to improve organism recovery. F. tularensis can also sometimes be seen through direct tissue or secretion examination using dark field microscopy.

There are no commercial test kits for tularemia, so serologic antibody testing is commonly used. A fourfold or greater rise in antibody titers between the acute and convalescent phases' sera is the criteria for diagnosis. Because it is often difficult to obtain convalescent phase serum, a single titer of greater than 1:160 in a patient who has been sick for a week is good evidence of disease. It is important to note that lipopolysaccharide-directed antibody responses can be detected as early as 5 days after symptom onset and up to a decade after infection (the peak is between 1 and 2 months).

The differential diagnosis for each type of tularemia is broad and is described in Table 67.1.

Typical Disease Course and Complications

Clinical signs and symptoms of Tularemia depend on the clinical syndrome. However, initial symptoms can be nonspecific and may include an abrupt onset of fever (38°–40°C), lymphadenopathy, ulcer or papule, and nausea and vomiting, making a diagnosis easy to miss. Incubation time is generally 3 to 5 days but can range from 1 to 14 days. Descriptions of clinical syndromes are listed in Table 67.2.

Organisms

Microbiology

Three currently recognized species of Francisella exist. The main species responsible for human disease, F. tularensis, also contains three recognized subspecies, which vary in virulence and geographic distribution. Major microbiological features that all species possess include the following: small size, lightly staining, pleomorphic, gram-negative coccobacillus, aerobic, nonmotile, non-sporulating, weakly catalase positive, oxidase negative, thin and lipid-rich capsule, usually requires a sulfhydryl for growth (such as cysteine), grows in commercial blood media but not standard agar, and visible growth takes approximately 2 to 5 days. It is easily confused with Haemophilus or Actinobacter. It is not easily seen by light microscopy in tissue samples, but visualization is possible. Details about each species and subspecies can be found in Table 67.3.

Primary and Secondary Organisms

Primary reservoirs of F. tularensis include rabbits (in North America, Europe, and Japan), aquatic rodents (eg, beavers and muskrats), voles, rats, squirrels, lemmings (in the former Soviet Union, Sweden, and Norway), and mice (eg, meadow and field mice generally seen in the former Soviet Union). Primary

Table 67.1 Differential Diagnoses of Suspected Tularemia Syndromes[a]

Syndrome	Differential
Glandular	*Yersinia pestis, Bartonella henselae, M. tuberculosis*, and other *Mycobacterium* species; *Sporothrix schenckii, S. aureus, S. pyogenes, H. ducreyi, C. trachomatis, Treponema pallidum* (secondary), genital herpes
Ulceroglandular	*Bacillus anthracis, Orf* virus (a *Parapoxvirus*), *Pasteurella multocida, Treponema pallidum* (primary), *Spirillum minus, Rickettsia akari, Orientia tsutsugamushi* (formerly *Rickettsia tsutsugamush*), *Staphylococcus aureus, Streptococcus pyogenes*
Pneumonic	Community-acquired bacterial pneumonia: • *Mycoplasma pneumoniae* • *Chlamydia pneumoniae* • *Legionella pneumophila* or other *Legionella* species • *Chlamydia psittaci* • Other bacterial agents (eg, *S. aureus, S. pneumoniae, H. influenzae, Klebsiella pneumoniae, Moraxella catarrhalis*), *Bacillus anthracis, Yersinia pestis, Coxiella burnetii, Mycobacterium tuberculosis* or Viral pneumonia: • Influenza • *Hantavirus* • *Human respiratory syncytial virus* • *Cytomegalovirus*
Oculoglandular	Adenoviruses, *Bartonella henselae, Coccidioides immitis*, herpes simplex virus, Pyogenic bacterial infections, *Sporothrix schenckii, Treponema pallidum, Mycobacterium tuberculosis*
Oropharyngeal	*Streptococcus pyogenes*, Epstein-Barr virus, Adenoviruses, *C. diphtheriae*
Typhoidal	Brucellosis, fungal infections, endocarditis, *Leptospira interrogans, Legionella pneumophila, Plasmodium* species, *Coxiella burnetii* WITH SEPSIS *N. meningitidis*, other gram-negative bacteria, staphylococcal or streptococcal Toxic Shock Syndrome

[a]Adapted from Dennis DT, Inglesby TV, Henderson DA, et al. Tularemia as a biological weapon: medical and public health management. *JAMA*. 2001;285(21):2763–2773.

vectors of *F. tularensis* include ticks (eg, Lone Star, Rocky Mountain, American dog ticks, and *Ixodes* species), mosquitoes (eg, *Aedes cinereus* and *A. excrucians*), and biting flies (eg, deer fly). *F. tularensis* is also thought to persist for years in different environments in symbiotic relationship with amoebae.

Life Cycle

F. tularensis is transmitted to humans in a number of ways, including animal and insect bites, direct contact with infected animals, ingestion of bacteria, inhalation, and laboratory exposure. Human-to-human transmission has not been documented.

Once inside a target, *F. tularensis* multiplies largely within macrophages. It is a facultative intracellular pathogen, which enters the macrophages through phagocytosis. Once macrophage apoptosis occurs, bacteria are released and infect other cells, which propagates the cycle of infection. The pathogenesis of *F. tularensis* is still being investigated. Multiple virulence factors have been identified and studied in depth.

Treatment

Contained Casualty

In a situation where medical professionals can treat individuals in a normal fashion, IV or IM antibiotics are preferred over oral forms. Supportive care is also critical in patients who develop signs of systemic disease; some patients may even require critical care, including respiratory support. First-line treatment includes streptomycin or gentamicin, doxycycline, and ciprofloxacin. See Table 67.4 for dosing.

Mass Casualty and Post-Exposure Prophylaxis

In the event of a bioterrorist attack, during which the health care system may not be able to accommodate individual administration of IV or IM treatment, PO antibiotics can be used. In this case, the same

Table 67.2 Clinical Syndromes of Tularemia[a]

Syndrome	Symptoms	Laboratory Findings	Complications and fatality rates
Glandular and Ulceroglandular	• Painful skin lesion that ulcerates at inoculation site (only in ulceroglandular, not seen in glandular) • Painful lymphadenopathy • Constitutional symptoms • Other various skin lesions	• White blood cell count usually on the high side of the normal range • Elevated liver enzymes may be seen	• Lymph node suppuration • Secondary pneumonia • Sepsis • Full recovery may take several months • 1%–5% case fatality rates have been reported, usually associated with type A[b]
Pneumonic	• Similar to atypical community-acquired pneumonia, unresponsive to conventional antibiotics • Constitutional symptoms • May be rapidly progressive • May see other various skin lesions	• X-ray findings include patchy subsegmental opacities; hilar adenopathy; pleural effusions; and, less commonly, cavitations, cardiomegaly, mass, or miliary pattern. • White cell count usually on the high side of the normal range • Elevated liver enzymes may be seen • Sputum gram stain not usually helpful in making a diagnosis	• Lung abscess • ARDS (acute respiratory distress syndrome) • Fibrosis • Granulomas • Sepsis • Meningitis • Pericarditis • Full recovery may take up to months • Fatality ~2%–3% in one case series, usually associated with type A
Oculoglandular	• Multiple yellow conjunctival nodules • Ulcerations of the conjunctivae • Chemosis • Periorbital and facial edema • Tender cervical lymphadenopathy • Constitutional symptoms • History of eye trauma or exposure • May present with Parinaud's syndrome (A group of eye movement abnormalities and pupil dysfunction)	• Generally unremarkable • Gram stain of ocular scrapings may demonstrate organism, but unlikely	• Lymph node suppuration • Sepsis • Fatalities rare
Oropharyngeal	• Fever • Constitutional symptoms • Pharyngitis/tonsillitis (exudative) • Oral ulcerations • Stomatitis • Cervical lymphadenopathy • Concomitant pneumonia • Dental abscess	• Generally unremarkable • Possible elevation in WBC count • Possible elevation in sedimentation rate	• Sepsis • Lymph node suppuration • May take months to recover • Fatalities rare
Typhoidal	• Fever • Constitutional symptoms • Prostration • Dehydration • Gastrointestinal symptoms • Skin lesions	• WBC count on high side of normal range • Possible elevated liver function tests • Microscopic pyuria may occur	• Secondary pneumonia • Sepsis • Rhabdomyolysis • Acute renal failure • May take months to recover • Fatalities rare

[a]Adapted from: Dennis DT, Inglesby TV, Henderson DA, et al. Tularemia as a biological weapon: medical and public health management. *JAMA.* 2001;285(21):2763–2773.
[b]See Table 67.3 for definitions of Type A and Type B *tularensis.*

Table 67.3 Species and Subspecies of *Francisella*[a]

Species	Subspecies	Geographic Distribution	Relative Virulence	Pathogenic Features	Comments
F. philomiragia			Low	Rarely associated with human disease, difficult to identify by conventional methods (only 20 case reports in the literature)	Associated with immune defects, such as steroid use, chronic granulomatous disease, and near-drowning episodes
F. tularensis	*tularensis AI*	United States (central)	Very high	Demonstrates citrulline ureidase activity and produces acid from glycerol fermentation	Common vectors—Lone Star tick, American dog tick
	tularensis AII	United States (west)	Medium	Demonstrates citrulline ureidase activity and produces acid from glycerol fermentation	Common vectors—Rocky Mountain wood tick and deer fly
	holarctica (sometimes referred to as tularensis B)	Northern hemisphere	High	Does not demonstrate citrulline ureidase activity, or acid production from glycerol fermentation	
	medostiatica	Asia (central)	High		
	novicida	Global	Low	Generally causes illness only in immunocompromised hosts	

[a]Adapted from Oyston P. *Francisella tularensis*: unravelling the secrets of an intracellular pathogen. *J Med Microbiol*. 2008;57:921–930. doi:10.1099/jmm.0.2008/000653-0.

regimen is recommended for both treatment and prophylaxis. Doxycycline and ciprofloxacin are the first-line recommendations. See Table 67.4 for dosing.

Vaccines

A live attenuated vaccine has been studied in depth for decades with largely negative results. Although immune response can be measured after vaccine administration, it is not predictive of virulence. Killed bacteria, which also elicit antibody production (but no cell-mediated immune response like the live attenuated vaccine), have shown little or no benefit in human studies.

Other Key Issues

Bioterrorism

Considered a category A bioterrorism agent, *F. tularensis* could easily be used as a weapon. Characteristics that render it useful for this purpose include the following: it is highly infectious, requiring as few as 10 organisms for inoculation in some cases; it occurs widely in nature; it is easily grown in the lab; and it can be aerosolized and dispersed over large areas with relative ease. The most likely form of intentional infection would be aerosolized bacteria. Clinical symptoms would include those of pneumonic tularemia (see Table 67.2). Oculoglandular, glandular, and oropharyngeal infection could also occur from exposure to eyes, broken skin, and/or oral mucosa, respectively.

If used in a bioterrorist attack, it is likely that a more virulent strain would be used. Therefore, shorter incubation times would be expected (although the incubation period could still range from 1–14 days). Urban areas would be the most likely targets, and patients without risk factors would begin contracting the disease. Antibiotic resistance should also be considered in the case of a bioterrorist attack in which patients deteriorate despite the use of recommended antibiotics.

Table 67.4 Tularemia Treatment Recommendations by The Working Group on Civilian Biodefense[a]

Patient Category	Recommended Therapy
Contained Casualty	
Adults	Preferred choices: Streptomycin 1g IM twice daily (10 days) Gentamicin 5 mg/kg IM or IV once daily (10 days) Alternative choices: Doxycycline 100 mg IV twice daily (14–21 days) Chloramphenicol 15 mg/kg IV 4 times daily (14–21 days) Ciprofloxacin 400 mg IV twice daily (10 days)
Children	Preferred choices: Streptomycin 15 mg/kg IM twice daily (should not exceed 2 g/day) (10 days) Gentamicin 2.5 mg/kg IM or IV 3 times daily (10 days) Alternative choices: Doxycycline (14–21 days) If weight ≥ 45 kg: 100 mg IV If weight < 45 kg: give 2.2 mg/kg IV twice daily Chloramphenicol 15 mg/kg IV 4 times daily (14–21 days) Ciprofloxacin 15 mg/kg IV twice daily (10 days)
Pregnant Women	Preferred choices: Gentamicin 5 mg/kg IM or IV once daily (10 days) Streptomycin 1 g IM twice daily (10 days) Alternative choices: Doxycycline 100 mg IV twice daily (14–21 days) Ciprofloxacin 400 mg IV twice daily (10 days)
Mass Casualty and Post-exposure Prophylaxis	
Adults	Preferred choices (14 days): Doxycycline 100 mg orally twice daily Ciprofloxacin 500 mg orally twice daily
Children	Preferred choices (14 days): Doxycycline If ≥ 45kg: give 100 mg orally twice daily If < 45 kg: then give 2.2 mg/kg orally twice daily Ciprofloxacin 15 mg/kg orally twice daily (max dose 1 g/day)
Pregnant Women	Preferred choices (14 days): Ciprofloxacin 500 mg orally twice daily Doxycycline 100 mg orally twice daily

Abbreviations: IM, intramuscularly; IV, intravenous.

[a]Adapted from Dennis DT, Inglesby TV, Henderson DA, et al. Tularemia as a biological weapon: medical and public health management. *JAMA.* 2001;285(21):2763–2773.

Suggested Readings and References

1. Dennis DT, Inglesby TV, Heznderson DA, et al. Tularemia as a biological weapon: medical and public health management. *JAMA.* 2001;285(21):2763–2773. doi:10.1001/jama.285.21.2763. http://jama.jamanetwork.com/article.aspx?articleid=193894 and http://www.bt.cdc.gov/agent/tularemia/tularemia-biological-weapon-abstract.asp

2. Staples JE, Kubota KA, Chalcraft LG, Mead PS, Petersen JM. Epidemiologic and molecular analysis of human tularemia, United States, 1964–2004. *Emerg Infect Dis.* 2006;12(7). http://dx.doi.org/10.3201/eid1207.051504. doi:10.3201/eid1207.051504.

3. Oyston P. *Francisella tularensis*: unravelling the secrets of an intracellular pathogen. *J Med Microbiol.* 2008;57:921–930. doi:10.1099/jmm.0.2008/000653-0. http://jmm.sgmjournals.org/content/57/8/921.full

4. Ellis J, Oyston P, Green M, Titball R. Tularemia. *Clin Microbiol Rev.* 2002;15(4):631–664. http://cmr.asm.org/content/15/4/631.full.

5. Hornick R. Tularemia revisited. *N Engl J Med.* 2001;345:1637–1639. doi:10.1056/NEJM200111293452211. http://www.nejm.org/doi/full/10.1056/NEJM200111293452211

6. Cowley S, Elkins KL. Immunity to *Francisella*. Front Microbiol. 2011; doi:10.3389/fmicb.2011.00026. http://www.frontiersin.org/Cellular_and_Infection_Microbiology_-_closed_section/10.3389/fmicb.2011.00026/full

7. US Department of Labor, Occupational Safety & Health Administration, Safety and Health Topics. Tularemia. http://www.osha.gov/SLTC/tularemia/index.html

8. http://www.cidrap.umn.edu/cidrap/content/bt/tularemia/biofacts/tularemiafactsheet.html

Section XV

Antibiotic Resistance

Chapter 68

Antibiotic Resistance

Eili Y. Klein

Introduction

Antibiotics are an integral part of modern medicine. In the hospital, approximately 60% of all patients receive at least one dose of an antibacterial drug. Annually more than 260 million antibiotic prescriptions are filled in pharmacies across the country.[1] Antibacterial resistance, which has become a global epidemic, threatens the ability of physicians to treat infections and increases the probability of mortality for patients. Decreased antibiotic efficacy also threatens to reverse medical gains, particularly in advanced surgical procedures (such as organ and prosthetic transplants), which are dependent on antibiotic effectiveness. However, even simple procedures bring tremendous risk when antibiotics lose their effectiveness, as antibiotic prophylaxis has become a standard means of controlling surgical site infections.

Recent estimates suggest that, at a minimum, more than two million Americans are infected with antibiotic-resistant infections annually, resulting in more than 23,000 deaths each year.[2] Many of these infections are acquired in the hospital, although other health care settings, particularly long-term care facilities, are also a significant source of resistant infections. The history of antibiotic resistance has consistently been one where resistance first emerges in hospital settings and then spreads to the community. [3] Particularly when antibiotic-resistant community-associated infections first emerge, they can be difficult to identify and treat appropriately because individuals often have limited risk factors that would otherwise raise suspicion for resistant organisms.

A major contributor to the burden of antibiotic resistance is methicillin-resistant *Staphylococcus aureus* (MRSA), which has been estimated to kill anywhere from 10,000 to 20,000 Americans every year,[4] although other pathogens—such as carbapenem-resistant *Klebsiella pneumoniae*, vancomycin-resistant enterococci, resistant *Acinetobacter* species, and resistant *Streptococcus* species[2]—have also been noted to cause significant morbidity and mortality.

Beside increased morbidity and mortality, there is a tremendous cost to the health care system. The treatment of antibiotic-resistant infections is estimated to result in more than 8 million additional hospital days at a cost of $21 to $34 billion annually.[5] Although these numbers are significant, they fail to capture the full extent of the individual costs that patients pay as a result of these resistant infections, including (1) increased time in the hospital; (2) longer recovery times; and (3) increased out-of-pocket costs due to the longer hospital stays and due to the additional cost of the newer, more expensive antibiotics needed to treat resistant pathogens.

Antimicrobial Stewardship

There is a strong link between antibiotic use and resistance.[1] In fact, most patients have been shown to harbor antibiotic-resistant bacteria after taking antibiotics.[6] Despite the significant morbidity and mortality associated with antibiotic-resistant infections and the link between increased antibiotic use and resistance, a large fraction of antimicrobial use continues to be inappropriate. This is particularly true for acute respiratory tract infections, which include nonspecific upper respiratory tract infections (URIs), acute bronchitis, sinusitis, pharyngitis, otitis media, and pneumonia. URIs account for the majority of outpatient antibiotic use. Approximately 60% of patients visiting a physician for an URI receive antibiotics, even though the available evidence strongly demonstrates that the majority of these infections are viral in origin and are, therefore, unlikely to benefit from antibiotic treatment. Inappropriate use of antibiotics in the treatment of skin and soft tissue infections as well as urinary tract infections (UTIs) is common as well.

The disadvantages of inappropriate antibiotic use go beyond antibiotic resistance and the cost of the drugs. Additional disadvantages include medication side effects, allergic reactions, and secondary infections, such as *Clostridium difficile*, which have been estimated to result in approximately 140,000 emergency department visits annually,[7] or approximately 1 out of every 2000 antibiotic prescriptions. Serious side effects have also been documented for some drugs, including an increased of serious arrhythmia (with QT prolonging antibiotics). Patient discomfort due to less severe side effects of antibiotics (eg, diarrhea, colitis, gastro-esophageal reflux, nausea, or headache) can be substantial. As described above, reductions in inappropriate prescribing would yield significant benefit to patients on an individual level as well as the health system as a whole.

History of Antibiotic Resistance

The risk of antibiotic resistance is as old as the discovery of antibiotics. Alexander Fleming, in his 1945 Nobel Prize acceptance speech, warned of the danger of resistance emergence, having seen how easily it could emerge in the lab. Only 2 years later, resistance to penicillin in *S. aureus* hospital isolates was described. These resistant infections were first found in hospitals in London but soon spread to other hospitals and into the community. By the early 1950s, resistant infections had become a global pandemic.[3]

The rapid introduction of new antibiotics, including methicillin, reduced the initial problem of penicillin resistance. However, the first reports of MRSAs were published in 1961, just 2 years after the introduction of methicillin. MRSA was first detected in the United States in the late 1970s. By the mid-1980s, it had become a global hospital pandemic.[3] Community-associated (CA) strains of MRSA (CA-MRSA), which are believed to have evolved independently of hospital strains,[3] were first reported in the late 1990s when otherwise healthy children with no risk factors for MRSA were noted to be dying of overwhelming infection.

Between 1999 and 2005, the number of MRSA hospitalizations more than doubled from a rate of 3.95 per 1,000 hospitalizations to 8.02 per 1,000 hospitalizations, driven largely by a surge in skin and soft tissue infections.[4] Since 2005, the rate of MRSA hospitalizations has held approximately constant or decreased slightly[8]. However, the emergence of CA-MRSA led to seasonal patterns of resistance. CA-MRSA infections (primarily skin and soft tissue infections) are more common in the summer. Hospital-associated (HA) strains (HA-MRSA) is more common in the winter, primarily due to increased rates of HA-MRSA pneumonia.[8] These differences matter from a clinical perspective, as CA-MRSA strains are generally resistant to fewer antibiotics.[9]

It is unclear whether or not CA-MRSA strains will replace HA-MRSA strains in coming years. Mathematical models suggest that heterogeneities in hospitalization rates and antibiotic use will allow both strains to coexist with differing antibiotic susceptibility patterns. [9] However, current evidence has suggested that CA-MRSA strains are continuing to displace HA-MRSA strains.[10]

Other Threats

Although MRSA continues to be one of the most significant antibiotic-resistant pathogens in terms of mortality and the overall number infections,[2] new pathogens (eg, carbapenem-resistant Enterobacteriaceae [CRE]) are increasing in clinical significance. Although encompassing a wide range of potential pathogens, the most common health care associated Enterobacteriaceae are *Escherichia coli*, *Klebsiella* species, and *Enterobacter* species. CRE is particularly troubling for clinicians because there are limited options for treating these infections; thus, CRE infections in health care settings have mortality rates of 40% to 50%. Although CRE is a significant threat in the hospital, what is more troubling is a rising incidence of CRE in non-acute-care settings,[11] which may be indicating the arrival of a community-based epidemic. CRE is not the only pathogen with limited appropriate antibiotics available for treatment. Vancomycin, for example, is one of the last resorts for treating numerous pathogens, including MRSA. Although vancomycin-resistant *S. aureus* (VRSA) has been described, it has not yet become a widespread problem; but its emergence would significantly reduce a physician's ability to treat these infections.

Besides emerging threats, treatment of numerous common infections has become more difficult due to the emergence of resistance. A good example is gonorrhea, which causes high morbidity. Whereas penicillin was an effective treatment for decades, in recent years, strains of *Neisseria gonorrhoeae* with high-level resistance to ceftriaxone have been reported.[12] Resistant UTIs represent another common clinical entity whose treatment has become more complex. Nationally, in 2011, there were nearly 600,000 hospitalizations for UTIs. This represents approximately a 35% increase since 2001 when there were only about 430,000 UTI hospitalizations. This rise in hospitalizations over the last 10 years has likely been driven by the rising rates of resistance to many of the most common antibiotics for treating *E. coli* UTIs[13] (see Figure 68.1).

Global Threats

Antibiotic resistance is not only a problem of developed countries. In recent years, antibiotic use and resistance have been rising rapidly in developing countries, particularly India and China, but also in African countries.[14] This is a serious issue, as global travel allows a resistant pathogen to move across the globe in mere hours. For instance, New Delhi Metallo-beta-lactamase-1, a gene that confers resistance to a wide-range of beta-lactam antibiotics, including the carbapenems, is believed to have originated in India in 2009. This gene has spread around the world rapidly and is now a major problem in developed countries.

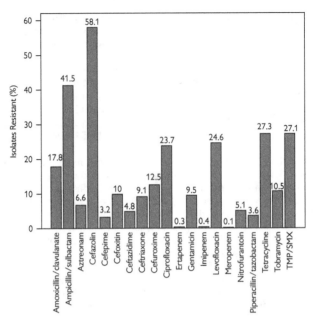

Figure 68.1 Percentage of *E. coli* isolates resistant to common antibiotics in 2012.
Source: The Surveillance Network Database–USA (TSN; Eurofins-Medinet).

Developing countries also face resistant pathogens that are not generally a problem in the United States at this time. Multidrug-resistant tuberculosis (MDRTB) strains (that have developed resistance to nearly all therapeutic antibiotics) likely represents the most significant threat. MDRTB may spread easily to the United States; in the past MDRTB strains have caused outbreaks in the United States. With increases in medical tourism and the increasing connectivity of the global economy, threats from MDRTB and other antibiotic-resistant pathogens will only increase.

Misaligned Incentives

In the past several years, the US Food and Drug Administration (FDA) has approved three new antibiotics to fight MRSA skin and soft tissue infections (telavancin, dalbavancin, and tedizolid), and a fourth will likely be approved soon. Despite this, most antibiotics in use today were developed decades ago, and there are few antibiotics under development, particularly for infections caused by gram-negative bacteria. The rate at which new antibacterial agents have been introduced has fallen steadily for the last 40 years, due in part to the high cost of bringing a new drug to market, which has been estimated to cost between $92 million and $1.8 billion. Moreover, the vast majority of compounds tested for therapeutic application never become an FDA-approved pharmaceutical.

In addition to the cost and uncertainty of bringing a drug to market, revenues from antibiotics are generally less than that of "blockbuster" drugs. For example, in 2005, Pfizer reported revenue of more than $12 billion for Lipitor and revenue of only about $2 billion for Zithromax (generic name azithromycin), which at the time was one of the most frequently prescribed antibiotics. This disparity is driven largely by the individual usage patterns for these drugs: whereas antibiotics are generally only taken for 7 to 10 days, a drug like Lipitor is often taken for a lifetime. The emergence of resistance has further diminished the incentives to develop new drugs, as doctors often reserve new antibiotics for when they are necessary, which reduces the gains that a pharmaceutical company can make before the patent on its drug expires.

There have been efforts to improve incentives for development in the past several years, including passage of the Generating Antibiotic Incentives Now Act, which extends the patent of antibiotics that treat serious or life-threating antibiotics. However, there have been few attempts to entice pharmaceutical companies to push for limiting antibiotic resistance. One reason for this is that the categorization of drugs into classes (and thus patents) is based on the chemical structure of the active molecule of the antibiotic rather than the mechanism that allows for bacterial resistance.[15] Thus, newly patented antibiotics may have a similar or shared chemical risk for bacterial resistance even if the structures of their chemically active molecules are "different" as defined by intellectual property law.

Because several competing pharmaceutical firms can produce antibiotics within a single antibiotic class, no single firm possesses a strong incentive to appropriately limit the use of its antibiotic in order to conserve the future effectiveness of the antibiotic class as a whole (an example of the economic theory of the tragedy of the commons). Patent expiration also serves as a direct disincentive to limiting inappropriate antibiotic prescriptions, as pharmaceutical companies have an incentive to sell as much of a drug as possible before their patent expires and generic formulations enter the market.

Summary

Prior to the discovery of penicillin, a scratch complicated by infection could potentially result in an agonizing death. The widespread use of antibiotics has since changed the medical landscape that we live in, but the emergence of resistance threatens a return to the reality of simple infections leading to significant morbidity and mortality. The past decades have suggested that there is no single factor that can eliminate this risk. However, we must work to reduce the inappropriate use of antibiotics while at the same time increasing incentives for the development of new antibiotics.

Suggested Readings and References

1. Sun L, Klein EY, Laxminarayan R. Seasonality and temporal correlation between community antibiotic use and resistance in the United States. Clin Infect Dis. 2012;55:687–694.

2. Centers for Disease Control and Prevention (CDC). Antibiotic Resistance Threats in the United States, 2013. Atlanta, GA: Centers for Disease Control and Prevention; 2013.

3. Chambers HF, DeLeo FR. Waves of resistance: Staphylococcus aureus in the antibiotic era. Nat Rev Microbiol. 2009;7:629–641.

4. Klein E, Smith DL, Laxminarayan R. Hospitalizations and deaths caused by methicillin-resistant Staphylococcus aureus, United States, 1999–2005. Emerg Infect Dis. 2007;13:1840.

5. Roberts RR, Hota B, Ahmad I, et al. Hospital and societal costs of antimicrobial-resistant infections in a Chicago teaching hospital: implications for antibiotic stewardship. Clin Infect Dis. 2009;49:1175–1184.

6. Costelloe C, Metcalfe C, Lovering A, Mant D, Hay AD. Effect of antibiotic prescribing in primary care on antimicrobial resistance in individual patients: systematic review and meta-analysis. BMJ. 2010;340:c2096. doi:10.1136/bmj.c2096.

7. Budnitz D, Pollock DA, Weidenbach KN, et al. National surveillance of emergency department visits for outpatient adverse drug events. JAMA. 2006;296:1858–1866.

8. Klein EY, Sun L, Smith DL, Laximarayan R. The changing epidemiology of methicillin-resistant Staphylococcus aureus in the United States: A national observational study. Am J Epidemiol. 2013;177:666–674.

9. Kouyos R, Klein EY, Grenfell B. Hospital-community interactions foster coexistence between methicillin-resistant strains of Staphylococcus aureus. PLoS Pathog. 2013;9:e1003134.

10. Diekema DJ, Richter SS, Heilmann KP, et al. Continued emergence of USA300 methicillin-resistant Staphylococcus aureus in the United States: results from a nationwide surveillance study. Infect Control Hosp Epidemiol. 2014;35:285–292.

11. Braykov N, Eber MR, Klein EY, Morgan DJ, Laxminarayan R. Trends in resistance to carbapenems and third-generation cephalosporins among clinical isolates of Klebsiella pneumoniae in the United States, 1999–2010. Infect Control Hosp Epidemiol. 2013;34:259–268.

12. Unemo M, Golparian D, Nicholas R, et al. High-level cefixime-and ceftriaxone-resistant Neisseria gonorrhoeae in France: novel penA mosaic allele in a successful international clone causes treatment failure. Antimicrob Agents Chemother. 2012;56:1273–1280.

13. May L, Klein EY, Rothman RE, Laxminarayan R. Trends in antibiotic resistance in coagulase-negative staphylococci in the United States, 1999 to 2012. Antimicrob Agents Chemother. 2014;58:1404–1409.

14. Laxminarayan R, Duse A, Wattal C, et al. Antibiotic resistance?the need for global solutions. Lancet Infect Dis. 2013;13:1057–1098.

15. Laxminarayan R, Powers JH. Antibacterial R&D incentives. Nat Rev Drug Discov. 2011;10:727–728.

Index